Epilepsy and Psychiatry

Epilepsy and Psychiatry

Edited by

E. H. Reynolds

MD FRCP

Consultant Neurologist, Bethlem Royal, Maudsley and
King's College Hospitals; Hon. Senior Lecturer, University
Department of Neurology, Institute of Psychiatry and
King's College Hospital Medical School, London

M. R. Trimble

MB BSc MPhil MRCP MRCPsych

Consultant Physician in Psychological Medicine, National
Hospital, Queen Square, London and Senior Lecturer in
Behavioural Neurology, University of London

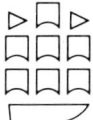

CHURCHILL LIVINGSTONE
EDINBURGH LONDON MELBOURNE AND NEW YORK 1981

CHURCHILL LIVINGSTONE
Medical Division of Longman Group Limited

Distributed in the United States of America by
Churchill Livingstone Inc., 19 West 44th Street,
New York, N.Y. 10036, and by associated companies,
branches and representatives throughout the world.

First published 1981

ISBN 0 443 02311 5

**British Library Cataloguing in Publication
Data**

Epilepsy and psychiatry
  1. Epilepsy
  I. Reynolds, E. H.   II. Trimble, M. R.
  616.8.53   RC372

Library of Congress Catalog Card Number 81-7729

Filmset by Speedlith Photo Litho Ltd, Manchester
and printed in Great Britain by
Butler & Tanner Ltd, Frome and London

Preface

The relationship between epilepsy and mental disorder has been a source of great interest and controversy since the earliest literature on the 'sacred disease'. Older ideas of supernatural intervention, of inevitable lunacy or mental deterioration, have given way in this century to a more balanced view which recognises that the majority of epileptic patients are mentally normal. However, as with all disorders of cerebral function, there is an increased prevalence of psychological disorders due probably, in varying degrees, to seizures, associated cerebral pathology, heredity, chronic anticonvulsant therapy and powerful psychosocial influences, not least the prejudice which stems from the older, deeply rooted historical attitudes. Widely varying opinions even in this century have more recently gradually given way to more scientifically based studies of the prevalence, nature, causes and treatment of various kinds of psychopathology associated with epilepsy. Much of this research has been in the United Kingdom where there is a tradition of interest in the many problems and facets of epilepsy stretching back to Jackson, Gowers and beyond. We therefore thought it an appropriate time to bring together in a comprehensive textbook on the psychiatry of epilepsy the experience of many British authors actively engaged in this field. Epilepsy has always straddled the fields of both neurology and psychiatry. Indeed it has been the differing perspectives and concepts of these two disciplines which has fuelled many of the controversies on this subject. We have therefore included neurologists, neurophysiologists, neuropsychiatrists, a social worker, as well of course as psychiatrists among the authors.

It is in some ways surprising that this gap in the psychiatric literature has not been filled before. The study of epilepsy has always illuminated neurology as exemplified by Gowers, the centenary of whose classic work *Epilepsy and other chronic convulsive diseases* is celebrated by the publication of this volume. There are many reasons to suspect that the study of the psychiatric disorders associated with epilepsy could also shed light on many other aspects of psychiatry, as discussed in several chapters in this book. We hope therefore that the publication of this volume will stimulate wider interest in a subject which stands squarely on the bridge between neurology and psychiatry.

1981

E. H. Reynolds
M. R. Trimble

Contributors

Brian Barraclough FRACP
Senior Lecturer, Department of
Psychiatry, University of Southampton

T. A. Betts MB ChB DPM MRCPsych
Senior Lecturer in Psychiatry, University
of Birmingham; Consultant Psychiatrist
to the Queen Elizabeth and General
Hospitals, Birmingham

Stephen W. Brown MA(Cantab.)
MA(Nottm.) MB BChir
Research Registrar, University
Department of Neurology, Institute of
Psychiatry, London; Honorary Registrar
in Psychiatry, Maudsley Hospital,
London

George Burden OBE BSc(Econ.)
Dip.Mental Health
Retired; lately Education Secretary,
British Epilepsy Association, and
Secretary General, International Bureau
for Epilepsy

John A. Corbett MB FRCPsych MRCP
DPM(Acad.) DCH
Consultant Physician, Bethlem Royal and
Maudsley Hospitals, London

George W. Fenton MB FRCP(Edin.)
FRCPsych MRCP(Lond.) DPM(Eng.)
Professor of Mental Health, The Queen's
University of Belfast, Northern Ireland

Peter Fenwick MB BChir(Cantab.)
DPM MRCPsych
Consultant Neuropsychiatrist to the
Epilepsy Unit, Bethlem Royal and
Maudsley Hospitals; Consultant
Neurophysiologist, Department of
Clinical Neurophysiology, St Thomas'
Hospital; Senior Lecturer, Institute of
Psychiatry, London

Richard H. E. Grant MB BS DCH
Director, the David Lewis Centre for
Epilepsy, Alderley Edge, Cheshire;
Advisor in Epilepsy, Manchester Area
Health Authority (Teaching)

John Gunn MD Acad DPM(Lond.)
FRCPsych
Professor of Forensic Psychiatry,
Institute of Psychiatry, London;
Consultant Psychiatrist, Bethlem Royal
and Maudsley Hospitals, London

Sir Denis Hill MB BS FRCP
FRCPsych
Emeritus Professor of Psychiatry,
Institute of Psychiatry, London
University

Janet M. M. Lindsay MD FRCPsych
DPM
Consultant in Administrative Charge,
Park Hospital for Children, Oxford

C. Ounsted DM FRCP FRCPsych
DPM DCH
Consultant Physician, Park Hospital for
Children, Oxford

Maurice Parsonage BSc MB FRCP
DCH
Director, Neuropsychiatric Unit
and Special Centre for Epilepsy,
Bootham Park Hospital, York; formerly
Senior Consultant Physician,
Neurological Department, General
Infirmary, Leeds and Senior Clinical
Lecturer in Neurology, University of
Leeds

Sir Desmond Pond MD FRCP
FRCPsych
Professor of Psychiatry, the London
Hospital Medical College, London

E. H. Reynolds MD FRCP
Consultant Neurologist, Bethlem
Royal, Maudsley and King's College
Hospitals, London

Gregory Stores MA MD MRCP
MRCPsych DPM
Consultant in Neuropsychiatry, National
Epilepsy Centre, Park Hospital for
Children; Clinical Lecturer, Department
of Psychiatry, University of Oxford

David C. Taylor MD MRCP
FRCPsych
Professor of Child and Adolescent
Psychiatry, University of
Manchester

Brian Toone MB BS MRCP MPhil
MRCPsych
Consultant Psychiatrist, Department of
Psychological Medicine, King's College
Hospital; Hon. Consultant Psychiatrist,
Bethlem Royal and Maudsley Hospitals,
London

M. R. Trimble MB BSc MPhil MRCP
MRCPsych
Consultant Physician in Psychological
Medicine, National Hospital, Queen
Square, London; Senior Lecturer in
Behavioural Neurology, University of
London

Denis Williams CBE MD DSc FRCP
Honorary Consulting Physician, National
Hospital, Queen Square, and St George's
Hospital, London

Contents

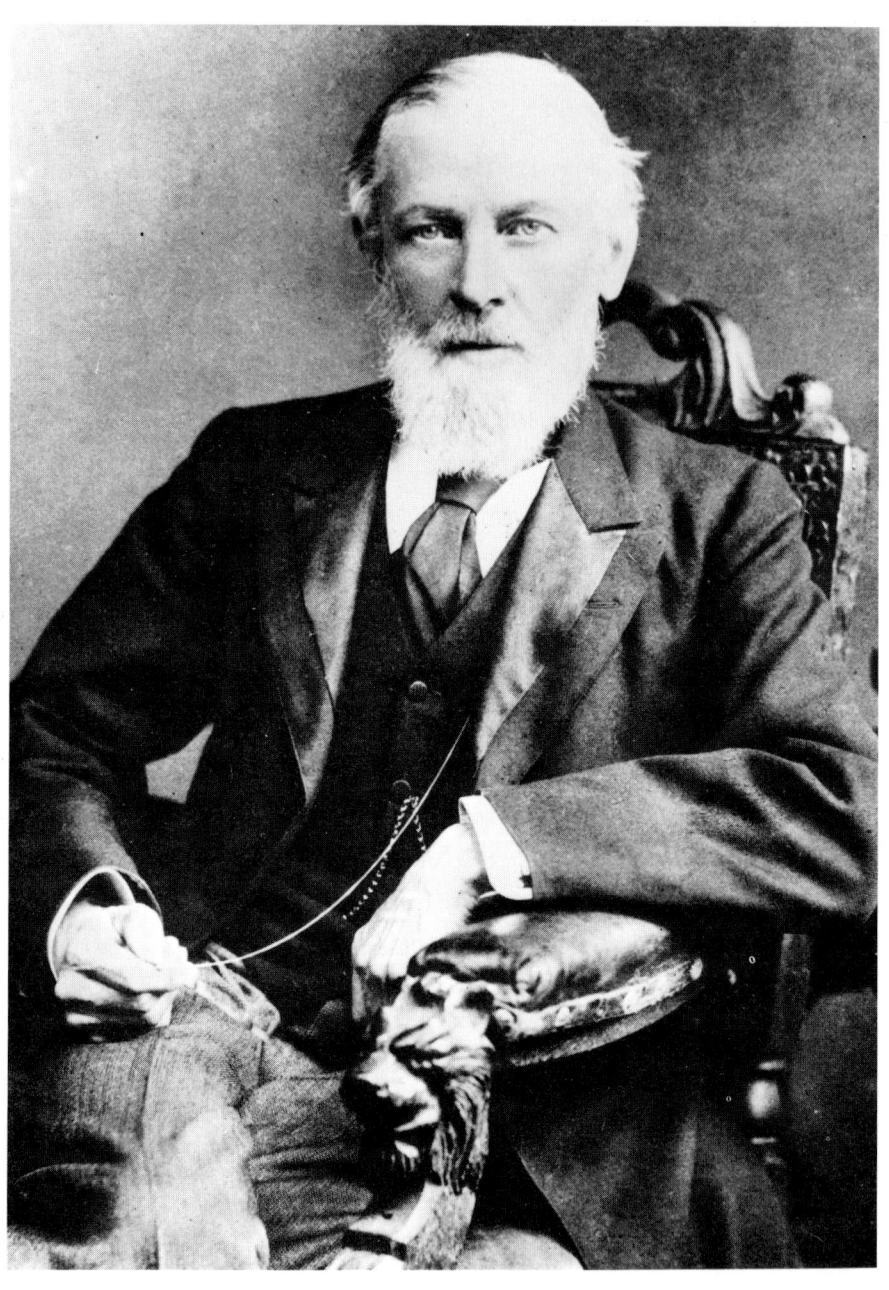

Sir William Richard Gowers (1845–1915)
By courtesy of the Wellcome Trustees

Historical note on
Sir William Gowers

William Richard Gowers was born in Hackney, London, in 1845, of humble origins. He qualified at University College Hospital at the age of 22, and three years later was appointed medical registrar at Queen Square, where he was to work for the next 40 years until his retirement. At the age of 27 he was appointed to the staff of the hospital. Of slight stature, he had an awkward gait and a strident voice. His speech was often caustic and these superficial characteristics tended to repel people, particularly as he often seemed rather cold and aloof. It is said that he was admired rather than liked, for he stood out in an age of strong personalities by reason of his individuality and brilliance, his marvellous powers of clinical observation, his meticulous concern with detail and his exceptional skill in the logical marshalling of facts in coming to an opinion. Throughout his career he was intensely absorbed in the recording, in a very neat short-hand, of clinical phenomena—often pausing while making an examination to record something he had observed. The accuracy of his observations made him famous. He was a skilled artist, and personally illustrated many of his books. His drawings and engravings were exhibited at the Royal Academy on a number of occasions.

Despite a large private practice which he carried on from his home in Queen Anne Street, he gave much of his time to Queen Square and soon became internationally recognised as a great teacher. William Osler, for example, attended his outpatient clinic to see and hear for himself. Gowers' habit was to speak his thoughts aloud when examining a patient. Therefore his students could follow his observations, listen to his self-questioning reasoning and arrive with him at the diagnosis. His outpatient clinics and ward rounds were thronged to the limit with physicians and neurologists from many countries.

Critchley (1949) in his *Biographical appreciation* of Gowers, has provided much detail on the life of this remarkable man. The antithesis between the personalities and achievements of Gowers and Hughlings Jackson, his senior by a few years, has often aroused comment. Jackson was easy-going and warm-hearted where Gowers was intolerant and difficult. Jackson the philosopher was ever seeking to understand the principles lying behind neurological phenomena, while Gowers was the great naturalist, clinical observer and teacher. These two never collaborated, but they always treated one another with great respect and courtesy. Despite the fact that Gowers was a lone wolf—he never had a collaborator—he made many life-long friends, among them Russell Reynolds, William Jenner,

William Osler, James Taylor, Victor Horsley and Risien Russell.

His writings were prolific. In 35 years of active clinical life he published, in short and long articles (and most of his lectures at Queen Square were published), over 250 papers and books. His classic work on *Epilepsy and other chronic convulsive diseases*, published in 1881, has its centenary honoured by this book. His *Borderlands of Epilepsy* was published in 1907, and his most influential work, the *Manual of diseases of the nervous system*, was published in two volumes in 1886. These works were translated and published in many countries throughout the world. Critchley (1949), who considered Gowers one of the greatest clinical neurologists of all time, points out the great contribution he made to the descriptive concepts of neurological disorders. We owe to him the terms 'amyotatic', 'abiotrophy', 'knee jerk' and 'fibrositis'. He first described vaso-vagal attacks, progressive lenticular degeneration, myasthenia gravis, paramyoclonus multiplex, Schilder's disease, musicogenic epilepsy, sleep paralysis, geniculate herpes, dystrophia myotonica and many others. He died, after some years of illness, in 1915.

1981   Denis Hill

Historical review

To the ancient Greeks it was obvious that epilepsy was the most sacred and the most psychological of all diseases. Only a God could throw a sane normal man to the ground, deprive him of his senses, convulse him and then restore him to normality. Hippocrates (b. 460 B.C.) taught otherwise, writing that epilepsy like other diseases has a natural cause, and is no more sacred or divine than they are. It was due to ignorance and wonder that men so regarded it, because epilepsy is not like other diseases. Hippocrates also definitely ascribed epilepsy to a disorder of the brain, perhaps due to lack of air, and he suggested that those who doubted this should examine the brains of epileptics. At that ancient time there was also the belief that some diseases are regulated by the celestial bodies, where Gods presided. Even Galen (b. A.D. 131), although he was a biologist who believed that the immediate causes of epilepsy were 'humoral' or toxic, held that the moon regulated the occasions of fits, which returned when the moon was full. For this reason in the Graeco-Roman world the term 'lunatic' was restricted to epileptics. They were distinguished from 'maniacs' or mad people because the latter were possessed by demons, not by Gods — hence the term 'demoniac'. But the epileptic could be both lunatic and maniac, if in addition to his fits he was also mad. It seemed that the time when the fits occurred was one when the patient was particularly liable to invasion by demons.

Although the Greeks ascribed epilepsy to divine intervention, later opinion alternated with the view that demons rather than Gods were responsible and this gained ascendancy by the time of the Christian gospel writers, and is alluded to in the miracles of Jesus. A man brought his son, suffering from fits to Jesus who asked him how long he had suffered, and was told since childhood, and that often 'It had cast him into the fire, and into the waters, to destroy him. When Jesus saw that the people came running together, he rebuked the foul spirit, saying unto him : Thou dumb and deaf spirit, I charge thee, come out of him, and enter no more into him. And the spirit cried, and rent him sore, and came out of him and he was as one dead; insomuch as many said, He is dead. But Jesus took him by the hand, and lifted him up, and he arose.' (St. Mark, Ch. 9, v. 17–27)

It seems probable that people with epilepsy did not generally suffer the persecutions and massacres which were inflicted on the mentally ill throughout Europe during the late middle ages. Possibly this was due to the Hippocratic tradition, but also to the fact that so many great men of genius had been epileptic.

W. G. Lennox (1960) listed 72 men of genius who were reported to have epilepsy at some time in their lives. It is also probable, because of its antique history and the great place epilepsy has had in medical thinking from the time of the Greeks, that almost until the present time epilepsy 'per se' has been given a separate category as a form of mental disorder in nosological classifications. It is only in the present century that the distinction between it and epilepsy with psychosis, or epilepsy with personality disorder or dementia has been made. In the 13th century St. Thomas Aquinas (1225–1274), who like Plato differentiated between conditions of supernatural origin and those of natural origin, placed epilepsy among the latter, and thus reasserted Hippocratic teaching.

At the time of the Renaissance and later, there was an attempt to classify mental disorders according to alleged causes — generally the humoral pathology of Galen, and individual symptoms and syndromes ceased to appear. The confusion of ideas, partly medical, partly philosophical which characterised attempts at classification in the 17th and 18th centuries is even shown by the illustrious Pinel who classified epilepsy as a 'neurosis' along with asthma, ileus, whooping cough, tetanus, rabies and the neuralgias. But he regarded 'neurosis' as a 'functional disease of the nervous system' (Menninger 1963).

THE WORK OF PSYCHIATRISTS AND NEUROLOGISTS IN THE 19TH CENTURY

The work of psychiatrists as keepers, apothecaries, superintendents or physicians of institutions where the insane were confined was well recognised and established even in the 17th century, and by the late 18th a few occupied prominent positions as physicians in medicine itself. It was not however until the mid-19th century that the specialities in medicine and surgery as we know them today, began to appear. Modern neurology began in France with Duchenne (1806–1875), Charcot (1825–1893), Pierre Marie (1853–1940) and Dejerine (1849–1917). In England the first neurological hospital in the world was opened in 1859 in Queen Square, (as the National Hospital for the Paralysed and the Epileptic), and among its brilliant staff were Russell Reynolds (1828–1896), William Gowers (1845–1915) and Hughlings Jackson (1834–1911). By the latter part of the last century the approaches to the problems of epilepsy by psychiatrists and neurologists were essentially different, and more important they seem to have had little influence on one another. Psychiatry was dominated by general theories about the nature of mental disorders, which included epilepsy, and such theories were comprehensive and holistic. On the other hand the first neurologists who were extremely interested in epilepsy, were concerned with a detailed analysis of all the phenomena of epileptic fits, the different types and the associated clinical phenomena. The psychiatric aspects, and the problems of dementia, psychosis and personality disorder were not matters with which they had much acquaintance. Indeed psychiatrists' experience was largely determined by the patients for whom they cared in the institutions where chronic epileptics were confined; and the neurologists' experience was limited to the outpatient department, the hospital ward, the laboratory and the private consulting room. It is therefore necessary to consider neurological and psychiatric developments separately. It is only in the modern period that any reconciliation has occurred.

PSYCHIATRIC THEORIES IN THE 19TH CENTURY

Epilepsy until recent times was accepted as a major category of mental disorders, and classified with them. By the mid-19th century there were two contrasting views about the nature of mental disorder. Following the 18th century systematists, who took their approach from Sydenham, mental disorders were seen as numerous, discrete, specific and of different species. Very elaborate classifications had emerged of different disease entities. During the nineteenth century there was an attempt to simplify and to reduce plurality to a few main categories and this culminated at the end of the century in the great work of Kraepelin. In the first editions of his textbook epilepsy was classified as a 'neurosis', following the ideas of Pinel a century earlier; but in the seventh edition it is separated and given a category of its own, distinct from psychopathic personalities (which included the 'born criminal') and mental disorders resulting from constitutional predisposition. In the last edition (1915) there are still 17 categories in all.

The opposing view of mental disorder was that it was unitary, a single disorder but having varying stages of severity. It was conceived as a progressive and developmental tendency, starting with what we would term neurotic symptoms, and then progressing perhaps to 'confusion' and finally to dementia. H. Neumann (1859) who promulgated this view in Germany, was supported according to K. Menninger (1963) by his contemporary in England, Hughlings Jackson, who advocated the ordering of mental diseases according to the degree of dissolution of functions of the nervous system (Stengel 1963). It is known that Jackson's writings influenced Freud, who saw in the concept of dissolution, what he himself termed regression. Modern adherents of the unitary concept include Karl Menninger and Henri Ey, the former following Freudian theory, the latter Jacksonian. In the unitary concept epilepsy is seen either as a regressive phenomenon, or one of dissolution, due to disinhibition from higher centres. In the U.S.A. Adolph Meyer at first introduced and espoused the Kraepelinian classification, and then adopted a more unitary concept of 'ergasia' in which epilepsy for example was conceived as a form of 'psychobiological reaction' of the organism to the stresses of life.

A near ally of the unitary concept was B-A. Morel in France, another contemporary of Neumann and Jackson. In 1857 he formulated his degeneracy theory of insanity which was to prove very influential in psychiatry, and particularly for ideas about epilepsy, which lasted well into this century.

The degeneracy theory
It is necessary to emphasise the pervasive and long-lasting influence — baleful as we now view it in retrospect, of the degeneracy theory of mental disorder, which included epilepsy, which B-A. Morel set forth in 1857. It had much in common with the unitary hypothesis. The theory was that much mental disorder, including

epilepsy, was the result of a progressive hereditary degenerative strain, running from one generation to the next, and progressively becoming more severe in its manifestations in each generation, until as a result of idiocy the strain is wiped out. Evidence of this degeneracy could be seen, it was alleged, not only in frank insanity, but also in weakness of character, moral defects, epilepsy and mental deficiency. Moreover there were identifiable physical stigmata of degeneration, particularly in the formation of the ears. Lombroso (quoted by Hibbert 1963) was later to assert that the unitary bond between the moral imbecile and the criminal was epilepsy. All born criminals were epileptics, although not all epileptics were born criminals. Also not all geniuses were epileptic, although many had been. The concept of the 'born criminal' found its way into Kraepelin's early classification of mental disorders.

In Morel's theory of hereditary degeneracy the ultimate prognosis for the individual was dementia, and for the family extinction through idiocy. Morel was the first to coin the term, dementia praecox, which was adopted by Kraepelin at the end of the century. He also accepted that the disease ended in inevitable deterioration.

Early in the last century, both in England and in Germany, terms such as 'congenital brutality', 'moral imbecility' and moral diseases of the mind came to be used. In 1891 the term 'psychopathic inferiorities' was introduced in Germany. In England the terms 'insane neurosis' and 'epileptic neurosis' came to be used (Maudsley 1873).

Henry Maudsley in his book *Body and mind* accepted Morel's theory. He wrote:

'Morel made the interesting observation which is certainly well founded, that the epileptic neurosis may exist for a considerable period in an undeveloped or masked form, showing itself not by convulsions, but by periodic attacks of mania, or by manifestations of extreme moral perversion, which are apt to be thought wilful viciousness.'

and later:

'The epileptic neurosis is certainly most closely allied to the insane neurosis, and when it exists in its masked form, affecting the mind for some time before convulsions occur, it is hardly possible to distinguish it... . The difficulty of doing so is made greater, inasmuch as epilepsy in the parent may engender the insane neurosis in the child, and insanity in the parent, the epileptic neurosis in the child. A character which the insane neurosis has in common with the epileptic neurosis is, that it is apt to burst out in a convulsive explosion of violence.'

Henry Maudsley was almost certainly the most influential psychiatrist of his time in this country. But his acceptance of the general theory of Morel is duplicated again and again in the writings of eminent psychiatrists in Europe and in the U.S.A. No less a man than E. Bleuler, who replaced dementia praecox by the concept of schizophrenia in 1911, accepted it. So too, in modified form, did D. K. Henderson as late as 1950 in his well-known textbook of the period.

Perhaps the most influential adherents to the Morel theory in the field of epilepsy were L. Pierce Clark in the U.S.A., and later Stauder in Germany. Clark, working with institutionalised epileptics, in 1917 strongly supported the concept of the epileptic personality, stating that the personality and consequently the seizures themselves came from a constitutional hereditary psychopathic make-up.

Stauder (1938) claimed support for the theory based on the results of the Rorschach test, since discredited.

From all this, and the writings of many other authors there developed such concepts as the epileptic or 'epileptoid' character and the idea of epileptic or psychic equivalents, which became confused with psychomotor epilepsy, a term coined, according to Bailey (1958), by Van Gieson in 1902 and taken over by the Gibbses and Lennox in 1938 to describe a certain EEG pattern, which they at first misinterpreted.

The consequences of this approach to epilepsy which dominated the scene for nearly 100 years were two-fold. The first was the enormous stigma which attached to the epileptic, making him a man apart. By destiny he was seen as mad and bad, liable to explosive and unpredictable attacks of violence and insanity, perhaps murder or at least moral depravity. In every aspect of life he was doomed to adaptive failure, and there was the risk, even the certainty in some minds, that the end for him was one of intellectual, moral and social deterioration — dementia in fact. The second was that it was no longer appropriate or necessary to investigate the independent phenomena of a behavioural or psychological nature from which many epileptics, particularly the institutionalised ones, suffered. They were all encompassed in the theory of the epileptic neurosis and were seen as natural reactions of the sufferer to the exigencies of life.

The influence of Morel can be traced well into our own century. In the 1930 edition of William Osler's famous *Textbook of medicine*, revised by McCrae, he quotes Pierce Clark's account of the epileptic personality as showing 'egocentricity, supersensitiveness, emotional poverty, and an inherent lack of adaptability to normal social life.' It was stated that chronic alcoholism in the parents is a potent cause of epilepsy, and in the case of the insane epileptic occurred in over 50 per cent of cases. It was also stated that the mental condition of the epileptic is often seriously impaired, that post-epileptic symptoms were important, including trance-like states, automatism, and attacks of mania in which the patient is often dangerous and sometimes homicidal.

As late as 1950, A. J. Lewis in his section of Price's textbook of medicine had not entirely abandoned the Morel theory for he wrote that: 'There is ground for regarding this impulsive, pretentious, fawning, and snarling way of some epileptics as partly a variable expression of their constitutional predisposition (to which the motor seizures are likewise due), and partly as a reaction to their situation.' But he held that many cases of severe epilepsy are free not only from dementia but also from these traits. He also recognised epileptic equivalents, which took the place of a convulsion, and could take the form of a furor, a twilight state, or a fugue in which the patient wanders with subsequent amnesia. Epileptic patients were also held to suffer from swings of mood, towards anger, depression or shallow sentimentalism.

Also in 1950, the seventh edition of the well-known psychiatric textbook by Henderson & Gillespie appeared. D. K. Henderson had in his Salmon Lectures of 1939 described three main types of psychopathic disorder. One of the sub-types of the predominantly aggressive group was the epileptoid character. In this Henderson followed Pierce Clark in believing that it could exist without, or in advance of actual fits. But the epileptoid character was a disorder of idiopathic not symptomatic epilepsy, and therefore of the hereditary or constitutional predisposition. He stated that this form of psychopathic disorder, the epileptoid character, could lead to a state of altered consciousness amounting to an 'affect' or psychic epilepsy. Since in such states the patient could be impulsive and homicidal, the concept had medico-legal significance. In view of the important role in British psychiatry which Henderson was to take, his views became influential, and were used extensively in the report of the Royal Commission on Capital Punishment (1953).

Finally, before closing the account of the historical aspects of epilepsy, seen from the point of view of the psychiatrist of former times, it is relevant to refer to the monograph prepared for WHO which E. Stengel published in 1960. In this he surveyed some 27 classifications of mental disorders, then being used throughout the world. In 1960 the International Classification of Diseases published by WHO, as well as the American Psychiatric Association, had made the distinction between epilepsy 'per se', and epilepsy with deterioration or psychosis. Epilepsy 'per se' was no longer a mental disorder, but this was not the case in other national classifications, as for example in Canada, France, Germany, Holland, Denmark, the USSR and Japan; nor was it always in the individual classifications of distinguished psychiatrists throughout the world, e.g. Kleist, K. Schneider, Essen-Möller, C. G. Jung, and Sjögren. It is indeed surprising that only 20 years ago, in so many countries, and in the opinion of so many internationally well-known psychiatrists, epilepsy alone as the ancients believed over 2000 years ago, was still regarded as a mental disorder. Since 1960 the U.K. for official purposes has used the ICD — the ninth revision of which appeared in 1978. In this epilepsy 'per se' as a mental disorder finds no place, but epileptic confusional and twilight states are classified under the heading of 'transient organic psychotic conditions' — forms of acute confusional state; it occurs again as a chronic organic psychotic condition, as dementia in epilepsy, and also as a chronic epileptic psychosis.

THE WORK OF EARLY NEUROLOGISTS

The pioneers who led the way towards modern understanding of epilepsy were not psychiatrists (except Hans Berger), but neurologists. The different experience which neurologists had, and the reasons for it, have already been described. But unlike psychiatrists, neurologists were concerned with the careful detailed descriptions of epileptic seizure phenomena, their relation to one another, to physiological understanding of the nervous system and the relation between the type of seizure and brain pathology. Many, perhaps the majority of patients with epilepsy whom they saw in clinical practice seemed mentally normal to them, but they were intrigued by the psychic and behavioural phenomena which often preceded, accompanied or followed fits. Russell Reynolds (1861) for example, the senior to Gowers and Hughlings Jackson at Queen Square, did not accept the Morel theory about degeneracy. He claimed that from his own experience nearly 40 per cent of epileptics showed no defect of mental health. For the first time he drew a clear distinction between idiopathic, essential or cryptogenic epilepsy on the one hand, and symptomatic epilepsy on the other — the result of general or local brain disease, or of diseases of systemic origin. He was careful to select the idiopathic cases for this enquiry.

Gowers (1907) also found most epileptics mentally normal, and in his book the *Borderlands of epilepsy* there is little reference to psychiatric disorders. He was more concerned with the differential diagnosis of syncope, vaso-vagal attacks, migraine and vertigo. Nevertheless he wrote that the frequency of seizures was greater, the intervals between shorter in those who showed mental failure, than in those who did not. This was not the view of Hughlings Jackson (according to Lennox 1960) who believed that it was not the frequency or severity of convulsions which caused mental damage, but rather the frequency of brief absences, vertiginous feelings, pauses or stoppages of consciousness — which were called 'petit mal', which were more injurious. The confusion between what we now term pure petit mal (3/second spike and wave attacks), and the rather similar 'psychic seizures' or absences of temporal lobe epilepsy remained for many years and was not resolved until the advent of the EEG. Hughlings Jackson (1931), who was a scientific philosopher less interested in prognosis than in the physiological pathology of epileptic phenomena, gave the first scientifically accurate definition of what epilepsy is — 'occasional, sudden, excessive, rapid and local discharges of grey matter'. Jackson believed that the cause of epilepsy lay in defective cell nutrition, a view he shared with Hippocrates. He described focal cortical epilepsy, still called Jacksonian, and of course uncinate fits. He also suggested that epilepsy could occur at three different levels of the nervous system — an idea which was to influence the work of Wilder Penfield later. For Jackson however the highest level fits started in the 'organ of mind', which is the anatomical substratum of consciousness — mainly the frontal and prefrontal cortex, and gave rise to generalised seizures. As an evolutionist he conceived that disinhibition from paralysis of higher centres could lead to discharges in lower centres. He also stated that where an expected discharge in the higher centres failed to occur, this led to mental disturbance and bad temper. Jackson also conceived of 'inward fits', not affecting the sensory-motor system, and was convinced that automatisms or psychic seizures are only the sequelae of fits which are not observed (Lennox 1960). In describing uncinate epilepsy he again drew attention to the focal origin in the brain of a group of clinical manifestations, among which he included hallucinations and illusions, disturbances of mood and other psychological phenomena.

In 1880 Sommer showed that a specific area of the hippocampus was often severely damaged in epileptics. A general Ammon's horn sclerosis had been recognised as a common lesion in epileptics for many years, but the correlations between autopsy findings and the behavioural and psychological characteristics, as well as the type of seizures from which the patients had suffered in life, were not made until the modern era.

There is no doubt that for many years the psychological and behavioural phenomena, now generally associated with temporal lobe epilepsy, had been recognised but were thought to be either the results of an abortive convulsive seizure or an 'attenuated' seizure — that is to say a variant of a convulsion or petit mal. Such terms as 'larval mental epilepsy' and 'intellectual grand mal' and 'intellectual petit mal' began to appear in the middle of the last century.

Throughout the period beginning with the work of the brilliant group at Queen Square and only ending with the modern era which followed the Second World War, there was confusion of ideas about many of the phenomena which relate to the psychiatric aspects of epilepsy.

'Epileptic equivalents'

The term 'equivalent', which was commonly used in the first half of the present century, is probably of much earlier origin (Lennox 1960), and has had an unfortunate history. Neither Gowers nor Jackson used it, but the latter's discovery of uncinate epilepsy, which later led to the recognition of psychic seizures as true epileptic manifestations, clouded the argument. The question was whether psychic experiences and automatic behaviour, or disturbances of affect or mood could occur in the epileptic patient in the *absence* of actual epileptic discharge, or whether only as a consequence of it, as Jackson believed. That they could, gave rise to the idea of the 'equivalent' and was used in various contexts to explain prolonged disturbances of mood in the inter-ictal period, or brief episodes of altered psychic experience or disturbed behaviour. The term persisted into the EEG era with such terms as psychomotor equivalent, but the word equivalent was soon dropped by the Gibbses. Nevertheless as late as 1951, Schwab in his textbook on electroencephalography gave as synonyms for psychomotor seizures — automatisms, psychic equivalents, rages and fugues. To many however the term equivalent was an absurdity. A phenomenon was either epilepsy or the consequence of epilepsy or it was not. Kinnier Wilson (1935) was sure that these psychic equivalents were in fact epilepsy itself.

Much the same arguments were applied to 'epileptic mania' (furor). This condition, now rather rare, had been recognised at least since the 18th century and has always had medico-legal significance since in the attack the patient is often extremely dangerous and homicidal. As Hunter & Macalpine (1963) relate, English juries for over 200 years have nearly always found the accused insane. Hughlings Jackson (in Taylor 1931) is reported to have thought that in such cases there were abnormal discharges — but in the 'organ of mind', and these discharges were different from those during the epileptic seizure. The organ of mind was for him, as previously stated, the frontal and prefrontal cortex. It was generally agreed however that 'furious maniacal' attacks usually occurred in relation to the actual occurrence of seizures, and not in the interictal periods.

'Hystero-epilepsy'

The subject of hysteria will be dealt with in detail later in this book (see Chapter 9), and reference here will only be given to the confusion which existed in the medical and popular mind over the distinction between epilepsy and hysteria, and the alleged relationship between the two, which existed over many centuries. Lennox (1960) gave a good account of the historical background to this subject. Hysteria today is certainly different from former times. Conversion hysteria has become increasingly rare. The attacks of mental confusion, 'dancing mania', extreme excitement and stupor, even 'coma' as if dead, bizarre postural behaviour such as the 'arc de cercle' of the hysterical convulsion are now rarely if ever seen; but hysterical convulsions still occur and their differentiation from epileptic convulsions may be difficult to establish, particularly in nurses and other observers, trained in the care of patients with epilepsy.

Hysteria has an ancient history, similar to epilepsy. While the latter according to Hippocrates was a disorder of the brain, the former was concerned with the uterus and was therefore thought to be a disorder of women only. The uterus was held to be a mobile organ, which in the hysteric moved up the abdomen to embarrass the functions of the intestines, the heart and even the carotid arteries. As a result abdominal symptoms were thought to be common in the hysteric, as were disturbance of the heart rhythm, of respiration and even the brain, through interference with its blood supply. Treatment therefore consisted in physically preventing the uterus from moving upwards. This was done by weights, by manual pressure on the abdomen, or by tight binding with bandages.

Both the hysterical attack — whatever its form — and the epileptic fit could be precipitated by emotionally disturbing circumstances, and as is now appreciated both could occur in the same patient. The fact that hysterical behaviour could lead on to an epileptic convulsion, gave rise to the concept of hystero-epilepsy which was to bedevil thinking until the modern era. The 'suffocation of the mother' (globus hystericus) as hysteria was called, was conceived as the result of uncontrolled passions, and epilepsy was only the final result of such disorder. Disordered and uncontrolled passion was held to be 'an omnibus psychosomatic concept of aetiology' (Hunter & Macalpine 1963), which only gave way with the rise of organic pathology in the 18th and 19th centuries. Thomas Willis (1621–1675) often regarded as the father of neurology, vindicated the uterus as the cause of hysteria, which he regarded as a cerebral disorder. The 'fit' for Willis was the epitome of hysteria and he therefore classified it as a convulsive disorder. It remained so until the time of Charcot (1825–1893), but by this time the afflicted organ was no longer the uterus, but the ovary which it was believed was hyperaemic in the hysterical patient. Freud, who spent time in Charcot's clinic, was the first to throw psychological light on the nature of hysteria.

THE MODERN ERA

The modern era, the age of enlightenment for patients with epilepsy, began after Adrian & Mathews (1934), at a meeting of the Physiological Society in Cambridge, confirmed and made scientifically respectable Hans Berger's human EEG which he had discovered more than 30 years before. Within 5 years, just prior to the Second World War, a flood of information about epilepsy was leashed upon the world. One must contrast the Harvard studies, carried out by Lennox and E. & F. A. Gibbs with those at Montreal where Jasper, Erickson and Penfield worked. Notable too was the work of Grey Walter in London and later Bristol during the war. By 1949 the approaches of the Harvard workers, concerned with the clinical correlates of EEG patterns, approximated to those of the group in Montreal, which were also supported by the group working on epilepsy at the Maudsley Hospital. The localisation in the brain of epileptic discharges, and their association with lesions, was seen to be more important than anything else in determining the character of the seizures, particularly their auras or type of onset. To a considerable extent too it seemed that this had a bearing on the personality disorder of the patient, if one was present. The observations and ideas of Hughlings Jackson were fully vindicated. The concept of temporal lobe epilepsy, of which uncinate epilepsy was one form, was born in 1949. The nature and the origins of lesions in the deep structures of the temporal lobe became an absorbing interest, and neurosurgeons led by Percival Bailey and Wilder Penfield in North America and Murray Falconer in London turned their attention to them.

It seemed that from the point of view of personality and the psychiatric disorders of epilepsy, a sharp distinction could be drawn between pure petit mal, which Penfield called centrencephalic epilepsy, and focal cortical epilepsy of which temporal lobe epilepsy was one example. H. Gastaut in Marseilles, and the group at The Maudsley Hospital, London which D. Pond and the writer led, paid particular attention to the psychiatric associations in these different types of epileptic patients. It became apparent in several centres in different countries that 'genuine', essential or idiopathic epilepsy was from the psychological point of view the most benign. By contrast it seemed that the serious psychiatric consequences of having epilepsy, depended upon the existence of pathological lesions, where they were in the brain, and whether they were focal or diffuse. It became apparent that most institutionalised epileptic patients, with varying degrees of subnormality of intelligence and neurological defects, were the victims of severe diffuse brain pathology, rather than the epilepsy which these lesions provoked. A different group were the patients with chronic paranoid hallucinatory psychoses, first described in detail by Slater et al (1963) and called 'schizophrenia-like' by them.

There is little doubt that the idea of inherent degeneracy of the epileptic leading inevitably to psychosis and dementia has been finally put to rest. So too in a different way has the idea of the inherent epileptic personality antedating the fits. Emphasis became increasingly placed on excessive drug treatment, frequent attacks of status, social isolation, and rejection by society. The social and occupational aspects of epilepsy received increased attention. The study of epilepsy both in man and in the experimental animal has now become the outstanding bridge between neuroscientists from different disciplines on the one hand, and social scientists, including psychologists, on the other. The list of those who have contributed, and continue to contribute to greater understanding is now very long.

References

Adrian E D, Mathews B H C 1934 The Berger rhythm: potential changes from the occipital lobes in man. Brain 57:355–385

Bailey P 1958 The problem of temporal lobe epilepsy. In: Baldwin M, Bailey P (eds) Temporal lobe epilepsy. C C Thomas, Springfield, Illinois

Clark L Pierce 1917 Clinical studies in epilepsy. Quoted by Lennox W G Epilepsy and related disorders, 2 vols. Churchill, London

Gowers W R 1907 The borderland of epilepsy. Churchill, London

Henderson D K 1939 Psychopathic states. Norton, New York

Henderson D, Gillespie R D 1950 A textbook of psychiatry, 7th edn. Oxford University Press, London

Hibbert C 1963 The roots of evil. Weidenfeld & Nicolson, London

Hunter R, Macalpine I 1963 Three hundred years of psychiatry 1535–1860. Oxford University Press, London

Jackson J H 1931 Selected writings of John Hughlings Jackson, vol 1. In: Taylor J (ed) On epilepsy and epileptiform convulsions. Hodder & Stoughton, London

Lennox W G 1960 Epilepsy and related disorders, 2 vols. Churchill, London
Lewis A 1950 Psychological medicine, Section 20. In: Price F W (ed) A textbook of medicine. Oxford Medical Publications
McCrae T 1930 Osler's principles & practice of medicine, 11th edn. Appleton-Century, London
Maudsley H 1873 Body and mind, 2nd edn. Macmillan, London
Menninger K 1963 The vital balance. Viking Press, New York
Morel B-A 1857 Traité des dégénérescences physiques, intellectuelles et morales de l'espèce humaine et des causes qui produisent ses variétés maladaptives, vol 1. Ballière, Paris
Neumann H 1859 Lehrbuch der Psychiatrie. F Euke, Erlangen
Reynolds J R 1861 Epilepsy: its symptoms, treatment and relation to other chronic convulsive diseases. Churchill, London (quoted by Hunter R, Macalpine I 1963)
Royal Commission on Capital Punishment 1949–1953 Cmd 8932 HMSO
Schwab R S 1951 Electroencephalography. W B Saunders, London
Slater E, Beard A W, Glitheroe E 1963 The schizophrenia-like psychoses of epilepsy, I–V. British Journal of Psychiatry 109:95–150
Sommer W 1880 Erkrankung des Ammonshornes als ätiologisches Moment der Epilepsie. Archiv für Psychiatrie und Nervenkrankheiten, Berlin 10: 631–675
Stauder K H 1938 Konstitution und Wesensanderung der Epileptiker. G Thieme, Leipzig
Stengel E 1960 Classification of mental disorders. Bulletin of the World Health Organisation 21:601–663
Stengel E 1963 Hughlings Jackson's influence on psychiatry. British Journal of Psychiatry 109:348–355
Taylor J (ed) 1931 On epilepsy and epileptiform convulsions. Hodder & Stoughton, London
Wilson S A Kinnier 1935 The epilepsies. Handbuch der Neurologie, vol IX. Springer, Berlin, p 1–84

Psychiatric disorders of epilepsy: classification and phenomenology

INTRODUCTION

The classification of psychiatric illness is always difficult and frequently controversial, as illustrated by the historical review and critique by Kendell (1976). However, the system introduced by Pond (1957) provides the best available framework upon which to build. More recently, Betts et al (1976) have described a useful method of classifying the epileptic psychosis. The presumed site (or sites) of origin within the brain of the seizure discharge (or discharges) causing the fits has important theoretical implications for the psychiatrist. Hence, it is essential to present a classification of the epilepsies themselves before proceeding to discuss the psychiatric disorders of epilepsy.

Classification of the epilepsies

Following the introduction of electroencephalography to the investigation of the epilepsies and the pioneering work of Penfield & Jasper (1954), it has become usual to classify the epilepsies according to the presumed site (or sites) of origin within the brain of the seizure discharge. To achieve uniformity of terminology, in 1964 the International League Against Epilepsy prepared a classification which was recommended by the International League Against Epilepsy, World Federation of Neurology, World Federation of Neurosurgical Societies, and the International Federation of Societies for Electroencephalography and Clinical Neurophysiology. The revised version (Gastaut 1969) has now achieved international usage, though yet another revision is currently being undertaken by a commission of the International League Against Epilepsy. The present international classification divides the epilepsies into three main categories, which are as follows:

1. Generalized epilepsies: the EEG discharge causing the fits is generalized from the onset and arises synchronously from either all or most of the grey matter of both hemispheres. It is accompanied by generalized, bilaterally synchronous spike and wave complexes in the EEG.

The generalized epilepsies can be subdivided into the following groups:

a. primary: where there is no brain disease and the causation is predominantly genetic.

b. secondary: where there is brain disease, usually of a diffuse nature acquired early in life. Occasionally, the secondary generalized epilepsies can be secondary to a primary cortical focus located on the mesial surface of the hemisphere or the orbital frontal areas.

c. undetermined generalized epilepsies, which cannot be assigned to either of the first two categories, usually because the EEG data is insufficient to permit subclassification.

2. Partial epilepsies: in contrast, the partial epilepsies originate from a focal epileptogenic discharge arising in a local area of cerebral cortex or related subcortical structures. However, it should be remembered that the seizure, though it may have a focal onset, can later spread to involve both hemispheres and become generalized. The partial epilepsies are regarded as being the result of acquired focal cerebral pathology, though it must be admitted that in many patients the evidence for a focal pathological lesion depends entirely on the seizure pattern and the EEG findings, without any other confirmatory neurological deficits either in the history, on examination, or following special investigation.

While the abnormal neuronal discharge remains localized and involves only one hemisphere, it may elicit a conscious sensation or series of sensations which the patient learns to recognize as a warning or aura. The character of the aura is determined by the function of the neuronal systems involved and is a manifestation of dysfunction of such systems. The aura is thus not a warning but the initial event of the seizure. Motor phenomena can also occur as the initial events of a partial seizure. Partial seizures often spread bilaterally and develop into generalized seizures (secondary generalization). The generalization may occur so rapidly that focal features are not observable clinically and no aura will be experienced. Partial seizures with onset in 'silent' areas of cortex like the frontal lobe usually have no aura. Similarly, one in five patients with temporal lobe epilepsy present with generalized convulsions without aura.

3. Unclassifiable epilepsies: those epilepsies which cannot be classified either for lack of clinical or EEG information, because they do not fit into the other two categories, or because they present a mixed picture with features of both partial and generalized epilepsy.

Classification of seizures
An international clinical and electroencephalographic classification of seizures is also available for use, being formulated by similar principles to those used in classifying the epilepsies. Seizures are subdivided into the following categories (a) partial seizures (seizures beginning locally), (b) generalized seizures (bilaterally symmetrical and without local onset) (c) unilateral seizures (d) unclassified epileptic seizures (due to incomplete data).

Partial seizures are further subdivided into the following two groups according to the type of clinical phenomena.

1. partial seizures with elementary symptomatology (simple partial seizures): attacks without impairment of consciousness accompanied by motor or sensory symptoms due to activation of one or more cortical or special sense areas of one hemisphere and corresponding to the functional representation of the areas involved. e.g. motor Jacksonian attacks, somatosensory seizures, etc.

2. partial seizures with complex symptomatology (complex partial seizures): attacks with disturbance of highest level functions of one or more cortical areas

often with impairment of consciousness, i.e. seizures with cognitive, affective or psychosensory symptomatology, automatism or compound (mixed) forms.

Generalized seizures are numerous and varied in manifestation. They include absence (petit mal) seizures, bilateral massive epileptic myoclonus, infantile spasms, clonic seizures, tonic seizures, tonic-clonic seizures (grand mal attacks), atonic and akinetic seizures. The various types of seizure are described in detail by Gastaut (1969).

CLASSIFICATION OF THE PSYCHIATRIC DISORDERS OF EPILEPSY

Before proposing a classification of the psychiatric disorders of epilepsy it is necessary to exclude certain categories of clinical problem. Isolated fits do occur from time to time in mentally ill patients. Generalized convulsions sometimes are a feature of acute catatonic states and also chronic schizophrenia. Grand mal attacks do develop during drug and alcohol withdrawal states. Finally, major seizures do occur from time to time in patients on phenothiazine and tricyclic antidepressant medication as a result of the epileptogenic effects of those drugs. Such patients should not be given the diagnostic label of epilepsy. Epilepsy is by definition a chronic brain disorder characterized by recurrent seizures. Thus epilepsy should only be used to include those patients with seizures which recur over a period of time.

Desmond Pond, in his 1957 paper, classified the psychiatric disorders of epilepsy into three main categories. These are as follows:

1. Disorders due to the brain disease causing the fits
2. Disorders directly related to the seizures
3. Those disorders whose occurrence is unrelated in time to seizure occurrence; namely the interictal disorders. I shall discuss each of these groups of disorders separately.

The disorders due to the brain disease causing the fits

These can be subdivided into those cases with diffuse cerebral dysfunction and those with focal cerebral lesions.

Diffuse cerebral dysfunction

This includes the following categories:

1. mental handicap, where the seizures and intellectual impairment are both a reflection of underlying cerebral pathology; between 20 and 50 per cent of mentally retarded patients have epilepsy, the prevalence of fits increasing with the severity of the mental handicap (Corbett et al 1975, Corbett & Pond 1979, Chapter 11).

2. the specific epileptic syndromes, of which seizures are a constant feature but are only one of a number of symptoms and signs of an organic brain syndrome, e.g. infantile spasms (West's syndrome), Univerrich-Lundberg disease, subacute sclerosing leucoencephalitis (SSLE), the Lennox-Gastaut syndrome. These disorders are associated with global intellectual impairment, which in many cases is progressive.

3. organic brain syndromes, in which seizures may occur as a symptom but are not a constant feature of the clinical picture, e.g. Alzheimer's disease (major convulsions are common in the terminal phase), arteriosclerotic dementia (fits occur in 20 per cent of cases).

4. psychotic syndromes of unknown or uncertain aetiology: psychoses, in which recurrent fits are a not uncommon finding and appear to be a manifestation of underlying, but as yet unidentified, brain dysfunction causing the psychosis. These begin before puberty and fall into the ninth International Classification of Diseases (ICD-9) category; psychoses with origin specific to childhood. The sub-divisions of this category are as follows:

a. infantile autism; a syndrome present from birth or beginning almost invariably in the first 30 months. Responses to auditory and sometimes visual stimuli are abnormal and there are usually severe problems in the understanding of spoken language. Speech is delayed and if it develops, is characterized by echolalia, the reversal of pronouns, immature grammatical structure and inability to use abstract terms. There is generally an impairment in the social use of both verbal and gestural language. Problems in social relationships are most severe before the age of 5 years and include an impairment in the development of eye-to-eye gaze, social attachments and co-operative play. Ritualistic behaviour is usual and may include abnormal routines, resistance to change, attachment to odd objects and stereotyped patterns of play. The capacity for abstract or symbolic thought and for imaginative play is diminished. Intelligence ranges from the severely subnormal to normal or above. Performance is usually better on tasks involving rote memory or visuospatial skills than on those requiring symbolic or linguistic skills.

b. disintegrative psychosis: a disorder in which normal or near normal development for the first few years is followed by a loss of social skills and of speech, together with a severe disorder of emotions, behaviour and relationships. Usually this loss of speech and of social competence takes place over a period of a few months and is accompanied by the emergence of over-activity and stereotypes. In most cases, there is intellectual impairment, but this is not necessarily part of the disorder. The condition may follow overt brain disease such as measles encephalitis, but it may occur in the absence of any known organic brain disease or damage.

c. atypical childhood psychosis: this shows some, but not all, of the features of infantile autism. Symptoms may include stereotyped repetitive movements, hyperkineses, self-injury, retarded speech development, echolalia and impaired social relationships. Such disorders may occur in children of any intelligence level but are particularly common in those with mental retardation. Such psychotic syndromes in children with epilepsy are rare, apart from infantile autism in which fit occur in 29 per cent (Rutter et al 1970, Wing 1975).

d. non-psychotic personality change, personality and behaviour disorders: where diffuse brain dysfunction plays an important causative role. In such patients it is often difficult to determine the extent to which the initial brain damage causes the psychological difficulties and the degree to which such factors as the repeated anoxic effects of recurrent major seizures, the psychological and social consequences of being an epileptic and the depressant effects of the anticonvulsant medication are important in the aetiology. Like most psychiatric disorders, it is probable that the pathogenesis results from a complex interaction of multiple factors; biological, psychological and social, the relative importance of any one factor varying from one individual to another.

Focal brain disease
Brain tumours are not uncommonly accompanied by both mental and seizure manifestations, though only the chronic, relatively benign tumours are of interest to physicians dealing with chronic epilepsy. In rapidly progressive space-occupying lesions, fits tend to be a relatively minor component of the quickly deteriorating clinical picture. Other localised brain lesions as well as tumours may cause focal brain syndromes, involving the frontal, temporal or parietal lobes. These can cause disorders of behaviour, personality and cognitive function and are described in detail by Lishman (1978). It seems reasonable to include also the HHE syndrome (hemiconvulsion-hemiplegia-epilepsy). This is a syndrome consisting of a unilateral convulsive seizure or a unilateral convulsive condition in early childhood followed by transient or permanent hemiplegia and, after a variable free interval, by the subsequent development of epilepsy, usually partial in nature. This is frequently associated with some degree of mental handicap and behaviour disorder is common.

As well as the focal brain syndromes presenting with clinical symptoms or behavioural change, one needs to include the specific focal cognitive deficits, which are often subclinical and only detected by psychometric testing, e.g. the memory, verbal and non-verbal learning deficits associated with temporal lobe lesions, the card sorting test impairments in frontal lobe dysfunction, language deficits in dominant hemisphere lesions and the complex deficits associated with parietal lobe pathology (Lishman 1978).

Disorders related in time to seizure occurrence
These can be divided into prodromal (pre-ictal), ictal and postictal events. Prodromal symptoms during the few days or hours immediately preceding the occurrence of a fit are often reported, particularly in institutionalized epileptic patients; irritability and dysphoria seem the most commonly found. This type of behaviour or mood change usually improves following seizures, and is found in about 20 per cent of institutionalized patients.

Psychiatric disturbances directly due to seizure discharge include complex partial seizures, petit mal and psychomotor status. Complex partial seizures occur when the seizure onset is localised to one part of the brain and the initial seizure manifestations involve higher level mental processes. Such seizures are predominantly of temporal lobe origin, though forced thinking or a recurrent compulsive thought entering the mind to the exclusion of all other thoughts seems to occur with lesions involving the posterior portion of the frontal lobe.

The term 'complex' implies an organized, high-level cerebral activity. Hence complex partial seizures are manifest by complex, psychological symptoms such as automatic behaviour, illusions, hallucinations, and changes in affect, memory or ideation (Gastaut & Broughton 1972). There is an alteration in the content of consciousness which, as the seizure evolves, may lead to an alteration in the level of consciousness manifested by unresponsiveness, confusion and amnesia. The hallucinations of complex partial seizures differ from those somatosensory or special sensory experiences which occur in elementary partial seizures. The latter consist of crude and undifferentiated sensations, which to the patient do not duplicate any previously experienced sensation. In contrast, the hallucinations of complex partial seizures are 'formed', in the sense that they constitute a fully developed, recognizable sensory experience which occasionally may be the memory of an actual experience (Daly 1975). It is important to note that this altered content of consciousness constitutes an intrusion upon the patient's on-going stream of awareness. No matter how vivid, complex or 'real' the ictal experience, the patient recognizes that it is an experience imposed upon him. His consciousness is 'split', and he can often remain an objective observer of these events intruding upon his stream of consciousness. Hughlings Jackson termed this phenomenon 'mental diplopia'.

The international classification recognizes the following six categories of complex partial seizures:

1. with impaired consciousness only
2. with cognitive symptomatology
3. with affective symptomatology
4. with psychosensory symptomatology
5. with 'psychomotor' symptomatology (automatism)
6. compound forms (the simultaneous or sequential occurrences of any of the above symptoms).

As Daly (1975) points out, the symptomatology of complex partial seizures can be ranked in a hierarchy of increasing complexity of subjective experience beginning with psychosensory symptoms to affective symptoms and finally cognitive symptoms. Since impaired consciousness and automatisms only occur when the ictal discharge becomes generalized (Jasper 1964), these phenomena will be considered last.

Psychosensory symptomatology
These subjective phenomena are either hallucinations, sensory perceptions in the absence of a stimulus, or illusions, distorted perceptions of actual sensory stimuli.

Formed hallucinations
Formed hallucinations probably result from seizure discharges in secondary (association) rather than primary sensory cortical areas. In certain regions these association areas are adjacent to each other. Hence multimodal hallucinations may occasionally occur.

Visual hallucinations. Seizures arising in the primary visual cortex produce crude sensations of light or darkness — for example small circles or ellipses of white or coloured light (Penfield & Jasper 1954, Brindley 1973). In contrast formed visual hallucinations may range from simple, static, monochromic but recognizable objects to intricate, multicoloured progressing scenes. Daly (1975) describes the following static examples — simple image of a tree, unfamiliar static landscape with mountains, a man carrying a cane accompanied by a dog, a complex scene of the patient as a small girl seated on a sofa in a large living room beside her mother looking out through two large bay windows on to a snowy winter landscape and expecting to depart on a journey. Occasionally a seizure may arise in primary visual cortex and then spread into association cortex first giving an unformed hallucination progressing to a formed one. Penfield & Jasper (1954) report a patient seeing irregular coloured triangles replaced by the hallucination of a robber coming after him with a gun. While recognizing the unreality of these experiences, patients often comment on the consistency from episode to episode. Definite ictal memories are rare. Mulder & Daly (1952) describe a 44 year old man with a gunshot injury of the right temporal lobe. He experienced his first attack while picking potatoes with his brother and brother-in-law. This attack consisted of a brief sensation of dizziness as he stooped over. He then stared in a daze for several seconds but continued to work. Subsequent attacks consisted of dizziness associated with a vivid still-life version of the potato patch in which the first attack occurred. The scene was exceptionally vivid and complete and lasted a few seconds. Several years later these episodes were followed by generalized convulsions.

Auditory hallucinations. These parallel visual hallucinations in their variety and complexity. Examples are as follows: a voice calling the patient's name; a lullaby being sung; a band playing, etc.

Vertiginous hallucinations. Commonly these consist of a sensation of rotation or linear displacement. A small number of patients experience more complex sensations, e.g. a 'floating' sensation (Smith 1960).

Olfactory hallucinations. Most are unfamiliar indescribable odours with either a pleasant or unpleasant quality. On rare occasions a recognizable odour occurs, e.g. a vivid smell of peaches or lemons. Olfactory reminiscences similar to visual or auditory memories can occur as a rare finding.

Gustatory hallucinations. These usually parallel the basic sensations of taste namely acid, bitter, salty or 'metallic'. Formed gustatory hallucinations are very rare.

Somatosensory hallucinations. As Penfield & Jasper (1954) point out, formed or complex somatosensory hallucinations do not occur.

Multimodal hallucinations. In some patients hallucinations may involve more than one modality, e.g. an hallucination of a little black woman actively involved in cooking, accompanied by a horrible smell (Taylor 1931). A more complex hallucinatory experience is autoscopy, defined by Lukianowicz (1958) as a complete hallucination of one's own body projected into external visual space. Such hallucinations can be accompanied by perceptual illusions and affective change (Daly 1975).

Illusions

As with formed hallucinations, ictal illusions can involve any sensory modality. In visual illusions, objects may appear to grow larger (macropsia) or small (micropsia). Objects may appear close or further away. Occasionally shapes may be distorted. Sometimes illusions and hallucinations may blend, e.g. large round stones appearing to become toads (Daly 1958). In the auditory modality sounds may appear fainter or louder, or to rise or fall in pitch. Sometimes they take on an echoing quality. Olfactory illusions may consist of a sudden intensification of smell. Gustatory illusions are rare. In contrast to formed somatosensory hallucinations, somatosensory illusions are common, e.g. a limb feels larger or smaller, it does not seem to belong to the patient or it seems detached and removed some distance from the patient's body.

Affective symptomatology

Any recognizable emotion may occur as an ictal event. The quality varies from a crude undifferentiated welling up of feeling intruding on the patient's consciousness and unrelated to anything in the environment, an emotional change colouring other ictal experiences to highly refined feelings related to ongoing events in the environment (affective illusions).

Fear is the most frequent, usually brief in duration lasting only seconds. Pleasurable ictal experiences are rare (sudden feelings of ecstasy, elation, happiness, serenity, relaxation, etc.), the most famous patient being Dostoyevsky, the Russian novelist. Depression is also uncommon as an ictal event. It is a more enduring emotion than fear or anxiety. Hence the emotion persists throughout the ictal phase of the seizure and may continue for hours or days after the postictal confusion has cleared up. Weil (1956, 1959) has observed ictal depression lasting from minutes to as long as ten days. Feelings of sadness, futility, and lonesomeness have been described; also 'homesickness', thoughts of death and suicide. Unpleasant emotions which cannot be identified by the patient as a specific feeling state, like fear, are also not uncommon, e.g. 'an unpleasant, indescribable emotion.' Anger is rare as an ictal emotion.

Eroticism is also rare as an ictal event. Frankly sexual emotions must be distinguished from somatosensory sensations in the genitalia. Unilateral paraesthesiae in the labia, scrotum or medial thigh have been described in patients with partial seizures with onset in the postcentral, parasaggital area of the contralateral hemisphere. Such localized genital sensations are not associated with erotic feelings. However, a few patients with definite ictal sexual feelings have been reported, e.g. a feeling of being hot all over as if having coitus, genital sensations similar to those of orgasm, a sensation of itching in the perineum and a feeling as if a hot poker was inserted into the vagina. Another ictal sexual event is the occurrence of behaviour mimicking sexual activity during an epileptic automatism, for which the patient is subsequently amnesic.

In some patients ictal hallucinatory experiences acquire an affective colouring. In other instances the ictal emotion may attach itself to an otherwise neutral experience. For example, Daly (1975) describes two patients who said that when their attacks began, any object at which they were looking, e.g. a telephone or a chair, suddenly developed a threatening or malevolent quality, which each recognized as totally inappropriate. If they shifted their gaze to any other object, it did not seem threatening and the fear would diminish. However, returning the gaze to the original object would result in an intensification of the fear, which was followed by unconsciousness and automatism.

Epileptic or gelastic seizure laughter should perhaps not be classed under the affective symptoms because there is usually amnesia for this and the laughter is classically affectless and hollow. Gelastic seizure laughter is characterized by its unpredictability, its lack of provocation and the relatively unaffected facial expression which accompanies it. Flushing is quite common, however, and at some stage during the attack consciousness is frequently lost and a convulsive seizure may develop. Ictal laughter must be distinguished from other forms of pathological laughter in which sudden uncontrolled attacks of mirth seize the victim, but for which there is usually memory and a realization of the inappropriateness of the laughter. This type of pathological laughter is usually associated with basal mesencephalic lesions (Daly 1975). Ictal laughter tends to occur in partial seizures of temporal or frontal lobe origin.

Cognitive symptomatology

Cognitive symptomatology consists of the following three symptom subgroups: (1) ideational (2) dysmnesic (3) other symptoms. The most common ideational symptom is the phenomenon of forced thinking, in which a thought forces itself upon the patient. The thought may be one already present in the subject's mind when the seizure occurs, which he is incapable of resisting or putting out of his head. More often it is an entirely new thought (parasitic idea) forced upon the patient at the onset of the seizure.

The thought may be subjective (metaphysical or even transcendental, such as the idea of death or immortality); objective (a fixation upon the ideational content of a phrase read or heard before the attack); or unidentifiable and even impossible to recall, the patient only able to remember that he was thinking very intently about 'something'. Very rarely, forced thinking may consist of a very rapid recollection of more or less protracted experiences from his past life. In addition to the phenomenon of forced thinking, ictal language disturbances can also be classed as ideational events.

Dysmnesic seizures are those in which there is more or less marked impairment of memory. Included in this category are ecmnesic hallucinations (in which previous experiences are recalled by the subject and 'relived' with great intensity — panoramic memories) which are rare. In contrast, illusions of memory are common. These phenomena are as follows: déjà-vu (a feeling of having already seen an object or person not seen before), déjà-entendu (a feeling of having already heard something, not previously heard) and déjà-vécu (a feeling of having already lived through an experience, not actually experienced before), jamais-vu (a feeling of never having seen before a familiar object or situation), jamais-entendu (a familiar sound or speech appearing strange or unfamiliar), jamais-vécu (a feeling of not having lived through an experience which has, in reality, happened before). Déjà-vu, déjà-entendu and déjà-vécu have in common an illusion of familiarity, while jamais-vu, jamais entendu and jamais-vécu are illusions of unfamiliarity or strangeness. These dysmnesic symptoms are termed non-perceptive or agnosic illusions by Gastaut (1973); i.e. an external object or internal event is perceived normally but poorly understood. These contrast with perceptive illusions, which are distorted perceptions of external stimuli.

Other ictal cognitive changes, which can best be classified as agnosic illusions, are the disturbances of time perception that some patients experience. Everything seems speeded up and rushing past or events seem to be happening more slowly than normal, like a slow motion film. Feelings of depersonalization and derealization can also be regarded as agnosic illusions.

Impairment of consciousness and psychomotor symptomatology (automatism)

In complex partial seizures, the content of consciousness can be grossly disturbed by the perceptual, hallucinatory and emotional experiences. Such experiences tend in themselves to impair attention and awareness. Hence the patient, though he may still be to some extent aware of what is going on, is less completely conscious of self and environment than normally. Clouding of consciousness can also occur as a primary event in the absence of other abnormal experiences and may be accompanied by confusion and amnesia. Such attacks must be distinguished from ictal dysphasic attacks as a result of left hemisphere discharge and also from simple absence seizures. Petit mal absences due to generalized spike and wave discharges are usually brief lasting 10 seconds or less and cease abruptly with immediate return to clear consciousness and resumption of normal behaviour. Complex partial seizures presenting with episodes of brief unconsciousness without aura or other lateralizing features are of longer duration, a minute or more, and recovery to clear consciousness is gradual with a brief period of confusion being common. Absence seizures often occur many times a day. Such high frequency is rare with complex partial attacks.

In association with the clouding of consciousness due to the partial seizure discharge, the patient may behave abnormally carrying out simple or complex movements without being aware of what he is doing. Such actions are known as automatisms. Behaviour automatism can occur either as the direct result of a seizure discharge or as a postictal event following any type of fit, especially after one or more generalized convulsions. The area most commonly involved in the initiation of an ictal automatism appears to be the periamygdaloid region. This includes the uncus, the amygdaloid nucleus, the central claustrum and the temporoinsular cortex deep in the anterior part of the Sylvian fissure.

However, Jasper (1964) has pointed out that stimulation of these structures will only produce automatic behaviour in about 50 per cent of cases. Automatism will not occur while the after discharge remains confined to the amygdala or hippocampus. There is always bilateral involvement of the amygdaloid-hippocampal structures with invariable spread to the mesial diencephalon and temporoparietal cortex. In many cases the frontal and central areas will be involved as well. Indeed automatic behaviour in some patients results from discharging lesions at sites other than the mesial temporal structures; namely the frontal, orbito-frontal and parietal regions or the mesial surfaces of the hemispheres (Geier et al 1976, 1977). Presumably, the discharging focus causes secondary activation of the periamygdaloid-hippocampal structures with rapid spread to the mesial diencephalon and subsequent projection back to the neocortex via the diffuse projection system of the upper brainstem. Ictal automatism can occasionally result from prolonged generalized spike wave discharge (petit mal automatism) or generalized frontotemporal theta/delta rhythms initiated by primary activation of the diencephalon (Jasper 1964).

Behaviour during epileptic automatism varies greatly from patient to patient and in the same individual on different occasions. The person's actions have a quasi-purposeful quality but are often inappropriate to the environmental situation. There is usually impairment of awareness and lack of responsiveness to the surroundings. Attacks lasting 10 seconds or less merely cause cessation of activity. More prolonged episodes of 20 to 30 seconds duration display stereotyped repetitive movements, e.g. chewing, swallowing, clenching fists, etc. Attacks which last several minutes are associated with more complex, variable but quasi-purposeful behaviour, e.g. undressing, wandering away, etc., which involves interplay with the environment and gradually merges into normal behaviour. The earlier stereotyped phenomena are a direct manifestation of the ictal discharge, while the later complex behaviour continues during the postictal phase of the attack. The majority of automatisms are brief; five minutes or less in 80 per cent and never over an hour. Serious violence during epileptic automatisms is rare. The relation between epilepsy and automatism has been reviewed in detail by Fenton (1972, 1980).

Many of the phenomena experienced during complex partial siezures, such as déjà-vu feelings, depersonalization, hallucinations, and affective changes occur in functional psychiatric illnesses. However, when occurring as ictal events they are paroxysmal in occurrence with sudden onset and rapid resolution. The duration is transient lasting minutes rather than hours, days, weeks, months or even years. The attacks are recurrent and have a stereotyped quality, each one being essentially similar to the previous ones. Sometimes the patient will comment that the sensations experienced are 'imposed upon' him, being quite different from normal feeling states. Further, careful questioning and observation will usually reveal some degree of alteration of consciousness during the attacks. In the functional psychiatric syndromes, these phenomena always occur in clear consciousness.

The other two ictal psychiatric disorders are petit mal and psychomotor status. Both are states of clouding of consciousness resulting from continuing generalised spike and wave complexes or local temporal lobe discharges respectively. These clouded states may last for hours or days. Petit mal status is a relatively common event, especially in children with epilepsy. In contrast, psychomotor status is extremely rare. It consists of recurrent episodes of automatic behaviour which may merge into a fugue-like state.

Postictal disorders
These are disorders which immediately follow one or more seizures, usually generalised convulsions. The common feature is clouding of consciousness due to post-seizure depression of cortical function and hence the EEG is usually dominated by diffusely slow frequencies within the theta and delta range with little or no normal activity being present. Such patients usually manifest behaviour associated with confusional states (clouded states, twilight states, fugue states) or automatic behaviour. Again, these are relatively short-lived, differing from the ictal events in lasting hours or days or occasionally one or two weeks, but rarely longer. Total recovery is the rule.

Interictal disorders unrelated in time to the seizures
The interictal psychiatric disorders of epilepsy are those whose occurrence is unrelated in time to seizure occurrence. The symptoms are present between attacks and often in the absence of seizures. It is assumed that the epilepsy and/or

the cerebral epileptogenic lesion have played a role in the genesis of the psychiatric disorder. Though the illness is unrelated in time to seizure occurrence, the onset, intensity and course of the illness may be influenced by fit frequency; most commonly by an exacerbation of epileptic attacks; less often and more controversially by a reduction in fit frequency.

There is much evidence that both adults and children with epilepsy have a higher prevalence of psychiatric disorder of a nature that cannot be directly related to seizure occurrence than would be expected in the general population. The work of Rutter et al (1970) surveying children between the ages of 5 and 14 years on the Isle of Wight has also demonstrated clearly that, in children at least, this is not simply due to a reaction to the stress of coping with a chronic illness. Rutter et al (1970) found that epileptic children had about three times as much psychiatric disability as those children with other chronic disorders affecting the peripheral rather than the central nervous system. The evidence concerning adults with epilepsy is much more equivocal. We await definitive studies of whole population samples.

It is a general rule that the interictal psychiatric disorders of epilepsy manifest the same range of mental state and behavioural phenomena as the functional psychiatric syndromes in the absence of epilepsy. There may, however, be some differences in detail. For example, it is claimed that there is a specific temporal lobe syndrome (Geshwind 1977, Bear & Fedio 1977) and a number of authors have suggested that there are qualitative differences between the schizophrenia-like psychoses of epilepsy and 'non-epileptic' schizophrenia; namely warmer affect, less personality deterioration, paranoid delusions with a religiose colouring, a relatively common occurrence of mystical delusional experiences and more common visual hallucinations than in 'non-epileptic' schizophrenia (Hill 1953, Pond 1957, Slater et al 1963). These apparent qualitative differences still require to be demonstrated by the use of quantitative mental state assessments like the Present State Examination technique. Finally it is necessary to point out that there is considerable unavoidable overlap on the proposed classification between the disorders due to brain disease category and the interictal disorder group. Indeed brain dysfunction frequently contributes to the causation of the interictal psychoses, personality and behaviour disorders.

The interictal psychiatric disorders of epilepsy can be classified as follows:

1. Disorders of childhood

a. neurotic disorders: these include anxiety and fearfulness, misery and unhappiness, sensitivity, shyness and withdrawal, relationship problems such as sibling rivalry but excluding aggressive behaviour. According to the ninth revision of the International Classification of Diseases (ICD-9), this syndrome has been given the term, disturbance of emotions specific to childhood and adolescence.

b. antisocial disorders: a syndrome characterized by behaviours such as defiance, disobedience, quarrelsomeness, aggression, destructive behaviour, tantrums, solitary stealing, lying, teasing, bullying and disturbed relationships with others; this syndrome is also known as unsocialized disturbance of conduct (ICD-9).

c. mixed (antisocial/neurotic) disorder: where there is considerable emotional disturbance as well as the antisocial behaviour; also known as mixed disturbance of conduct and emotions (ICD-9).

d. hyperkinetic syndrome of childhood (ICD-9): disorders in which the essential features are short attention-span and distractibility. Overactivity, impulsiveness, marked mood fluctuations and aggression are also common symptoms. Delays in the development of specific skills are often present and disturbed peer relationships are common.

e. psychosis with origin specific to childhood (ICD-9): this diagnostic category has already been described in the section concerning the disorders due to the brain disease causing the fits.

2. Disorders of adulthood

a. Non-psychotic disorders affecting personality. Personality is a descriptive label referring to the sum total of the relatively enduring or permanent traits, attitudes and patterns of behaviour which typify an individual, i.e. the sum of the person's noteworthy characteristics, intellectual, affective, physical, social traits, interests, values and beliefs, which give to each person both an individuality and a resemblance to his/her fellows. The effects of epilepsy on personality can be classified as follows:

(i) personality disorder; which is defined as deeply ingrained maladaptive patterns of behaviour generally recognizable by the time of adolescence or earlier and continuing throughout most of adult life, although often becoming less obvious in middle or old age (ICD-9). The personality is abnormal either in the balance of its components, their quality and expression, or in its total aspect. Because of this deviation the patient suffers or others have to suffer and there is an adverse effect upon the individual or on society. Personality disorder in people with epilepsy tends to occur in those with an early onset of seizures and multiple handicaps; not only biological, but personal and environmental as well.

(ii) personality change: an alteration in personality functioning in a person with a previously well-adjusted, 'normal' personality; due to focal or diffuse cerebral pathology, frequent fits, overmedication, a reaction to the stress of coping with the epilepsy or an interaction between all these factors.

(iii) behaviour disorder: a disturbance of one or more aspects of the individual's behaviour as a consequence of the fits, the treatment, underlying brain pathology and/or the psychological and social effects of having epilepsy. Behaviour disorder is most common in adolescents. The clinical features are similar to those of disturbed adolescents without fits and include irritability, moodiness and sometimes frank mood change with social withdrawal, quarrelsomeness and paranoid attitudes, temper tantrums and occasionally explosive aggressiveness, impulsiveness, restlessness, poor attention span, distractibility and lack of application, disturbed interpersonal relationships and sometimes delinquent behaviour.

b. the sexual dysfunctions: the most common being low sex drive and reduced libido but isolated case reports of sexual deviation such as fetishism, transvestitism and exhibitionism have been reported in association with temporal lobe epilepsy.

c. the psychoses: functional in form in a setting of clear consciousness with affective or schizophrenia-like symptoms. The affective and schizoaffective disorders are the most common (Pahla et al 1980, Perez & Trimble 1980), and tend to run an intermittent course with remissions and relapses. In contrast, the schizophrenia-like psychoses have a more chronic outcome. Betts et al (1976) classify the psychoses as follows:

(i) global disruption of personality: with disturbance of thinking, behaviour, emotional relationships, feeling and perception. This includes the schizophrenias and schizophrenia-like states.

(ii) primary disturbance of mood: depression or pathological elation and such secondary symptoms as depressive hallucinations or delusions.

(iii) organic psychosyndromes: including confusional states, changes in behaviour in relation to fit frequency or subclinical ictal activity. The organic psychosyndromes are, of course, disorders directly related to the epileptic activity within the brain, while the schizophrenias and affective states are interictal psychoses.

References

Bear D, Fedio P 1977 Quantitative analysis of interictal behaviour in temporal lobe epilepsy. Archives of Neurology 34:454–467

Betts T A, Merskey H, Pond D A 1976 Psychiatry. In: Laidlaw J, Richens A (eds) Textbook of epilepsy. Churchill-Livingstone, Edinburgh

Brindley G S 1973 Sensory effects of electrical stimulation of the visual and paravisual cortex in man. In: Jung R (ed) Handbook of sensory physiology, vol VII. Springer-Verlag, Berlin, Ch. 36

Corbett J A, Harris R, Robinson R G 1975 Epilepsy. In: Wortis J (ed) Mental retardation and developmental disabilities, Vol VII. Churchill-Livingstone, Edinburgh

Corbett J A, Pond D A 1979 Epilepsy and behaviour disorders in the mentally handicapped. In: James F E, Snaith R P (eds) Psychiatric illness and mental handicap. Gaskell Press, London

Daly D 1958 Ictal affect. American Journal of Psychiatry 115:97–108

Daly D D 1975 Ictal clinical manifestations. In: Penry J K, Daly D D (eds) Complex partial seizures and their treatment. Advances in Neurology, Vol II. Raven Press, New York

Fenton G W 1972 Epilepsy and automatism. British Journal of Hospital Medicine 7:57–64

Fenton G W 1980 Epilepsy and automatism. Journal of Irish Medical Association (in press)

Gastaut H 1969 Clinical and electroencephalographical classification of epileptic seizures. Suppl. Epilepsia 10:S2–21

Gastaut H 1973 Dictionary of epilepsy. W.H.O., Geneva

Gastaut H, Broughton R 1972 Epileptic seizures. Thomas, Springfield, Illinois

Geier S, Bancaud J, Talairach J, Bonis A, Szikla G, Enjelvin M 1976 Automatisms during frontal lobe epileptic seizures. Brain 99:447–458

Geier S, Bancaud J, Talairach J, Bonis A, Szikla G, Enjelvin M 1977 The seizures of frontal lobe epilepsy. Neurology 27:951–958

Geschwind N 1977 Current research. In: Blumer D, Levin K (eds) Psychiatric complications in the epilepsies: current research and treatment. McLean Hospital Journal, special issue, June 1977

Hill D 1953 Psychiatric disorders of epilepsy. Medical Press 229:473–475

Jasper H H 1964 Some physiological mechanisms involved in epileptic automatism. Epilepsia 5:1–20

Kendell R E 1975 The role of diagnosis in psychiatry. Blackwell Scientific Publications, Oxford

Lishman W A 1978 Organic psychiatry. Blackwell Scientific Publications, London

Lukinowicz N 1958 Autoscopic phenomena. Archives of Neurology and Psychiatry 80:119–220

Mulder D W, Daly D 1952 Psychiatric symptoms associated with lesions of the temporal lobe. Journal of the American Medical Association 150:173–176

Pahla A, Fenton G W, Driver M V, Fenwick P B C 1980 Epilepsy and psychiatric disorder (in preparation)

Penfield W, Jasper H H 1954 Epilepsy and the functional anatomy of the human brain. Little Brown & Co, Boston

Perez M M, Trimble M R 1980 Epileptic psychosis — diagnostic comparison with process schizophrenia. British Journal of Psychiatry 137:245–249

Pond D A 1957 Psychiatric aspects of epilepsy. Journal of the Indian Medical Profession 3:1441–1451

Rutter M, Graham P, Yule W 1970 A neuropsychiatric study in childhood. Heinemann, London

Slater E, Beard A W, Glithero E 1963 The schizophrenia-like psychoses of epilepsy. British Journal of Psychiatry 109:95–150

Smith B H 1960 Vestibular disturbances in epilepsy. Neurology 10:465–469

Taylor J (ed) 1931 Selected writings of John Hughlings Jackson, Vol 1. Hodder and Stoughton, London

Weil A A 1956 Ictal depression and anxiety in temporal lobe disorders. American Journal of Psychiatry 113:149–157

Weil A A 1959 Ictal emotions occurring in temporal lobe dysfunction. Archives of Neurology 1:101–111

Wing L 1975 The syndrome of early childhood autism. In: Silverstone T, Barraclough B (eds) Contemporary Journal of Psychiatry, special publication no. 9

Epildemiology of the psychiatric disorders of epilepsy

INTRODUCTION

Epidemiological studies always require:

1. an adequate definition of the cases to be studied; that is, a description which is reliable, valid and as far as possible easy to apply to the large number that is usually involved;

2. an appropriate population which can be surveyed by the methods for measuring the cases.

In discussing the epidemiology of the psychiatric symptoms of epilepsy, the difficulties are doubled if not squared in that the criteria for caseness are twofold: firstly, for epilepsy; secondly, for psychiatric disorder. It is therefore necessary to start with a short discussion of the epidemiology of epilepsy as a whole, which has to be followed by a discussion of the epidemiology of psychiatric symptoms before the two can be properly combined together.

EPIDEMIOLOGY OF EPILEPSY

Hauser (1978) has recently reviewed the main epidemiological studies of epilepsy and shown that the wide variation in rates in different studies is largely, if not entirely, due to different criteria of what consitutes an epileptic person. A single attack is not usually regarded as evidence for counting a person as having epilepsy, though this may be important for some purposes, for example heavy goods vehicle licences. Epilepsy is a clinical diagnosis, and there may be disagreement about the exact description of which attacks are to be regarded as epileptic and which not. In the end, as someone said a few years ago, a person becomes diagnosed as having epilepsy when a competent epileptologist says he is!

Nevertheless, in spite of the diagnostic difficulties, certain broad facts are generally acceptable. Annual incidence rates cluster around 30 to 50 per 100 000 population, and the rates for males are slightly higher than for females. There is general agreement that the incidence is high in the first year of life, falling throughout childhood to fairly low values, but with a rise again over age 60. The prevalence that results from this incidence works out at about between 3 and 6 per 1000 population. Surprisingly, even in the most intensively investigated cases the aetiology is not definitely known in about half of all cases. There are probably no significant differences between social classes, but socio-economic factors have not been adequately investigated.

From the epidemiological point of view a very accurate method of study is the long-term follow-up of particular groups or cohorts as they are now called. The advantage of this method is that it will uncover those who have dropped out through death or might disappear from a general population survey by long-term residence in a hospital or other institution. A rather more sombre picture than might be expected from most surveys emerges from such studies, though they are few in number. Harrison & Taylor's (1976) 25-year follow-up of early childhood onset epilepsy is one of the longest, and they show that 10 per cent had died (mostly within 1 or 2 years); 11 per cent were in institutions (mainly hospitals for the subnormal); 6.6 per cent were wholly at home (and likely to be hospitalised when parents or other relatives could no longer cope). These three groups made up a quarter, and another quarter had chronic epilepsy (of whom only half were self-supporting in the community) so only half were fit-free. It is, of course, well known that the prognosis of early onset epilepsy is much worse than late onset, so a cohort of those starting for example in adolescence, is likely to show a better long-term prognosis.

The main point to stress now is that there is a highly significant association with mental handicap, which I shall discuss later. Ross et al (1980) reported a 16-year follow-up of patients with epilepsy in the National Child Development study and the same point emerged. Sillanpää's (1973) even more gloomy follow-up must, I think, be due to his including epileptic children who nearly all had been hospitalised at some stage—one wonders what happens to simple febrile convulsions in Finland.

One other epidemiological point worth mentioning is the question whether the incidence of epilepsy is falling over the years, which hopefully it should do with better obstetric and perinatal care and fewer serious childhood problems such as infections. Only the figures from Rochester (Hauser 1978) are relevant, and they show an equivocal fall in childhood. Surprisingly no-one seems to have looked in Britain at, for example, general practice records. The total prevalence may well be actually rising since any possible fall in childhood is probably more than compensated for by the increasing number of elderly persons whom it is now clear have quite a high incidence of late onset epilepsy. Later life expectancy is difficult to determine accurately as epilepsy is frequently not mentioned on death certificates, even as a contributory cause of death, but it appears likely that there is an excess of deaths due to suicide, accidents and status epilepticus, which straightaway shows the importance of the psychiatric aspects.

However, Hauser, Annegers & Elveback (1980) have just reported a long-term follow-up of a cohort of patients with epilepsy, which is not altogether satisfactory as information was missing in a considerable number of cases. The increased mortality in many groups of epileptics seemed to be due to a variety of conditions. There was an excess of accidents, but status epilepticus was not mentioned as a cause of death and there was not an excess of suicide. This last finding may be related to lack of follow-up data on many of the longer-term cases.

EPIDEMIOLOGY OF PSYCHIATRIC DISORDER IN EPILEPSY

Turning now to the epidemiology of psychiatric disorder, we find, if anything, even more methodological difficulties. Self-administered questionnaires are perhaps less frequently used than they were, though they are still of value for rough screening of large populations. More reliance is now placed on structured interviews, especially standardised ones like the Present State Examination. The psychiatric aspects of epilepsy are particularly difficult to evaluate as the mental disturbances are often episodic; for example, postictal confusional states. Some may feel that it is not appropriate to include these in a psychiatric survey of epilepsy. At any one moment of investigation the ongoing psychiatric disorders unrelated temporally to attacks are, of course, much the most common in the general population, though perhaps not in epileptic patients admitted to hospital.

This last point brings out the great importance of specifying exactly what population is being studied. Most of the early studies and even some more recent ones, for example by Guerrant et al (1962), are based on in-patients or, at any rate, hospital attenders. Amongst others, Pond & Bidwell (1959) showed several years ago that the epileptic population seen in hospital is significantly different in a number of ways from those who are seen only by general practitioners in the community. The ideal epidemiological study of psychiatric symptoms in persons with epilepsy should therefore consist of a whole population survey (not omitting those in hospital) by standardised structured psychiatric interviews, and would include data obtained not only from the patient but also from relatives. Few studies reach this level: one is of epileptic school children in the Isle of Wight, by Rutter, Graham & Yule (1970). My own general practice study of 20 years ago could now be regarded as unsatisfactory, as the psychiatric assessment was relatively unstructured and carried out by a psychiatric social worker. She was in fact very knowledgeable of patients with epilepsy, having worked in my clinic for some years, and I do not think that the figures we obtained were noticeably biased. We also relied on the GP's diagnosis for primary case finding, and may therefore have missed a few not properly recorded — I know that in at least one practice, for example, we did not see some of the over-60s with late onset fits as they were misdiagnosed as having cerebrovascular attacks or what are nowadays called transient ischaemic attacks.

With all these provisos in mind, therefore, we may now turn to such information as can be regarded as reliable. It is convenient to consider children and adults separately as most of the published work does this and the studies of children are more common than of adults. We must consider first the standard work of Rutter, Graham & Yule (1970) which is part of their large survey of schoolchildren on the Isle of Wight. They found that the prevalence of psychiatric disorder as defined by interview and standardised questionnaires to parents and teachers was 8 per cent in the general population, nearly double in children with chronic medical handicap (like asthma) not involving the CNS and more than doubled again to one third in those with uncomplicated epilepsy. The latter figure is very similar to that I found in the relatively small number of children in my GP survey (Pond & Bidwell 1959). The prevalence rises to 50 per cent in epilepsy complicated by other neurological disorders mainly because of mental subnormality.

As regards adults, there have been many surveys of mental hospital in-patients and of outpatient attenders at neurological, psychiatric and special clinics for epilepsy, all of which, as would be expected, show a high percentage of mental disturbance in persons with epilepsy. Such reports are, however, of limited value as regards determining true prevalence since, as I have already said, my survey shows that non-attenders manifest fewer disturbances than hospital attenders—something, of course, that is true of many other conditions besides epilepsy. Hospital studies, however, may be of value if particular sub-groups or symptom-clusters are studied, all of whom (or at least the great majority) would expect to be seen there (e.g. status epilepticus or paranoid-hallucinatory psychoses).

As far as I know, the only two useful community studies are my own (Pond & Bidwell 1959) and that of Gudmundsson (1966) in Iceland. Gudmundsson's survey is of value as regards the prevalence of psychiatric disturbance in adult patients with epilepsy, since not only did he personally examine most of them but also he was able to compare the prevalence rates with a general psychiatric survey of the Icelandic population by Helgason (1964). He finds that 10 per cent of the men are neurotic, which is the expected rate, but one quarter of the women show neurotic symptoms which is substantially higher. Another quarter of the group show the 'ixoid' personality—a rate which is much higher in the men than in the women. A much smaller number show the 'ixothym' personality, and exactly half the group are regarded as having a normal personality. Pond & Bidwell (1959) thought that 29 per cent of their group showed psychological difficulties, but pointed out that this was an underestimate since a number of the cases were not personally interviewed by the psychiatric social worker. Half the group showed neurotic symptoms, so that about 15 per cent of the whole group of epileptics showed neurotic symptoms—a figure remarkably close to that obtained by Gudmundsson (1966) and probably hardly higher than that to be expected to occur in the general population. It is not possible to compare figures for any other diagnosed group, though it is of interest to note that the English survey diagnosed the so-called epileptic personality in 11 patients, which is nearly 5 per cent of the whole group, while Gudmundsson found that 8 per cent of his group would be regarded as psychotic. 7 per cent of Pond and Bidwell's group had been in a mental hospital before or during the survey year, and they estimated that about 10 per cent of the whole group would probably have some period of in-patient psychiatric care at some stage. 4.5 per cent of Gudmundsson's group had been admitted to mental hospital, though over 7 per cent of them had been 'psychotic' at some time.

The relationship between type of personality change and type of epilepsy is, of course, complex and few figures are available, even to confirm or deny the special psychological disorders associated with temporal lobe epilepsy. Moreover, apart from this latter group there is disagreement on what other forms of epilepsy are meaningful to investigate. Perhaps simple febrile convulsions is one group, and here the general impression is that they suffer from no significant increase in psychological disturbance. Petit mal may be another group; it is a rare condition and a random sample hard to reach for proper psychological study. As regards temporal lobe epilepsy, some figures may be extracted from Gudmundsson's (1966) paper and from my own GP study (Pond & Bidwell 1959) though neither paper specifically discusses this issue.

In Gudmundsson's study 50 per cent of his patients with temporal lobe epilepsy had psychological difficulties, and only 24 per cent of those without temporal lobe epilepsy as diagnosed clinically. Rather less than half of his patients had an EEG, and of the EEGs taken half were normal. Of the rest it is possible to compare temporal lobe foci with the generalised EEG changes: the former have a slightly higher rate of neurotic and ixoid disturbances. In Pond & Bidwell's survey (1959) the patients with temporal lobe epilepsy had slightly more employment difficulties than the non-temporal ones, though the difference was hardly significant. However, using the crude index of hospitalisation in a mental hospital, the temporal lobe epileptics have a significantly higher rate, nearly 20 per cent of them having been in hospital, whereas there were only 7 per cent in the whole group. It is of interest that this apparently small group of patients with temporal lobe epilepsy constitute half of all those who had been in mental hospital, thus underlining their significance as regards the problem of epilepsy in mental hospitals.

An important recent long-term follow-up of temporal lobe epilepsy beginning in childhood is by Lindsay, Ounsted & Richards (1979) (Chapter 15). TLE beginning in childhood does not, of course, include all such cases seen in adult life — in fact only a quarter began under the age of 15 in the large series of Currie et al (1971). The Oxford group find that nearly one quarter were subnormal but of the rest, 70 per cent were psychiatrically healthy, an improvement over the high rate of disorder found when they were last surveyed in childhood. 10 per cent had developed a paranoid-hallucinatory psychosis (in which group there was only one female and none had a unilateral right-sided EEG focus) and from the natural history known so far of this disorder, a few more cases of psychosis would be expected in later years, for which men with left-sided foci seem at particular risk. The authors also make the point that treated neurotic and depressive illnesses seemed uncommon, but again more cases are likely as the sample ages.

As a working hypothesis, therefore, one may say that the prevalence of general neurotic disorder is probably about 15–20 per cent, much as would be expected in any sample of subjects with a chronic medical disability that carries with it also psychosocial disabilities. To this number must then be added about the same number with problems peculiar to epilepsy resulting from the associated CNS damage, drug effects and the episodic ictal–related alterations of consciousness. There is also an increased tendency to paranoid hallucinatory psychosis for reasons that are not clearly related to the CNS disorder. Finally, about 10 per cent of the group are likely to be educationally subnormal or worse, according to Pond & Bidwell, which is not dissimilar from 7 per cent of Gudmundsson's 1966 group having IQs below 75. This is about five times the expected rate from Helgason's survey of the same population.

References

Currie S, Heathfield K W G, Henson R A, Scott D F 1971 Clinical course and prognosis of temporal lobe epilepsy. Brain 94:173–190

Gudmundsson G 1966 Epilepsy in Iceland. Acta neurol scand Suppl 25:43

Guerrant J, Anderson W W, Fischer A, Weinstein M R, Jaros R M, Deskins A 1962 Personality in epilepsy. C C Thomas, Springfield, Illinois

Harrison R M, Taylor D C 1976 Childhood seizures: 25-year follow-up. Lancet 1:948–951

Hauser W A 1978 Epidemiology of epilepsy. In: Schoenberg, B S (ed) Neurological epidemiology: principles and clinical applications. Advances in Neurology 19:313–339 Raven Press, New York

Hauser W A, Annegers J F, Elveback L R 1980 Mortality in patients with epilepsy. Epilepsia
   21(4):399–412
Helgason T 1964 Epidemiology of mental disorders in Iceland. Acta psychiat scand Suppl 142
Lindsay J, Ounsted C, Richards P 1979 Long-term outcome in children with temporal lobe
   epilepsy. III Psychiatric aspects in childhood and adult life. Devel. Med. Child Neurol
   21:630–636
Pond D A, Bidwell B H 1959 A survey of epilepsy in 14 general practices. II Social and
   psychological aspects. Epilepsia 1:285–299
Ross E M, Peckham C S, West P B, Butler N R 1980 Epilepsy in childhood: findings from the
   National Child Development Study Brit med J i:207–210
Rutter M, Graham P, Yule W 1970 A neuropsychiatric study in childhood. Clin. Dev. Med. 35.
   Spastics International Press in association with Heinemann Medical Books, London
Sillanpää M, 1973 Medico-social prognosis of children with epilepsy. Acta paed scand Suppl 237

Problems of learning and behaviour in children with epilepsy

INTRODUCTION

This topic is of considerable practical importance as well as research potential. For both purposes, however, it is necessary to carefully define the basic concepts involved and to disentangle the many possible causal factors.

Such care has rarely characterised discussion of behavioural aspects of epilepsy. Particularly during the 19th century, global clinical impressions of mainly brain damaged, institutionalised patients with uncontrolled convulsive seizures were generalised to other types of patient. As noted in Chapter 1, it was believed that recurrent seizures were evidence of constitutional degeneracy which would lead to physical, mental and moral deterioration and that nothing could be done to halt this progression. Unfortunately, this sort of belief persists to some extent in the notion of 'the epileptic personality' which is still used freely by doctors, social workers, teachers and others. Tizard (1962) considered very carefully the idea that all people with epilepsy share common personality characteristics and concluded that there was no convincing evidence of this at all. Although her study was carried out over 15 years ago, no new evidence has been produced to the contrary.

In contrast to the impressionistic approach characterised by generalisations from ill-defined groups of patients, is the attempt to carefully define and measure particular aspects of behaviour in specific sub-groups within the epileptic population. This approach attempts to distinguish between the behavioural effects of recurrent seizures themselves and other aspects of the patient's situation such as drug treatment and the psychological and social circumstances at home, school or work. This more discriminating approach has a long history and could be seen as starting with the investigations by a physiologist, W. G. Smith, working at the London County Asylum at Claybury in Essex at the start of the century (Smith 1904). In a somewhat controlled study, Smith found that although epileptic patients performed worse than normals on some psychophysiological tasks, on others their performance was equal to that of the controls. Unfortunately, the example set by Smith was not followed by psychologists even though he presented his interesting findings to the British Psychological Society in 1903. Impressions and generalisations about people with epilepsy prevailed. For example, Tylor-Fox (1924) said that epileptic children suffered from 'lack of concentration and inadequate recent memory' and Burt (1937) referred to their 'typical slowness of mental reaction'. Although these formulations were expressed in terms of apparently circumscribed functional deficits, precise testing of these functions does not seem to have been carried out by any of the authors. Years later, Gwynn Jones (1953) still concluded that there were few valid results in the literature because of inadequate research techniques.

Not until the studies by Halstead (1957) was there a real attempt at more sophisticated psychological assessment of the intelligence of children with epilepsy taking type of schooling and physical handicap into account. Halstead also considered in a preliminary way type of epilepsy and emotional upset as important variables. He was also aware of the possible adverse influence of anti-epileptic drugs on intellectual function. However, it is only in the last few years that such factors have begun to be studied in any detail. The present account is a summary of such findings in children.

Peri-ictal disturbances of behaviour will not be discussed as these are considered elsewhere (Chapter 2). Emphasis is placed on children of school age, as they are the most investigated group, although the behavioural problems of many children may well originate earlier in life or intensify with adolescence. Both periods of pre-adult life are particularly under-researched as far as behavioural aspects of epilepsy are concerned. To some extent problems of learning and behaviour will be merged as they are often intimately related although their precise relationships may be difficult to define (Rutter 1974). Treatment or wider aspects of management often follow from the demonstration of the causal factors involved.

Extent of the problems

The frequency of even severe problems of learning and behaviour in children with epilepsy is unknown. An immediate limitation to such knowledge is the difficulty of identifying the different forms of seizure disorder especially in children. Pond (Chapter 3) illustrates the problems involved in the epidemiology of epilepsy and in establishing prevalence rates. The figures usually quoted for children are likely to be an underestimation as they are based mainly on convulsive forms of epilepsy. Where determined attempts have been made to include all forms (with the exception of febrile seizures), estimates as high as 2 per cent have been made (Rose et al 1973). Very low prevalance rates are quoted in some surveys of school children with epilepsy, such as that by Holdsworth & Whitmore (1975) in which a figure of 1.9 per 1000 is given, suggesting that many children with seizure disorders do not come to adequate medical or educational attention.

The wide variations in earlier estimates of behavioural problems in children with epilepsy is clearly shown in the review by Rutter et al (1970). The actual figures in these studies mean very little and certainly comparisons cannot be justified because of the differences in criteria and methods of assessment. The same is true of more recent investigations (Rutter et al 1970, Ross & Evans 1972, Holdsworth & Whitmore 1975, Green & Hartlage 1971, Pazzaglia & Frank-Pazzaglia 1976). What does seem to emerge consistently is that, although many children with epilepsy behave normally at school, proportionally more of them do have learning difficulties and behavioural problems compared with non-epileptic children. In other words, children with epilepsy as a group are at special risk for developing such complications to their lives. The question arises how more precise predictions of risk can be established.

TYPES OF DISORDER AND THEIR ASSESSMENT

As mentioned earlier and emphasised elsewhere (Chapter 2), it is not appropriate to refer to 'the epileptic personality' or to use the other stereotype notions implying inevitable and commonplace deterioration of mental state in people with epilepsy. More precise and empirically derived concepts are needed for discussion to be meaningful and of clinical value. Such precision is not easy in the present state of psychological and psychiatric enquiry. The key concepts of 'learning problems' and 'behavioural problems' need to be clarified.

Learning problems

'Learning problems' has been used as a rather ill-defined and all-embracing rubric, particularly in North American discussions of 'minimal brain dysfunction' which itself is a blanket term embracing a spectrum of different types of disorder, most of them of doubtfully organic origin. For describing primary cognitive dysfunction the concepts of 'educational under-achievement' or 'specific learning difficulties' are preferable although they also need clarification.

The judgement that a child is not doing as well at school as he might implies a comparison between his actual attainments and what can be expected of him in view of his age and basic intellectual ability. The statistical difficulties arising from this apparently simple formulation have been discussed by Rutter & Yule (1974). To allow for the imperfect relationship between mental age and attainments, the most satisfactory procedure is probably to use regression equations from which performance in a given subject is predicted on the basis of observed correlations in the general population between that subject, intelligence and chronological age. This use of multiple regression techniques not only allows the size of disparity between actual and predicted attainments to be ascertained, but also permits the probability to be calculated of observing a given discrepancy by chance.

In fact, this procedure has been employed very little. Yule (1973) describes its use in the original Isle of Wight investigations and subsequent follow-up studies in children with reading problems. A fundamental distinction was made in these studies between children whose poor reading level was part of the general intellectual handicap ('reading backwardness') and those whose reading level was disproportionately low compared with their overall intelligence ('specific reading retardation'). These two groups are different in various important respects (Rutter & Yule 1974) including neurological abnormality, sex ratio, associated problems and prognosis. Accounts of educational achievements in these terms has unfortunately been restricted to reading skills. In the Isle of Wight study which concentrated on 9–11 year old children, over twice as many of those with epilepsy showed serious specific reading retardation compared with non-epileptic children. Appropriate regression equations need to be compiled for other attainments including arithmetic ability. This would be particularly relevant to children with epilepsy as there is some evidence that as a group they are particularly hampered in the acquisition of such skills (Bagley 1970).

'Specific learning difficulties' means defects of verbal or perceptual skills, for example. It might be thought that here the definitions would be simple, but verbal abilities covers a variety of skills and perceptual abilities can be equally subdivided. Indeed, the structure of human abilities is still debated (Vernon 1971). 'Attentiveness' is a particularly important concept in relation to epilepsy as patients are often described as lacking in attention. In Holdsworth & Whitmore's (1975) study, 42 per cent of children with epilepsy attending ordinary school were described by their teachers as 'markedly inattentive'. What is meant by such statements is unclear if the problem behaviour is not specified precisely. In a study by Stores et al (1978), teachers' crude assessment of inattentiveness of children with epilepsy showed no correlation with other supposedly more precise measures including vigilance, activity levels and distractability. In assessment, psychologists should attempt to evaluate these various aspects of attentive behaviour as it remains an open question whether these processes are affected differentially in epilepsy.

Behavioural problems

In a similar way, it is important to be as precise as possible when describing other behavioural problems in children with epilepsy. For this purpose, the definitions of the multi-axial classification scheme for psychiatric disorders in childhood and adolescence (Rutter et al 1975) are particularly valuable. These definitions cover the various neurotic, antisocial, psychotic and other types of disturbed behaviour some of which, it is claimed, bear a close relationship to certain types of epilepsy. The diagnosis of depression is generally more difficult in children than in older subjects (Graham 1974). Special care is needed in the question of 'over-activity' which is also freely used to describe many children with epilepsy. Indeed, it is often assumed that over-activity is an inevitable accompaniment of brain dysfunction whereas it is more usually a reflection or component of conduct problems (Shaffer et al 1974). However, the term over-activity also covers many behaviours from the largely incessant gross motor over-activity of what might be called the 'true hyperkinetic syndrome' (Ounsted 1955) (fortunately a rare condition), to behaviour described by intolerant parents or teachers as over-active which on enquiry proves to be normal exploratory behaviour for the child's age. Other groups included in this blanket term include anxious, bored or over-stressed children (Bax 1972).

Careful clinical enquiry is the safest way of making a precise diagnosis but for screening purposes the Isle of Wight scales for teachers and parents (Rutter et al 1970) are useful. The teachers' scale has been used in an attempt to identify particular characteristics of school children with epilepsy (Hackney & Taylor 1976). The Conners' scales, also for parents and teachers (ECDEU 1976) and designed for the assessment of drug effects, provide scores on anxiety, conduct problem, inattentiveness, over-activity and social isolation factors.

As many parents are often said to induce over-dependency in their epileptic children by being too protective, dependency is also of special importance in assessing the social consequences of epilepsy. Berg (1974) has produced evidence that different types of dependency can exist independently of each other. The Conners' scales and Berg's Dependency Questionnaire have both been used effectively in studies of the behavioural associations of different types of childhood epilepsy (Stores 1978a).

More detailed discussion of the measurement of childrens' behaviour, including psychosocial functioning, is to be found in Werry (1978).

Accurate assessment of the behaviour of infants and pre-school children remains particularly difficult. The question of whether temperamental characteristics can be identified at that early age is still debated and few attempts have been made to devise measures of such behaviour. Possible measuring instruments include the Carey Infant Temperament Questionnaire (Carey 1978) and the Behaviour Screening Questionnaire (Richman & Graham 1971).

DIVERSITY OF CHILDHOOD EPILEPSIES

Epilepsy is not a single entity. The term covers a very wide variety of different underlying conditions and types of seizure. The diversity of seizure types is reflected in the scheme promoted internationally in recent years (Gastaut 1970), which is already undergoing revision (Dreifuss 1980). At one extreme is the generalised tonic-clonic convulsion popularly associated with epilepsy; at the other extreme, seizures may consist of a brief subjective experience with little or no external manifestation. The precise sequence of subjective and objective events has to be known for the accurate classification of seizures which is important for the choice of treatment and in order to anticipate behavioural consequences.

Absences (Penry et al 1975) and complex partial seizures (Daly 1975) are of particular importance in child psychiatry because of their behavioural manifestations. Although they may share certain features, they are very different forms of seizure in terms of aetiology, response to treatment and behavioural associations. They can be distinguished from each other by certain simple clinical criteria (Penry et al 1975). Both can occur as forms of epileptic status to produce prolonged confusion, psychosis or apparent subnormality. Another important and apparently common form of childhood epilepsy, previously misclassified as temporal lobe epilepsy yet with a particularly good prognosis in contrast to many seizure disorders associated with temporal lobe lesions, is benign childhood epilepsy with centro-temporal (Rolandic) discharges (Heijbel & Bohman 1975).

The behavioural consequences of this range of seizure disorders are unlikely to be the same. The effects may be related to cause and type of epilepsy, as well as age of onset, seizure frequency or the natural history of the disorder and response to treatment. Generalisations in these circumstances are bound to be inaccurate and misleading.

FACTORS ASSOCIATED WITH PROBLEMS OF
SCHOOL CHILDREN WITH EPILEPSY

Although knowledge of the determinants of emotional and learning difficulties in school children with epilepsy is incomplete, it is possible to identify factors which are associated with such problems and which can form the basis of a diagnostic approach in individual cases.

The question arises how specific such factors are to epilepsy, calling for the special expertise and knowledge available in special epilepsy centres or clinics, or how far the same general principles can be applied to epileptic children as are practised in child psychiatry as a whole. Clearly, general factors do operate in many instances, such as constitutional predisposition, sex differences and socio-economic correlates of behaviour disorders, but other factors are intimately associated with the seizure disorder itself or its treatment.

1. Poor school attendance

Faced with a child who is under-achieving at school or socially disadvantaged there, it is important to exclude the simple possibility that much schooling has been missed through poor attendance. Although this is not usually the case (Rutter et al 1970, Holdsworth & Whitmore 1975), some children are frequently withheld from school or often sent home after an attack by over-cautious parents or teachers. In general, it is sufficient to allow the child to quietly recover from an attack and then allow him to continue with normal school activities rather than treat each seizure as an emergency.

2. Family problems

Convulsive seizures in particular, or the diagnosis of epilepsy itself (even in the more subtle types of seizure disorder) often have a disturbing effect on the attitude of parents to their affected child. After witnessing the first convulsion, many parents think their child has died and subsequent attacks bring with them the same threat. Sharing popular folklore, they may believe that they themselves are responsible for handing on or otherwise causing the condition, or that their child will become subnormal or insane.

Especially if full and repeated explanations and (where appropriate) re-assurances are not given, parents are likely to react with feelings of guilt, anger, hostility or less obvious forms of rejection or upset (Tavriger 1966, Voeller & Rothenburg 1973). Over-protection is common and unnecessary restrictions are frequently placed on the child's activities. There is some evidence that these attitudes instil excessive compliance and passivity in the child which limits academic achievement (Hartlage & Green 1972). Hartlage et al (1972) suggested that epileptic children are more dependent on their parents than children with more physically disabling handicaps such as cystic fibrosis. Emotional dependency in particular seems to characterise epileptic children with temporal lobe dysfunction (Stores & Piran 1978).

Epileptic childrens' self-image has been little studied. Their knowledge of epilepsy may well be fragmentary and misinformed. Older affected children are likely to share the general public's misconceptions about the nature and consequences of epilepsy, resulting in unnecessary anxiety and concern about the future. Withdrawal and isolation can have a serious affect on social skills and special help to overcome this may be required.

Having a child with epilepsy appears to impose special stresses on the family. Emotional distress seems to be more common in the mothers of epileptic children compared with mothers of children with other chronic handicaps (Rutter et al 1970). Parents may hesitate to use usual disciplinary measures in case seizures are provoked, or they may disagree and handle the child inconsistently. Fear that a seizure may occur, and embarrassment about public reaction, can severely limit a family's social activities. Other children in the family may be neglected emotionally because of the parents' preoccupation with their affected child. These problems are intensified in the unfortunate cases where epilepsy is combined with mental handicap or serious behavioural problems.

Improvement of these family problems is often difficult to achieve. Explanation, support and practical help has to be provided for the family as a whole. Social workers, psychologists or others familiar with such problems need to work closely with the child's doctor in order to have an overall view of the case. At present, this intensive help is rarely available outside special centres.

3. Difficulties at school

The child with epilepsy may well face similarly inappropriate and unhelpful attitudes at school from teachers and other children. Teachers may harbour all manner of misconceptions in the absence of adequate instruction in their training courses and, again, unnecessary restrictions may be imposed and recreational and other school activities curtailed on the assumption that physical or mental exertion may be harmful. The child can become an invalid or social outcast in the process, and may face ridicule or hostility from other children.

Both teachers and parents often believe that a child with epilepsy is intrinsically incapable of doing as well academically as unaffected children. Teachers tend to under-estimate the intellectual potential of children with epilepsy, basing their estimates on attainment levels which are often below their true ability (Bagley 1970). Low attainment may therefore be the result of under-expectation and lack of stimulation, even in intellectually gifted children. Boredom or more serious problems are likely to develop.

Schools must be closely involved in the investigation and management of a child's difficulties. This may well require repeated visits to the school by medical staff or the hospital psychologist, or attendance by teachers at hospital case conferences where possible. The same applies to educational psychologists who may not be any better informed than teachers.

4. Severity of seizure disorder

Severity can be measured in a variety of ways, all of which seem likely to affect behaviour adversely.

Fortunately, gross brain damage, severe developmental anomalies or degenerative conditions underly only a minority of seizure disorders, but where present are likely to reduce intellectual capacity and, in the case of focal lesions, may produce specific cognitive deficits. There are few, if any, convincing associations between specific conditions of which epilepsy may be a part and particular types of disturbed behaviour, but conditions involving physical handicaps, or which require prolonged, complicated or inconvenient treatment, are likely to be upsetting for the child and the parents alike.

Severity may also be judged in terms of the frequency of seizures or complications arising from individual attacks. Frequent convulsive seizures seem to impair cognitive development (Dikmen & Matthews 1977). These, or severe myoclonic or atonic attacks with falling or injury, are likely to be particularly upsetting although other attacks in which consciousness is preserved or altered (perhaps with frightening or otherwise unpleasant experiences as in many complex partial seizures) can be psychologically more harmful. The dramatic changes of behaviour and deterioration of abilities in non-convulsive types of status are particularly distressing to parents and, of course, convulsive status epilepticus carries with it the risk not only of severe brain damage but of death. Fortunately, head injuries, burns and other accidents occur in relatively few cases.

Age of onset is another aspect of severity. Early age of onset may itself suggest serious brain pathology, at least in some forms of neonatal seizures and in most forms of infantile spasms. Aetiology apart, there is some evidence (Dikmen et al 1977) that generalised convulsions which begin early in life carry a poorer prognosis for intellectual development than similar seizures which appear later. The precise nature of this relationship is unclear and could involve such factors as long exposure to drug treatment or disrupted education.

5. Type of seizure disorder

To some extent the likelihood of cognitive and other behavioural problems can be predicted if the child's type of seizure disorder has been carefully identified.

Cognitive impairment. There is some evidence that certain types of epilepsy are associated with specific defects of cognitive function. Verbal deficits may result if the seizure source is located in the hemisphere dominant for speech, or visuo-spatial problems if the non-dominant hemisphere is primarily involved (Fedio & Mirsky 1969). In contrast, sources of seizure discharge which are supposedly located in mid-line sub-cortical structures to produce generalised seizure discharge in the EEG have been associated with impaired attentiveness (Stores 1973), although, more recently, Wilkus & Dodrill (1976) have reported more widespread neuropsychological defects with this type of EEG abnormality.

The impairment caused by generalised seizure discharge was first studied by Schwab (1939) who demonstrated slowing of reaction times. Hutt and his colleagues (1977) showed that both clinical and 'sub-clinical' generalised spike and wave bursts can disrupt not only the registration of information but also its storage and recall, and that these effects depend on the complexity of the information as well as the rate at which the child has to work. Mirsky & van Buren (1965) demonstrated that the spike wave activity and associated inattention do not necessarily closely correspond in time and seem to depend on functionally independent mechanisms. It seems that the more generalised and bilaterally synchronous, the more regular and organised the spike wave complexes and the longer the duration of each burst, the more attention is disrupted (Mirsky 1969). Apart from the type of discharge, abnormalities of background rhythms may be important. For example, Dodrill & Wilkus (1976) have reported an association between even slight slowing of waking dominant posterior rhythms and impairment of abilities requiring simultaneous attention and complex mental operations.

Psychiatric problems. Although the high rates of psychiatric disorder found in children with epilepsy are likely to be associated with the social, psychological and other factors reviewed in this section, it seems likely that certain behavioural abnormalities are more intimately connected with brain dysfunction. Seizures arising in the temporal lobe have been particularly implicated in this way compared with generalised or other focal epilepsies. The subject was reviewed recently by Hermann & Stevens (1980) who pointed to the lack of suitable controls and other methodological problems in most of the studies. The reported associations are therefore more in the way of interesting possibilities in need of confirmation.

The particular types of disturbance linked with complex partial seizures (mainly of temporal lobe origin) in adults include personality disorders such as irritability, over-sensitivity, religiosity and extensive writing and drawing, as well as sexual abnormalities (usually hyposexuality) and psychotic states. Studies of epileptic children with temporal lobe abnormalities have also suggested an association with aggression or other forms of anti-social behaviour (Nuffield 1961, Ounsted et al 1966). Other preliminary reports have raised the possibility that certain personality features are related to the side of the temporal lobe abnormality. Comparisons of the findings in these studies is difficult because of the selected nature of some of the patient groups and the different ways in which behaviour has been assessed. Some claims are obviously incompatible. For example, aggression is sometimes linked with right temporal lobe abnormalities and on other occasions with left-sided lesions. An association has been claimed between right temporal lobe foci and affective psychosis, and between left-sided foci and schizophrenia-like illnesses (Hermann & Stevens 1980).

Recent studies have been carried out to identify those epileptic children attending ordinary school who were at most risk of learning and behaviour problems (Stores 1978a). Sub-groups were defined in terms of type of epilepsy, sex and drug treatment. Measures were taken of reading retardation, inattentiveness and dependency of various types and other aspects of behaviour. Although the main finding throughout these investigations was that the combination of male sex and epilepsy seems to be particularly disadvantageous, left temporal lobe dysfunction was repeatedly associated with a wide range of educational and behavioural problems.

6. Anti-epileptic drugs

Parents and teachers often worry that anti-epileptic medication will impair a child's performance at school. Although this concern is sometimes unjustified, it is undoubtedly true that careless use of drugs can seriously contribute to problems of learning and behaviour. Anti-epileptic drugs are an important part of treatment but, because of the injudicious use of such drugs, some children with epilepsy suffer more from their treatment than from their seizures. Sometimes behaviour improves strikingly when treatment is reduced or discontinued although, of course, this should always be carried out under strict medical supervision.

The possible effects on behaviour of individual anti-epileptic drugs have been reviewed in detail elsewhere (Stores 1975, Trimble & Reynolds 1976, Stores

1978b). Phenobarbitone and related drugs are still frequently prescribed for children even though they can have very serious adverse effects. Chronic phenobarbitone intoxication is well described in adults and older children who are likely to show confusion and obvious intellectual deterioration, but in younger children toxic effects may be less readily recognised and can cause serious developmental delay misinterpreted as permanent retardation (Cordes 1973). Lower blood levels of phenobarbitone are often associated with problems of 'over-activity', excitement, irritability, aggression and tearfulness. In a study by Wolf & Forsythe (1978), 42 per cent of children treated with phenobarbitone for febrile seizures developed a behaviour disorder compared with 18 per cent in an untreated group. Camfield et al (1979) have described a severe sleep disturbance in many children taking phenobarbitone for the same purpose. This group of drugs is best avoided wherever possible, certainly for children of school age.

The range of possible reactions to phenytoin is considerable with striking individual differences in response to treatment. The usual account of phenytoin intoxication (with its stress on cerebellar signs) ignores other intoxication syndromes that have been described more recently. Complete recovery does not always follow discontinuation of this drug. Various relatively insidious behaviour disorders have now been associated with blood levels of phenytoin apparently within the usually accepted optimum range. These include personality change, psychomotor slowing and intellectual deterioration (Reynolds & Travers 1974, Trimble & Corbett 1980), impaired motor skills (Dodrill 1975), and poor reading skills (Stores & Hart 1976). In addition, the possibly far-reaching effects on emotional well-being of physical change induced by drugs is well illustrated by phenytoin which has been associated with various cosmetic problems including coarsening of the skin and facial features (Falconer & Davidson 1973).

The behavioural effects of sodium valproate remain uncertain. Although some authors have claimed a beneficial effect on behaviour (which might well be accounted for in terms of improved seizure control or the withdrawal of harmful drugs), some children become over-active or aggressive during treatment. Over-sedation to various degrees has also been reported, although usually when the drug has been used in combination, especially with barbiturates (Browne 1980). Claims that valproate has a beneficial effect in psychiatric patients are conflicting.

Adverse behavioural effects in some patients have been attributed to all the other drugs used in the treatment of epilepsy. Careful surveillance is essential. Measurement of blood levels may be very informative especially where there has been poor control of seizures, where intoxication is suspected and whenever there is a change in the child's behaviour including deterioration in his school work. Some drug combinations are particularly hazardous, notably phenytoin and sulthiame which can readily produce phenytoin intoxication. The 'therapeutic' ranges of blood levels are only general guidelines, and the child's clinical condition is always more important than laboratory findings. During treatment, his physical state and behaviour need to be regularly re-assessed in order to detect adverse effects at an early stage. It is important to review previous treatment to anticipate the child's individual reactions which can vary considerably from one patient to another. The reputation that some anti-epileptic drugs have gained as psychotropic agents are mainly ill-founded (Stores 1978b).

7. Male sex

In general, school problems and disturbed behaviour are more common in boys than girls. In studies of epilepsy, however, the two sexes are not usually considered separately. Where they have been (Stores 1978a) interesting differences are seen as mentioned earlier. Different kinds of problems, including academic under-achievement as well as emotional problems, seem much more common in boys with epilepsy than in non-epileptic boys or epileptic girls. In the series of studies by Stores and his colleagues (1978a) these sex-related differences were not simply a reflection of behavioural sex differences in children as a whole. The combination of epilepsy and male sex seems to carry with it a special disadvantage perhaps for both biological and cultural reasons. For preventive purposes, boys with epilepsy can be seen as an especially high risk group.

Illustrative case

The cause of any one child's problems is rarely simple. The way in which several factors often combine is illustrated by the following case:

A.B. was 13 when referred to the Park Hospital for Children in Oxford. For ten years she had suffered frequent complex partial seizures, starting with a frightening abdominal sensation or feeling of dread, as well as mainly right-sided convulsions sometimes with urinary incontinence. Various drug treatments had been ineffective. Phenobarbitone had made her depressed and irritable, and phenytoin produced an acneiform rash and gum hypertrophy. Over the years she had become progressively more withdrawn. She was embarrassed at school and afraid to go out socially, fearing that she would have an attack and wet herself. She lived in a remote village with few friends of her own age and travelled to and from school by taxi rather than on a school bus which increased her feeling of isolation. Her parents, fearing for her safety, discouraged her from going out and she would spend weekends and holidays getting up late, sitting about the house or watching television for long periods. She had no interest in school work, her attainments were low even allowing for her modest intelligence, and she longed to leave school although without any career ambitions. On admission, she was a detached, embarrassed girl with a neglected appearance and pessimistic outlook on life in general, resentful of the social activities of other girls of her age.

Investigations revealed a calcified lesion in her left temporal lobe and a temporal lobectomy was subsequently carried out. The resected specimen contained an oligodendroglioma.

Her seizure frequency is now much improved. She has now left school but is unable to find a job. Attempts to improve her appearance and general demeanour and to increase her range of social activities have met with some success, but her life remains very narrow and inhibited. Although the neurological aspects of her situation have been a success, the legacy of ten years of psychological and social handicap remains and seems likely to limit her future adjustment considerably. Such problems might well have been lessened by adequate diagnosis and treatment at an earlier age.

ASSESSMENT, PREVENTION AND TREATMENT

With patients of any age it is essential to avoid merely labelling them 'epileptic' and prescribing anti-epileptic drugs. Unfortunately, this type of practice persists despite efforts to encourage a wider view of the person with recurrent seizures. Seizure disorders need to be assessed in terms of cause, type and severity. In treatment, the appropriate drug should be chosen and its effects (including possible adverse effects) monitored closely. Simplicity and other modern principles of prescribing are discussed elsewhere in this volume. Parents and older patients themselves need to be involved in repeated discussion of the many aspects of the problem.

Children diagnosed as having epilepsy should be considered at special risk of developing educational and emotional problems. The child's doctor should have a clear idea of the family situation including the parents' knowledge and attitudes towards epilepsy, their emotional state and that of any sibs, and the quality of family life. The school circumstances also need to be assessed in terms of teachers' attitudes and expectations, possible restrictions and friendships. Ideally, teachers, school doctors and educational psychologists would be informed enough to keep a special watch on the epileptic child's academic and social progress without being intrusive or over-concerned. If problems threaten, early intervention is required and referral (where possible) to a special epilepsy clinic for children. Psychologists have a central part to play in the investigation and care of children with epilepsy. Assessment should include not only general measures of intelligence but measurement of specific abilities and attainments.

Preventive possibilities in school are largely confined to early detection of problems and intervention. Resources to do so are, of course, limited. The attempts to identify sub-groups of epileptic children at highest risk are therefore important. From the studies mentioned, it appears that boys with epilepsy and children of either sex with left temporal lobe dysfunction are particularly prone to problems. Drug treatment is an additional risk for any child but barbiturates are particularly harmful.

Treatment possibilities have already been referred to in the previous section. There is no one special form appropriate for children with epilepsy. The whole range of psychiatric skills are required in order to care adequately for such children and their families. Often care has to be provided over long periods of time through childhood and adolescence. Where no suitable service exists for older patients, the children's hospital or clinic may have to continue to see their patients into adult life.

Adolescence may be a particularly troublesome time. Although some seizure disorders improve with age, others may intensify at puberty (for example in relation to the menstrual cycle) or drug treatment may need adjustment because of metabolic changes. The social consequences of epilepsy can be felt more acutely by the adolescent patient who is likely to be particularly sensitive about his condition or resentful about the limitations it imposes on his activities especially finding a job or driving.

Future developments
Certain recent trends in clinical practice and research promise improvements in the care of children with epilepsy who remain a neglected group compared with children suffering from other chronic disorders. Progress depends on more interest in epilepsy among professionals and in more information being acquired by those responsible for such children.

Diagnosis. Accurate diagnosis rests on careful clinical evaluation and appropriate EEG investigations (and not on sporadic, ill-directed standard EEG recordings). Used properly, EEG studies can be useful in a variety of ways for assessing behavioural aspects of epilepsy (Stores 1980a). Ambiguous categories such as 'grand mal' and 'petit mal' are inadequate. The more widespread adoption of the International Classification of Seizures (mentioned earlier) would help to make the choice of treatment more accurate and anticipation of associated psychological problems easier. Distinctions between seizures and other paroxysmal disturbances of behaviour is now more possible by means of intensive EEG monitoring systems, especially ambulatory monitoring which can be employed in real life situations (Stores 1980a).

Measurement of behaviour. The means used by psychologists to assess behaviour remain surprisingly limited in scope. Perhaps especially in the neuropsychiatric context, reliance is still placed on ill-standardised and multifactorial tests such as the Benton and Bender Gestalt Tests or even sub-tests of the Wechsler Scales. Impairment on these tests can be the result of various types of deficit. The diagnostic accuracy of such measures, in precise functional terms, is not surprisingly very poor. Assessment of behaviour in children (especially those of pre-school age) is even less satisfactory. As mentioned earlier, the measures worth considering have been reviewed by Werry (1978). Concepts of particular importance in epilepsy (such as 'inattentiveness' and 'dependency' as already discussed) need to be defined and appropriate measures devised. These problems, and at least preliminary indications of how they might be solved, were considered recently in a workshop on psychological assessment of people with epilepsy (Kulig et al 1980).

Psychological precipitants of seizures. Although this account has been concerned with ways in which seizures may adversely affect learning and behaviour, the converse possibility that psychological or environmental factors may influence seizure frequency is of great practical importance and interest. Information on this point has previously been difficult to obtain although the literature does contain some anecdotal or impressionistic accounts. The development of ambulatory EEG monitoring systems which permit long-term recordings in real life situations allows these possibilities to be explored much more effectively. The difficulty at present lies in obtaining sufficiently adequate and sensitive accounts of the child's activities and emotional state but preliminary attempts (Sato et al 1976, Stores 1980b) are encouraging.

References

Bagley C 1970 The educational performance of children with epilepsy. British Journal of Educational Psychology 40:82–83

Bax M 1972 The active and the over-active child. Developmental Medicine and Child Neurology 14:83–86

Berg I 1974 A self-administered dependency questionnaire (SADQ) for use with the mothers of school children. British Journal of Psychiatry 124:1–9

Browne T R 1980 Valproic acid. New England Journal of Medicine 302:661–666

Burt C 1937 The backward child. University of London Press, London

Camfield C S, Chaplin S, Doyle A B, Shapiro S H, Cummings C, Camfield P R 1979 Side effects of phenobarbital in toddlers: behavioural and cognitive aspects. Journal of Paediatrics 95:361–365

Carey W B, McDevitt S C 1978 Revision of the infant temperament questionnaire. Paediatrics 61:735–739

Cordes C K 1973 Chronic drug intoxication causing pseudo-retardation in a young child. Journal of the American Academy of Child Psychiatry 12:215–222

Daly D 1975 Ictal manifestations of complex partial seizures. In: Penry J, Daly D (eds) Complex partial seizures and their treatment. Advances in Neurology, no. 11, Raven Press, New York

Dikmen S, Matthews C G 1977 Effect of major motor seizure frequency upon cognitive-intellectual functions in adults. Epilepsia 18(1):21–29

Dikmen S, Matthews C G, Harley J P 1977 Effect of early versus late onset of major motor epilepsy on cognitive-intellectual performance: further considerations. Epilepsia 18(1):31–36

Dodrill C B 1975 Diphenylhydantoin serum levels, toxicity and neuropsychological performance in patients with epilepsy. Epilepsia 16:593–600

Dodrill C B, Wilkus R J 1976 Neuropsychological correlates of the electroencephalogram in epileptics. II The waking posterior rhythm and its interaction with epileptiform activity. Epilepsia 17:101–109

Dreifuss F G 1980 personal communication

ECDEU 1976 Assessment manual. National Institute of Mental Health, Rockville, Maryland

Falconer M, Davidson S 1973 Coarse features in epilepsy as a consequence of anticonvulsant therapy. Lancet 2:1112–1114

Fedio P, Mirsky A F 1969 Selective intellectual deficits in children with temporal lobe or centrencephalic epilepsy. Neuropsychologia 7:287–300

Gastaut H 1970 Clinical and electroencephalographical classification of epileptic seizures. Epilepsia 11:102–113

Graham P 1974 Depression in pre-pubertal children. Developmental Medicine and Child Neurology 16:340–349

Green J B, Hartlage L C 1971 Comparative performance of epileptic and non-epileptic children and adolescents. Diseases of the Nervous System 32:418–421

Gwynne-Jones H 1953 Experimental studies in the psychology of epilepsy. Revue de Psychologie Appliqué 3:209–277

Hackney A, Taylor D C 1976 A teachers' questionnaire description of epileptic children. Epilepsia 17:275–281

Halstead H 1957 Abilities and behaviour of epileptic children. Journal of Mental Science 103:28–47

Hartlage L C, Green J B 1972 The relation of parental attitudes to academic and social achievement in epileptic children. Epilepsia 13:21–26

Hartlage L C, Green J B, Offutt L 1972 Dependency in epileptic children. Epilepsia 13:27–30

Heijbel J, Bohman M 1975 Benign epilepsy of children with centrotemporal EEG foci: intelligence, behaviour and school adjustment. Epilepsia 16:679–687

Hermann B P, Stevens J R 1980 Interictal behavioural correlates of the epilepsies. In: Hermann B P (ed) Multidisciplinary handbook of epilepsy. Thomas, Springfield

Holdsworth L, Whitmore K 1975 A study of children with epilepsy attending ordinary schools. I Their seizure patterns, progress and behaviour in school. Developmental Medicine and Child Neurology 16:746–758

Hutt S J, Newton J, Fairweather H 1977 Choice reaction time and EEG activity in children with epilepsy. Neuropsychologia 15:257–267

Kulig B M, Meinardi H, Stores G 1980 Epilepsy and behavior '79. Lisse: Swets and Zeitlinger

Mirsky A F 1969 Studies of paroxysmal EEG phenomena and background EEG in relation to impaired attention. In: Evans C R, Mulholland T B (eds) Attention in neurophysiology. Butterworths, London

Mirsky A F, van Buren J M 1965 On the nature of the 'absence' in centrencephalic epilepsy: a study of some behavioural, electroencephalographic and autonomic factors. Electroencephalography and Clinical Neurophysiology 18:334–348

Nuffield E J A 1961 Neurophysiology and behaviour disorders in epileptic children. Journal of Mental Science 107:438–458

Ounsted C 1955 The hyperkinetic syndrome in epileptic children. Lancet 2:303–311

Ounsted, C, Lindsay J, Norman R 1966 Biological factors in temporal lobe epilepsy. Clinics in Developmental Medicine no. 22, Spastics International Medical Publications and Heinemann, London

Pazzaglia P, Frank-Pazzaglia L 1976 Record in grade school of pupils with epilepsy: an epidemiological study. Epilepsia 17:361–366

Penry J K, Porter R J, Dreifuss F E 1975 Simultaneous recording of absence seizures with videotape and electroencephalography. Brain 98:427–440

Reynolds E H, Travers R D 1974 Serum anticonvulsant concentrations in epileptic patients with mental symptoms. British Journal of Psychiatry 124:440–445

Richman N, Graham P J 1971 A behavioural screening questionnaire for use with three-year-old children: preliminary findings. Journal of Child Psychology and Psychiatry 12:5–33

Rose S W, Penry J K, Markush R E, Radloff L A, Putnam P L 1973 Prevalence of epilepsy in children. Epilepsia 14:133–152

Ross E M, Evans D 1972 Epilepsy in Bristol Secondary School children. Epilepsia 13:7–12

Rutter M 1974 Emotional disorder and educational underachievement. Archives of Disease in Childhood 49:249–255

Rutter M, Graham P, Yule W 1970 A Neuropsychiatric Study in Childhood. Clinics in Developmental Medicine Nos 35/36, Spastics International Medical Publications and Heinemann, London

Rutter M, Shaffer D, Shepherd M 1975 Multiaxial classification of child psychiatric disorders. WHO, Geneva

Rutter M, Yule W 1974 Specific reading retardation. In: Mann L, Sabatino D (eds) The first review of special education vol 2. Buttonwood Farms, USA

Sato S, Penry J K, Dreifuss F G 1976 Electroencephalographic monitoring of generalised spike and wave paroxysms in hospital ward and at home. In: Kellaway P, Petersen I (eds) Quantitative analytic studies in epilepsy. Raven Press, New York p 237–251

Schwab R S 1939 Method of measuring consciousness in attacks of petit mal epilepsy. Archives of Neurology and Psychiatry 41:215–217

Shaffer D, McNamara N, Pincus J H 1974 Controlled observations on patterns of activity, attention and impulsivity in brain damaged and psychiatrically disturbed boys. Psychological Medicine 4:4–18

Smith W G 1904 A comparison of some mental and physical tests in their application to epileptic and to normal subjects. British Journal of Psychology 1:240–260

Stores G 1973 Studies of attention and seizure disorders. Developmental Medicine and Child Neurology 15:376–382

Stores G 1975 Behavioural effects of anti-epileptic drugs. Developmental Medicine and Child Neurology 17:647–658

Stores G, Hart J 1976 Reading skills in children with generalised or focal epilepsy. Developmental Medicine and Child Neurology 18:705–716

Stores G 1978a School children with epilepsy at special risk of educational and other behavioural problems. Developmental Medicine and Child Neurology 20:502–508

Stores G 1978b Anti-epileptics (anticonvulsants). In: Werry J (ed) Pediatric psychopharmacology — the use of behaviour modifying drugs in children. Brunner/Mazel, New York p 274–315

Stores G, Piran N 1978 Dependency of different types in school-children with epilepsy. Psychological Medicine 8:441–445

Stores G, Hart J A, Piran N 1978 Inattentiveness in school-children with epilepsy. Epilepsia 19:169–175

Stores G 1980a Ambulatory monitoring in the diagnosis of epilepsy. In: Parsonage M J (ed) Aspects of epilepsy. Research and Clinical forums 2:141–148

Stores G 1980b A study of factors associated with the occurrence of generalised seizure discharge in children with epilepsy, using the Oxford Medilog system for ambulatory monitoring. In: Proceedings of 12th Epilepsy International Symposium, Copenhagen, September 1980 (in press)

Tavriger R 1966 Some parental theories about the causes of epilepsy. Epilepsia 7:339–343

Tizard B 1962 The personality of epileptics: a discussion of the evidence. Psychological Bulletin 59:196–210

Trimble M, Reynolds E 1976 Anticonvulsant drugs and mental symptoms. Psychological Medicine 6:169–178

Trimble M, Corbett J 1980 Behavioural and cognitive disturbances in epileptic children. Irish Medical Journal 73 Supp. 21–28

Tylor-Fox J 1924 The response of epileptic children to mental and educational tests. British Journal of Medical Psychology 4:235–248

Vernon P E 1971 Analysis of cognitive ability. British Medical Bulletin 27:222–226

Voeller K K S, Rothenberg M B 1973 Psychosocial aspects of the management of seizures in children. Pediatrics 51:1072–1082

Werry J S 1978 Measures in paediatric psychopharmacology. In: Werry J S (ed) Paediatric psychopharmacology. Brunner/Mazel, New York, p 29–78

Wilkus R J, Dodrill C B 1976 Neurophysiological correlates of the electroencephalography in epileptics. I Topographical distribution and average rate of epileptiform activity. Epilepsia 17:89–100

Wolf S M, Forsythe A 1978 Behavior disturbance, phenobarbital and febrile seizures. Pediatrics 61:728–731

Yule W 1973 Differential prognosis of reading backwardness and specific reading retardation. British Journal of Educational Psychology 43:244–248

The emotions and epilepsy

INTRODUCTION

Not much short of half a century ago, whilst engaged in the measurement of autonomic nervous activity in response to painful stimuli and other factors, I suggested that the enquiry should be extended to the emotions, but was told quite explicitly that as emotions cannot be measured, 'they are not scientific'. Whilst this view has not curbed my interest in the effects of emotional disorder on the development and persistence of intermittent neurological disturbances, it may have restricted my writing upon the topic. Until recently the climate of opinion has been such that it has not been seemly to include such topics in medical scientific journals, in which the artificial distinction between what are called the science and the art of medicine has been made absolute. There has in the last decade been a shift of interest, among young doctors noticeably, on both sides of the Atlantic, away from purely scientific enquiry in the laboratory to the application of the results interpersonally between doctor and patient in the ward or consulting room. This trend too has quite probably contributed to the vastly growing interest in psychiatry on the part of young medical men and women who, as students, had not achieved the full satisfaction of the zeal with which they had entered upon their vocation from the unintentionally rigid application of scientific data to the individual patient under study.

In the medical literature, attempts have been made to rationalise the two components of medical practice, components more easily seen in family practice and psychiatry than in other fields, in the use of the phrases 'soft data' and 'hard data', phrases which are much in use, especially amongst psychiatrists. But the quantitative tabulation of personality traits, feelings and responses which present the former in the guise of the latter has rather belittled the human and humane relationship between the patient and the observer at an academic level, anyway.

Certainly for me the transition from academic enquiry into the nature of the epileptic event to the care of patients was encouraged by growing certainty that what the patient with epilepsy thinks and feels about his affliction and what society does about it are of compelling importance — important most of all in modifying the fit pattern, for better or for worse. Granted a first physiological reason why one person has epilepsy and another not (whether this reason is structural or metabolic) the factors which most determine the continuity of fits despite appropriate medical treatment relate generally to the patient's life and to his own feelings towards his illness, as well as the feeling or lack of feeling of others. In other words, emotions not only come into the problem, they often dominate it.

The physical causes of epilepsy having been sought first in the clinical interview and then with the help of the special departments, an appraisal of the patient's life pattern and attitudes and especially of his attitude to the fact of epilepsy become essential. During the interview the physician must see all the consequences of having epilepsy through that patient's own eyes, distorted though they may be by misconceptions, ignorance, mood disorder, or misunderstanding of others at home or abroad. If he can 'get under his skin' the physician will be constantly surprised by what he learns and will be considerably helped, too. Now this effort in anamnesis, and what this entails, cannot be constrained into a scientific paper of the conventional sort. Clinical interpersonal skills cannot be learnt by reading alone, but they can be acquired by apprenticeship before being extended and polished by experience. It is with this in mind that this essay is being written, so I do not propose to quote the considerable literature relating to this important subject except to mention the monographs by Pond (1961) in his Goulstonian lectures, or that of Taylor (1972) which covers an important aspect of the subject, whilst I have covered much of what we know about emotions occurring during the ictus in Brain (1956). A contemporary parallel survey has been made in the Symposium in the Royal Society of Medicine entitled *Emotional support for cancer patients and their families* (1980).

The interrelations of the emotions and epilepsy will be presented in a personal way, the way we do at the bedside rather than in the lecture theatre. It would be better for you to be in at the consultation but that is not possible, for even an audience of one there is too public. As I write, a co-editor of this volume is helping a patient of mine who has major emotional disorders related to the fact of epilepsy, and has admitted her to hospital. Her gratitude was qualified by the remark—natural enough and fully understood—'but it wasn't the same with the other doctors listening.'

The physician's knowledge of the emotional consequences of having epilepsy comes from the intimate understanding of one patient only, the patient-of-the-moment, but through time there are thousands of those, and generalisations gradually emerge; but to each one of these thousands there is only one patient-of-the-moment. He is the one whom I really wish to keep before us.

The fact of having epilepsy

We are talking about 'a continuing liability to repeated attacks', so by the time the diagnosis is made the patient either knows that the liability is continuing or that sad fact is slowly being realised by him. He has faith in his doctor, who in referring him to the consultant or the hospital has eulogised his choice—he usually does. The care then shown and the investigations which are undertaken are impressive, and the anticonvulsants have certainly not been given with any implication that they might not be effective. The instructions given about his way of life—moderation in all things, and so on—have been absorbed and in varying degree applied by the patient and his family. Yet despite all this there is one recurrence and then another. The reasonable hopes fostered by his trusted advisors have been confounded. Soon the patient finds himself in an impossible situation, for he has to live as though he will never have another attack, and yet not be surprised if he does. The alternative would be to adopt an invalid, protected life with none of the minor risks which make for major happinesses and consequent contentment. It is only the inadequate, inferior person who can succumb to this second course, but most battle against the pressures within the family and outside it to impose restraints upon them.

Living with the problem

To clear the air we must first consider those patients where there does not seem to be any problem at all. This is so in a large group of patients who are important to my thesis, but who by their personalities select themselves outside it. These are the stoics who solve or seem to themselves to solve this insoluble problem by adopting an attitude detached from it, and who in the clinical interview seem to have no emotional response to their quandary at all. The detachment they seem to achieve is away from the frustration and the defeat imposed upon their lives through the very fact of epilepsy. It has the pattern of the outworn hysteria of older psychiatric textbooks. It also, inherently, seems to have the same psychological mechanism, for it seems to solve the problem; but as a general rule it makes it, the epilepsy itself, worse.

These people aver that the occasional fit, the chewed tongue, the incontinence in public, the lapse in conversation and the misunderstandings of their peers do not matter a bit. And yet you and I know how much they would matter to us, and that is the measure to be used. They quite boldly and even proudly proclaim that they have Epilepsy and seem to accept the consequences without gall, bitterness or distress. His Membership of the British Epilepsy Association is that of a Trades Union militant. They are the last to chide medicine or science in their promises to help or cure. They are 'good patients', though they do come back personally on the telephone or through letters with information from the medical press which may be just a pace ahead of their doctor's own reading. The most striking sign these patients show in consultation is the absence of affective response. They are bland, tolerant, courteous, and unruffled in demeanour in any way, having again in old terminology 'la belle indifférence'. In these, the attacks sometimes maintain a constancy of recurrence whatever the dose, content or combination of anticonvulsants, or at best there are short periods of remission or improvement with each change made.

The syndrome I have outlined in its obvious form is epitomised in a case history which follows shortly, but in its suppression of emotionality it is a relative state, which obviously pervades all those in adversity, in this instance the adversity being the effects of epilepsy. But in this essay we are considering emotions and epilepsy so that those whom this state involves are excluded from our consideration. They constitute however a large minority of the epileptic population, but it is a particularly important minority, for it includes so many of the otherwise normal patients whose epilepsy is recalcitrant to treatment. It includes especially the intelligent educated folk who have vocational ambitions, or perhaps it is just that in that group the psychological set is seen most vividly. Whilst these excellent people have limited expression of emotions, frustration may be allowed to show, and anger occasionally to explode, but little else. The patient I will describe is a particularly evident prototype of this group.

When he was 28, the captain of a large cargo ship started to have small attacks of blankness called by his family 'daydreams'. They have continued to the present, despite trial of most anticonvulsants as they have reached the market. He saw me six years after they began, and others in his seaport town had failed to control them (as I have too).

Fully investigated in The National Hospital before I saw him he was found to have a minimal right pyramidal disturbance. The right face is slightly the smaller, the right forefinger and second toe each being three millimeters shorter than its opposite. Motor function is normal, as are the reflexes and no other neural deficit is present, but there is a little flattening of the left fronto–parietal area of the skull. An electroencephalogram then showed abnormal slow waves more evident in the left frontal area. He is right-handed, his IQ is 135 whilst on medical treatment. Air encephalography, angiography and later a CAT scan were all normal. On two occasions at his request the advisibility of craniotomy had been investigated, discussed and rejected.

As a person he seemed to have been blessed in appearance, demeanour, ability and personality. In an exasperated letter he wrote 'to conclude: I am no neurotic invalid. I am a 6'6" second row forward who plays all sports. An extra master with a teacher's certificate who, over the last few years, has flown aircraft, commanded a hovercraft for a season, skippered a training ship, undergone survival courses and spent many days aboard small boats'.

He learnt about the attacks, of which he was ignorant, a year after their onset. He was then engaged to the only girl with whom he had made any attachment. They had had sexual intercourse. It was she who told him about the attacks, and a year later whilst still friends she had broken the engagement because, he said 'she was a simple soul and was so worried about them'. He has had no interest in any woman in the eight years since, is apparently pleased that he has no sexually directed feelings — 'it makes life so easy' — no libido at all, and has never since, he says, had an erection. He lives a very active physical life on small boats and teaching navigation on shore and at sea, and even joins in the usual healthy mess room smut with as much apparent enjoyment as the rest.

Through the years the short periods of amnesia and 'absences' have continued at about weekly intervals with from two a day to three weeks of freedom as the range, but they are interspersed by longer attacks lasting about a minute in which he grimaces and moves both arms and then feels unwell for half an hour. He knows he has these whilst he is unaware of the momentary absences. He has never had a major convulsion.

The maritime regulations preclude anyone with epilepsy from service. The patient's career was ended, he could not drive. He had a teacher's certificate, so obtained a post as navigation instructor on shore, but attacks in class brought that to an end. 'In no sense is any criticism implied to what follows — the marine staff have never been other than pleasant and helpful — but a snowball has been allowed to develop into an avalanche.'

Brief shore jobs followed each other; between them he maintained and crewed singlehanded a motorboat in the Pool of London, the Thames estuary and North Sea, living on board. The regulations being less strict he obtained a sea-going post as navigational instructor in a foreign based training ship with a Yugoslav captain and Iranian crew. 'I am back at sea and very happy with life. As regards my head problem, all is not well. Of course it was never a serious thing (a fact which made me feel rather guilty when seeking attention and still does so), and its untoward manifestation is minimal. I stiffen sufficiently to put my chair over sometimes. . . . . I am not concerned with the discomfort caused by these 'daily nightmares' but am starting to feel that my job is too much at the mercy of those I sail with.'

Alteration in maximal anticonvulsant treatment brings improvement for a couple of weeks but he now has at least one small attack a day and one more severe one each week.

The patient is much concerned about his vocational deterioration, active in searching for a new post when relegated from the former one, always busy at home or on the Thames, but trivialises his intractable epilepsy, is sympathetic with the doctors' failures, and always seems cheerful and at ease. I have never found any evidence in behaviour or in interrogation to suggest any emotional disorder. A psychiatrist found him well-adjusted and normal, and thought his asexuality might be drug-induced or a feature of the epilepsy. Endocrine studies were however normal and modification of treatment has made no differences.

His personality is that of an able dynamic perfectionist. Punctilious in his behaviour and appearance, the epitome of a naval officer, with charm, emotional detachment from his epilepsy as such, realistic about his wrecked romance and its promises, practical about his employment, but so contained withal as to be 'too good to be true'.

This is the archetype of the person with epilepsy, devoid of emotional consequences apparently, in whom the attacks continue recalcitrantly as 'stress symptoms', as may other recurring maladies such as migraine. I suspect that the persistent asexuality and impotence have a similar basis.

This solitary unit of the statistics, this patient-of-the-moment, epitomises all the other patients not included in the following pages, patients nevertheless who constitute major therapeutic problems, pharmacologically and psychotherapeuti-cally. Their defence against their difficulties also repels help.

THE EMOTIONS OF THOSE WITH EPILEPSY

The derogatory generalisation so often described by doctors in old institutions which led to the notion of an epileptic personality can best be described as a dull, grumbling paranoia against society at large, with aggression to those close to the problem. As a pathological entity it has had many knocks in recent years, and we know that whilst having epilepsy of necessity is likely to produce much the same feelings in many people, there is as wide a scatter of personality traits in those with epilepsy as in the population at large. This view must, however, be modified because epilepsy is invariably a symptom pattern of cerebral disorder, either primarily structural or primarily biochemical. Whilst it is general that those with constitutional epilepsy (who have classical petit mal with ubiquitous 3/second spike wave discharges in the electroencephalogram, generally without a focal onset) are in other regards, as people, entirely normal, many of the others whose epilepsy is related to structural brain disorder have associated disturbances of intellect, of personality, or defects of bodily function, though in both the emotional consequences of having epilepsy may be profound.

In the large second group we must try to separate the consequences of those shortcomings from the epilepsy itself, but of course total separation is as undesirable as it is impossible. An obvious example is that of the child of an abnormal birth who has behavioural disorder with rages, aggression and temporal lobe epilepsy. Accompanying the rages and underlying the aggression is an abnormal degree and quality of the emotion anger, an emotion abnormally evoked through the disturbed brain, as is the epilepsy. This is especially found in those with damage to a temporal lobe. The resulting disability with its two components, psychosocial and epileptic, is analogous to that in a patient with damage to a parietal lobe, whose disability is composed of a hemiparesis and focal convulsions, although here the consequences are more easily distinguished and are separable. It follows that the emotional consequences of having epilepsy alone are more easily studied 'in pure culture' in the first group of people with constitutional epilepsy without any contingent disturbances.

In both groups the consequences of epilepsy have been epitomised in the couplet by Adelaide Crapsley from *On seeing weather-beaten trees* —

Is it as clearly in our living shown
By slant and twist, which way the wind has blown.

The way the wind has blown is clear enough in the distorted life of a patient with uncontrolled epilepsy, but like the poet we may not recognise the kind of tree.

The consequences of the epilepsy

The affective disorders, mixed anxiety states, depressions with consequent high suicide rates of those with epilepsy follow the general pattern of the psychiatry of those with insoluble problems are dealt with elsewhere in this volume, and concern long-term moods rather than emotions per se. They are the illnesses dominating psychiatric practice in general, but because of the special qualities of the life disorder caused by epilepsy they tend to have special feeling tones related to the cognitive results of the disturbed life situations, for instance, the patients have reasonable feelings of personal and social insecurity, they feel perpetually frustrated, they may have anger against fate or their follows, and often experience or imagine misunderstanding. They also have unreasonable but pardonable feelings of bitterness, jealousy, or frank paranoia. Indeed, whilst we accept the occurrence of the schizophreniform psychosis in epilepsy which was described by Slater et al (1963), it is certain that in some or many of those patients the psychosis has been grounded in the emotional morass I have outlined. The paranoid depression seen in young adult epileptics which mimics early schizophrenia can be reversed by good medicine built upon understanding explanation, social help, and psychopharmacology. For the others, who sink into a state of chronic schizophreniform psychosis, it may well be that this situation is similar to that of the analogy of hemiplegia with focal fits referred to above, the psychosis being concomitant with the epilepsy, but not caused by it.

Let us escape from this topic by noting that it involves moods and not emotions alone, with the statement that in either case their content is unpleasant. As with the experience of pain, the emotions and moods secondary to epilepsy are never pleasant, though those arising within the attack itself may be (see below).

The emotions before the ictus

The comment that the emotions secondary to epilepsy are never pleasant is a banal truism is belied by the emotional precursors of a fit, whether predisposing or precipitating. Pleasure, especially in childhood, may precipitate a fit. This may be anticipatory pleasure as in the many children who have a convulsion whilst preparing to go home at the end of the school term or on the way to their first skiing holiday. It may be in the compound emotion called excitement which is contemporary with the event, as in a children's Christmas or birthday party. Or the immediate excitement called a thrill which is a compound of fear-pleasure induced by a sporting event. Here, the fit often happens during the event. When however the subject is involved in the physical action of the sport or the dance, or the competition, the convulsions generally follow the event in the tranquil aftermath, but no one knows why.

The unpleasant precursors of a fit generally involve the affect anxiety and the emotion fear or the complex emotion which is the opposite of pleasure–unpleasure or distress. Like the pleasant emotional precipitants these invariably have a circumstantial cause and the attack generally follows the causal event after an interval. A well known example is the isolated fit which happens in the lull after the State examinations; such fits are rarely encountered during the examinations or on the sports field, except in those with very frequent fits. Anticipatory fear leading to an attack usually has an intense circumstantial cause, as in punishment, minor surgical procedures, and the anticipation of pain. The effect of emotion is enhanced by suddenness, as with the news of a disaster. A young woman had her first fit when she heard that her husband had fallen from scaffolding—there and then—but then went on to have epilepsy. The compound emotion of unpleasantness cannot be given a single name for it has so many variations, so we say 'distress'. Of course the intermediate visceral changes resulting from the emotion may be operative, as with vasomotor instability or emotional overbreathing, but the suddenness of the ictus often seems to exclude such mechanisms.

These emotional precipitants are distinct from the natural secondary apprehension or fear that an attack may occur, or is imminent. They are also distinct from the emotions which sometimes occur within the ictus, and which have the same place phenomenologically as a visual or auditory hallucination within the attack, as local dysaesthesia, or ictal movement. These happen when the cortex and sub-cortex involved in the initiation of the emotion is overrun by the epileptic events. They can be considered to be hallucinations of emotion, and when they happen have their place in the Jacksonian march of events. They only seem to occur when the temporal and peritemporal cortex is the site of the event and as reference to the original paper shows, the area involved is the anterior part of the temporal lobe. They are dealt with in some detail in *The structure of the emotions reflected in epileptic experiences* (Williams 1956).

Within the ictus

Ictal emotions are generally unpleasant and of primitive nature. They are classed as fear, misery or sadness, pleasure, unpleasure and anger. They are described in 5 per cent of all ambulant epileptic patients who are seen. Fear was experienced in 60 per cent, sadness, or depression depending upon semantics, in 20 per cent, and the others equally in the remaining 20 per cent. Three-quarters of those who experienced fear had a focus of origin recognised in the electroencephalogram, the lesions, or from other Jacksonian features of the attack, in the anterior part of the temporal lobe, more commonly on the left side.

The emotion fear ranged from a strange, unnatural apprehension, of fear without an object, to stark terror. Autonomic changes associated with emotional change might accompany it, precede it, or be absent. Any other hallucinatory component of the ictus such as words or sights are pervaded by the fear. In addition the behavioural accompaniments of fear may be seen. Indeed, so-called cursive epilepsy occurs in such a state, and I suspect that in the attack the ictal running is evoked by the same spreading event; that is to say it is not the person who is running or the fear that is making the movements, but both have a common cause in the area of cortex traversed by the epileptic discharge.

One of the most consistent features of temporal epilepsy is amnesia for all or for part of the focal event, which is in contrast to parietal or occipital epilepsy. The patients who have focal clonic attacks or visual hallucinations can tell us about their experiences but with temporal epilepsy the ones who can do so are in the minority and, at risk of an eirism, they may have similar ictal experiences during their amnesia. These include most of the people who run in their attacks; people see them run but they themselves cannot remember the fear. This, too, probably explains why only a minority of people with temporal foci experience ictal emotions. Many illustrative case vignettes are given by Williams (1956). Variants of fear, including horror, occur and these pervade the whole experience too, but I must limit detail.

Sadness or depression will be felt when the origin of the attack is anywhere below the Sylvian fissure, have similar characteristics to those of fear, and may be accompanied by fear. As with fear, ictal sadness may accompany hallucinations, words, visceral feelings or activity, familiarity, and even pleasure (satisfaction). In considering ictal emotions, it seems important to keep in mind that the ictal spread is anarchic; it destroys the established order and spreads topographically rather than physiologically, disregarding accepted boundaries and pathways; hence the strangeness of the events and their association. The experience 'I smell a smell like the sound of blue thunder' was an experience in point.

Pleasure and its opposite are rare, and intensely pervade the hallucination giving experience of ecstatic vastness or eternity, a pleasurable smallness, a satisfaction, and so on, or at the other extreme total autoscopy. Here again the examples already described elsewhere are fascinating but beyond this essay. They of course abound in religious writings, and in the misunderstandings of mystics. The anecdotal essays on such instances are beyond the intention of this clinical paper.

The recognition of these ictal events is valuable, and not just for academic satisfaction. It helps to distinguish what in the illness is ictal and what due to continuing affective disorder. It enables psychological phenomena to be dealt with physiologically in the same manner as somatic ictal events are. And it widens our bridge of knowledge between the phenomena of physiology and psychology.

Postictal emotions

Emotions consequent upon a fit are commonplace. We all know of the disappointment, depression, dismay or anger at a recurrence. So often, though, the postictal emotional disorder which may last for days if a focal fit precedes a major convulsion, is intense and seems out of proportion to the physical consequences of the fit. Two reasons for this spring to mind. The first may be called natural—a further reminder of having epilepsy; the dislocation of immediate life pattern; the intense distress with muscle or joint pain, headache, and lacerated tongue; the further reminder of threats to security and the future; the attitude of friends and family—all natural enough. Suicide is some five times as common in epilepsy as in other patients (see Chapter 7), which should not surprise anyone.

The second reason is unnatural or ictal. Though the convulsion has passed, the whole brain is still suffering the consequences, analagous to the memory defect after curarised electropexy. And one of these consequences is the persistence of ictal mood disorder per se. The prime difference between an emotion and a mood is that in the normal, if such there be, the emotion does not long outlive the subject of its evocation. I suspect, for proof is impossible, that ictal sadness or depression initiated in the amnesia of the attack is common, and by definition the mood continues after the event. It is certain that the trailing black clouds have their beginning with emergence from the amnesia, and that they take days to pass in some patients.

TREATING THE EMOTIONAL DISORDERS OF EPILEPSY

The treatment is of the complex causes which have been touched upon already. The first goal of curing the fits having been missed, we can only help the unhelpable. Here the adjustment of the patient to his circumstance by personal interviews with objectivity, explanation, frankness, and practical advice is as important as knowledge of anticonvulsant treatment. This is within the knowledge of every psychiatrist and the scope of every physician. Although it is so important, it is so obvious that I will pass it by. It is the handling of a rather special form of affective disorder, bearing in mind that if the patient has enough to be depressed or anxious about, antidepressant or anxiolytics are not of much use, and certainly should not supplant the interview. Here the team is essential, first in the family, and then the friends, then the larger families of the form, the school, the employers, the social workers, the civil servants, and the voluntary organisations whose aim is to educate and advise all those at all levels. The ideal is that the patient himself should never seem to be being helped, but only the effects of his epilepsy. It is important to make this distinction to allow the patient to help himself with dignity, whilst accepting what can be done to help the epilepsy and the effects of the epilepsy upon him. The distinction is subtle but important.

Like us all, the subject of epilepsy is an ordinary person with special problems. We manipulate the social structure and other events to solve our problems with the help of others. His problems are different and greater. He must be shown that we know that he must welcome society's help in solving those problems as a responsibility which we accept, and not as a charity. It would be tedious of me to take the reader through the patient's life at home, in school, higher education, or special education, sexual development and intersexual misfortune, vocational training, vocational ambition and vocational hope, on (as I would hope) to successful marriage. This volume is about the psychiatry of epilepsy, and that is left to the capable pens of so many others.

I referred to the patient's rejection of help as a charity; charity (*caritas*) is a dirty word to citizens with fits; it is unfortunately anxious-*caritas* which disrupts his parental home, misplaced *caritas* which makes him different from his school friends, apprehensive-*caritas* which frustrates his vocational ambitions, but *caritas* of the real sort, that is, sharing or understanding he welcomes. It is that which makes the marriage of one with epilepsy such a success for he has found another who shares.

There is no one English word to match *caritas* — that may be because it has several shades of meaning, of course. In the King James Bible it is translated as 'charity', in the various contemporary ones as 'love'. The translation goes '*caritas* vaunteth not itself, doth not behave itself unseemly, is not puffed-up'. To the physician *caritas* (charity) is simply a state of mind, of attitude, thinking and action. His work is compounded of *scientia et caritas*; when I began medicine, *caritas* had to be dominant, for its *scientia* was then so limited, but whilst we have seen the phenomenal efflorescence of *scientia*, its flowering has often been at the expense of *caritas*, for they seem to be reciprocally valent, although so different. The first, *scientia*, is public and extra-personal, composed of facts available to all, whilst the second, *caritas*, is entirely personal and private, a 'state of mind', having so many attributes including the emotions, so perhaps the comment at the opening of this chapter that 'emotions cannot be measured and so are not scientific' may have some basis, after all; but that detracts not a whit from their importance to the physician in diagnosis, causation, and in treatment.

All this may be clear to the physician, but not to the patient. He is unable to see that the effects of his illness have extended far beyond the mere fact of fits, and as he sees it, he cannot accept that *caritas* vaunteth not itself, doth not behave itself unseemly, is not puffed-up. Even with what we know of epilepsy and its treatment, we can go far in helping the patient in reduction of the incidence of attacks as well as in his life pattern if we can place ourselves in the milieu at home and beyond of the patient before us. Helping his family and friends to understand as much as we do and to share our shortcomings helps the patient, too. The situation changes for the better, and consequently secondary feeling (or emotion) is altered, too. Here there is an important point to make. I have referred to the loving anxiety at home as anxious-*caritas*. This generally and naturally stems from the mother, though the father is of course much involved. The mother cannot logically deal with episodic unpredictable disturbances of behaviour or consciousness. They are beyond her ken, and often remain so. Emotionally they are a disaster. The anxiety taints the mother-child relationship and pervades the whole home. The consequences upon the child we know. The mother has the choice of behaving naturally, expressing her fears, and so making the situation worse, or of trying to act as if there were no anxiety, thus creating an artificial abnormal relationship. The first is probably the lesser of the two evils, but the grim fact is that the mother is trapped. She cannot do right, and as the child's home behaviour changes she feels instinctively that she is to blame. This blame makes things worse. In all this, the child does not *feel* an abnormal family environment; he simply lives it and helps to create it. There is simply the presence of that situation. It is the very reality of it, the is-ness which is so destructive and which potentiates the epileptic problem in the evocation of what we might consider stress-attacks. The child does not feel the stress, it simply biologically is there in the family. The security of family unity is eroded; there is the loneliness of covert anxiety. I stress this for there is the danger of thinking of the reality of the situation in a home with epilepsy in words which suggest feeling. There seems to be very little feeling in it, for the very reality of the situation subdues feeling and fosters change in behaviour. In such a home, his father dead, his mother guilty, though as yet undiscovered, Hamlet exlaimed: '*Seems*, my dear mother, nay it *is*'. This is what I have tried to convey, though less skillfully.

Much can be done by free discussion with the parents alone, then the child alone, and then with them together, to create understanding and sharing. Without that in such a home mere medication may be ineffectual. How often have we seen a child with epilepsy, living for a while with another family who care and understand but who have not the natural pervading anxiety of the parents, who for that time has ceased to have attacks, though they return when he is home again.

References

Pond D 1961 Psychiatric aspects of epileptic and brain-damaged children. Br. med. J. 2:1377–1382 and 2:1454–1459

Slater E, Beard A W, Glitheroe E 1963 The schizophrenia-like psychoses of epilepsy. Br. J. Psychiat. 109:95–150

Symposium 1980 Emotional support for cancer patients and their families. Proc. R. Soc. Med. 73:214–218

Taylor D C 1972 Mental state and temporal epilepsy. Epilepsia 13:727–765

Williams D 1956 The structure of emotions reflected in epileptic experiences. Brain 79:29–67

Depression, anxiety and epilepsy

INTRODUCTION

Of all the psychiatric conditions to be found in association with epilepsy, depression and anxiety in their various forms must be the commonest, and yet of all the conditions they are the least well recognised or described in the literature and seem almost taken for granted.

Study of the literature of the last 50 years suggests that depression is the commonest major psychiatric complication of epilepsy, and that neurotic illness, particularly anxiety, is generally more common in people with epilepsy than would be expected by chance. However, when one looks at both these statements closely and critically there are few figures to actually back them up, and much of the evidence is based on clinical impression and speculation. Few formal studies of the special properties of depression or anxiety in people with epilepsy have been made. Depression, for instance, is usually described as occurring in people with epilepsy as a kind of footnote or aside to studies on the prevalence of psychotic illness in epilepsy.

Review of those studies that have considered depression or neurotic illness in some detail, suggests that often no clearly defined operational criteria are used in the study, and a control population is not employed (Pond & Bidwell 1959, Gudmunsson 1966) or the study is based on relatively small numbers of patients (Flor-Henry 1969, Standage & Fenton 1975, Shukla & Katiyar 1980).

Indeed, one of the main problems in any review of the existing literature is that depression and anxiety have different meanings to different authors and anyway are capable of various definitions and relate to several different stages of epilepsy.

I will look first at the various relationships that exist between depressive feelings and epilepsy.

DEPRESSION

Clinically most psychiatrists distinguish between *depressive feelings* and *depressive illness*. In both there is a continued lowness of spirits, a sustained sadness. Depressive feelings are seen largely as understandable, as a reaction to circumstances. They can be mild or severe: if severe they may be accompanied by other psychological or physical phenomena. Some people are more prone to depressive feelings under stress or adverse circumstances than others: this relates to genetic and constitutional factors to some degree but also to a person's previous upbringing and life circumstances and the degree of emotional support he currently enjoys. Depressive feelings tend to respond to circumstance: if clearly reactive to some emotionally overwhelming event (like bereavement) powerful psychological restorative mechanisms exist, so that the victim eventually 'works through' his profound depressive feelings and returns to a normal mood (though such a return can be delayed or deviated if working through does not, for some reason, take place).

Depressive feelings, mild or severe, which cannot be understood or which seem to be totally out of keeping with the victim's circumstances, are seen as depressive illness. In addition to the sustained lowness of mood, characteristic physical and emotional symptoms occur, such as changes in weight and sleep pattern and the development of specific depressive delusions and even hallucinations. This kind of depression behaves like an illness. It has a characteristic distinguishable set of symptoms, it has a natural history, it begins to look as though it has a specific physiopathology, and it has specific and successful treatments. Constitutional and genetic factors are important determinants. Recovery is usual, recurrence common: there is a definite mortality rate (from suicide). Some victims, subject to recurrent bouts of depression, also have bouts of pathological elation (mania).

A clear distinction between depressive feelings (or reactive depression) and depressive illness (or endogenous depression) cannot be made. In some people reactive and endogenous factors co-exist: in others, because of the overlapping of symptomatology, a clinical distinction is impossible — here time and experience may be the only guides.

In Table 6.1, I present a classification of the relationships that may exist between depressive feelings, depressive illness and epilepsy.

Table 6.1 Depression and epilepsy

1. Depressive reaction to acquiring the label of epilepsy
2. Depressive reaction to social or family problems of epilepsy
3. Prodromal depressive feelings before a fit
4. Depressive feelings as an aura
5. Depressive feelings as an ictal experience
6. Postictal depressive feelings
7. Depressive twilight state
8. Epileptic depressive delirium
9. Endogenous depression unrelated directly to fits, but possibly to their decrease in frequency
10. Depressive symptoms occurring in association with other mental illnesses, particularly a paranoid or schizophrenic psychosis.

Most patients when given the diagnosis of epilepsy for the first time go through a painful period of adjustment, as they come to terms with the realities of their handicap. This adjustment is particularly difficult for people with epilepsy because of the social prejudice that exists against the illness, and the effect that having the illness will have on the patient's own family and relationships. A general description of this is given in Betts (1981), and it is sufficient to indicate here that most people and their families will go through a short or prolonged period of denial, emotional struggle and then depressive feelings as they come to terms with the condition. People need help during this period, particularly emotional support, from their family and their doctor. In addition to emotional support they also need information, but information given at the right time and in the right way so that it can be assimilated and understood. Unfortunately many doctors are unaware of the psychological skills needed to support and give information to patients who are frightened or unhappy, and in only a few medical schools is such instruction given (Sanson-Fisher & Maguire 1980).

The support and help of a social worker, particularly one experienced in epilepsy, who is able to visit the patient and family at home is invaluable for the patient as he works through his 'grief reaction' on learning the diagnosis of epilepsy. In my own department we are experimenting with special videotapes for patients, which in addition to providing information which the patient can see again and again — and with his family if necessary — also provide examples of the kind of reaction that families and others will have to the patient with epilepsy, and are used as triggers for discussion with patients and families about how best to deal with the problems and emotional reactions that epilepsy brings (Betts & Raffle 1980a,b, Betts 1980). The support of fellow sufferers in patient 'Action Groups' is also valuable.

A depressive reaction, rather like a grief reaction, to the knowledge that one has epilepsy is common, and with support can usually be worked through and the patient will come out of the other side of it to a condition of emotional stability and acceptance. Relatives need support as well, because both patient and the relative, in addition to any depressive feelings, may have profound feelings of guilt or anger, particularly if there is some known reason for the epilepsy, such as a head injury or a febrile convulsion. Such periods of emotional turmoil must not be treated medically (such reactions if treated by antidepressants or tranquillisers may actually become prolonged) but need to be supported and worked through using psychological treatments.

Even when a person comes to terms with his epilepsy, epilepsy can sometimes bring with it, particularly if intractable, a host of social and personal problems, in life-style, work, and personal relationships. If insurmountable these problems may also lead to the patient developing a depressive reaction and here again treatment techniques of social support, psychotherapy, and behavioural intervention may be more appropriate than chemotherapy. The problem of the differential diagnosis of such depressive feelings in this situation is dealt with in some detail elsewhere (Betts 1981), but it should be particularly remembered that in patients with intractable epilepsy, drug intoxication, particularly with phenytoin, can look very much like depression and the two need to be carefully distinguished.

In some patients depressive feelings, sometimes even resembling an endogenous depression, can occur as a regular prodromal phenomenon for hours, days or even longer before an epileptic fit (Williams 1956 and Chapter 5). Compared with other prodromal symptoms, such as irritability or excitability, they are probably not very common. It has been my clinical impression that patients with regular prodromal depressive symptoms, which are regularly followed by a tonic–clonic seizure, tend to be those patients in whom successful treatment of the fits is followed by a prolonged depressive illness. It used to be believed that such patients should be allowed to have an occasional spontaneous seizure to have a beneficial effect on their mood, but nowadays I think in such patients one should persist with anti-convulsant treatment because, even if a depressive illness does occur when the fits stop, the depression will eventually remit, particularly with antidepressant treatment.

Depressive feelings may have a more direct relationship to the seizure itself, either as a true aura before a tonic–clonic fit or as part of a partial complex seizure, or as a regular sequal to the ictus. Williams (1956) in 2000 personally seen patients with epilepsy found 100 who felt emotion as part of the attack. Of those, 61 had ictal fear, 21 ictal depression and 18 some other ictal emotion. Ictal or pre-ictal emotion might be hard to distinguish from normal emotion, but in Williams' words

'in all but one patient the epileptic emotion or mood was associated with other abnormal sensations. In about two thirds it was preceded, and in one third followed, by other ictal sensations, whilst in about one half it occurred in the very middle of the attack. This relationship as well as the description of the emotion felt and its total setting usually made the differentiation of natural from epileptic emotions quite clear'.

In other words ictal mood can be recognised because it may be bizarre or not feel 'right' or be occurring out of context and before, during or after its presence something else recognisably epileptic will be going on. This other epileptic phenomena may not be recognised or enquired for by an assessing doctor. In Betts (1981) I describe a patient with recurrent short-lived ictal guilt. Attempts at treating this with psychotherapy and religious counselling only stopped when a doctor bothered to ask her about other phenomena occurring during the guilt feelings and she described automatic voiding of urine: by this time her temporal glioma was inoperable.

Williams (1956) found, and my experience is the same, that 'depression as an ictal experience cannot be related to any one part of the brain'. He gives clinical descriptions of various types of ictal depressive experience: patients describe the ictal depression as 'feeling very sad' or as a profound depression 'with thoughts of death and the world' or of 'futility and misery'. One of Williams' patients had strong suicidal feelings and acted on them. In Betts (1981) I describe a patient who cut his throat whilst in an ictal depressive state.

Williams (1956) emphasises the occurence of short-lived dense depression as an immediate sequel of a convulsion as particularly striking, emerging from the postictal confusion and ending quite quickly. I have not encountered many examples of this myself but his description of peri-ictal depression (both before and after) being associated with 'a bad phase in the epilepsy' has a familiar ring, and I have several patients in whom exacerbations of depression (often with depressive delusions and hallucinations occurring in clear consciousness) and epilepsy occur together (and often disappear again if one waits). Some patients have a kind of depressive twilight state: Williams (1956) describes one such patient with recurrent two-day cycles of depression and altered brain function, and I have described (Betts 1981) a patient with continual left temporal spike wave activity who wandered miserably round her house unable to concentrate or cope until the temporal lobe abnormality suddenly stopped and she swiftly revived. More cases like this probably exist than are recognised.

There also exists a very small group of patients in whom a sudden increase in attack frequency leads not to the more usual confusional state or acute paranoid psychosis (see Chapter 10) but to a confusional state—characterised by forgetfulness and disorientation—accompanied by endogenous depressive symptoms (guilt, self-blame, unworthiness etc.) and in which any hallucinations have a depressive flavour (open graves, coffins, accusatory voices). I have not seen this elsewhere described in the literature, but have seen several examples of it in the last fifteen years. In all the patients the mental state returned to normal when the fit frequency returned to normal, suggesting that these were examples of a true depressive delirium. Clinically they remind me of the similar acute depressive confusional state with which hyperparathyroidism sometimes presents itself.

The occurrence of an endogenous type of depressive illness in people with epilepsy is generally considered to be common, although there is little hard factual evidence to support this. In Chapter 14 I review the literature on the relationship between mental illness and epilepsy as seen in mental hospitals over the last 50 years. In many of the earlier reports on the types of mental illness that people with epilepsy have in mental hospitals the occurrence of melancholia was described as the commonest. In a study of people with epilepsy admitted to psychiatric care in 1968/69, depression was certainly the commonest reason for admission (Table 6.2). (Betts 1974), and the patients in this study shared an interesting characteristic with

Table 6.2 Epilepsy admission study (Betts 1974)

Main psychiatric diagnosis (n = 72)	
Depressive illness (12 endogenous)	22
Brain syndrome (Dementia), intoxication, twilight stage etc.)	22
Personality disorder/psychopathy	15
Social distress	4
Paranoid psychosis	3
Phobic anxiety	3
Psychiatrically normal	2
Not known*	1

* Absconded before assessment

the patients described by Flor-Henry (1969), which was that the onset of depression seemed to be associated with a significant reduction in the patient's usual seizure frequency.

Gunn (1969) described depressive symptoms as being particularly common in people with epilepsy who were also in prison, and Mellor et al (1974) described children with epilepsy as being particularly prone to depression. It may be that the incidence of depression in epilepsy in centres which draw upon a selected population is less than in the unselected population of mental hospitals, although Toone & Driver (1980) describe affective psychosis (depression/mania) as being almost as common as a schizophrenic psychosis in their sample of 41 patients from the Maudsley Hospital.

Apart from the probable association between a decline (either induced or natural) in seizure frequency and the onset of depressive symptoms in people with epilepsy, it is uncertain whether endogenous depressive illnesses in people with epilepsy have any other unique characteristics, as little clinical description exists as to what they are like. It has been my own impression of 15 years' experience of mentally ill people with epilepsy that in patients recently admitted to hospital (rather than in the chronic inmates) depression and syndromes of organic brain impairment are about equally common as reasons for admission, and that when an endogenous type of depressive illness presents itself in someone with epilepsy it tends to be of sudden onset and sudden departure and may also fluctuate quite markely whilst it is present. Williams (1956) seems to have the same impression. Epileptic depression also seems rather resistant to conventional antidepressant treatment, and paradoxically may need electroconvulsive therapy to clear it.

One much-quoted study (Flor-Henry 1969) has suggested that depressive illness in people with temporal lobe epilepsy is particularly associated with right temporal lobe lesions. It is only when one reads this paper carefully that one realises that the now widely quoted and believed idea that right temporal (non-dominant) epilepsy leads to affective psychosis is based on observations made on nine epileptic patients, given the retrospective diagnosis of manic–depressive disorder, in which 44 per cent had a right temporal epileptic focus, 22 per cent a left and 33 per cent a bilateral one (i.e. four, two and three patients). It is not surprising that other authors have not really been able to confirm the right-sided hypothesis. I remain convinced, from observing my own patients, that, like ictal depression, epileptic depressive illness is not to be found in one area of the brain.

It should also be noted that the true prevalence of depressive illness in people with epilepsy has never been estimated, and indeed, because of its often fleeting nature, would be difficult to measure accurately.

In addition to depressive symptoms occurring in people with epilepsy as part of an endogenous depressive illness, there is little doubt that in patients with either a paranoid psychotic illness or a true schizophrenic illness occurring in association with epilepsy depressive symptoms are also common, and indeed this mixed kind of psychosis is being reported more frequently as more careful mental state evaluations are made on psychotic patients with epilepsy (Perez & Trimble 1980). It can be very difficult to tell sometimes whether one is seeing a depressive illness in which schizophrenic symptoms are also occurring, or whether one is seeing a true schizophrenic illness in which there is a large depressive component. In my limited experience of patients who show both depressive and schizophrenic symptoms at the same time, there is often a concomitant increase in attack frequency around the time of the onset of the psychotic experience and in some of these patients control of the epilepsy leads to a resolution of the psychosis. (In one such patient mixed manic and schizophrenic symptoms were accompanied by generalised spike and wave activity occurring over the right hemisphere, which disappeared when the psychosis abated).

The management of the depressive states in epilepsy starts with a careful assessment of the patient's symptoms, his epilepsy and his social and personal circumstances. Depressive symptoms that seem to be reactive either to the diagnosis of epilepsy itself, or to the life circumstances caused by the epilepsy, need social work intervention, supportive psychotherapy and possibly behaviour therapy: a search should also be made for possible drug intoxication.

Chemotherapy for depression should be avoided in people with epilepsy unless it is very clear that one is dealing with an endogenous type of depression.

When indicated antidepressant drug treatment for depressed people with epilepsy should be assessed with care, and has been reviewed by Trimble (1980 and Chapter 24). There is no doubt that some tricyclic antidepressant drugs (probably the best antidepressants) are potentially epileptogenic and in some patients have actually caused fits. It has been suggested that the newer antidepressant drugs such as viloxazine, nomifensine or mianserin should be used in the treatment of patients with epilepsy who are depressed, but the antidepressant efficiency of these drugs is still open to some doubt and viloxazine can readily produce phenytoin intoxication.

If the patient is severely depressed and does not seem to be responding fairly quickly to antidepressant medication there is no contraindication to the use of electroconvulsive therapy. A few patients in my experience will sometimes develop epilepsy for the first time during or after a course of ECT (probably due to some kindling mechanism), but ECT itself causes no problem in people with epilepsy and should not be withheld if there is good clinical indication for using it. Even when chemical or electrical treatment is offered for depression, the use of supportive psychotherapy and social work are still needed in the rehabilitation of depression.

One problem in the management of depression is, of course, that of suicide. Dr Barraclough in Chapter 7 describes the relationship between completed suicide and epilepsy, which seems to be of a more than chance association. It is also true that attempted suicide and epilepsy probably more commonly occur together than would be expected by chance (Mackay 1979, Hawton et al 1980). This relationship between attempted suicide and epilepsy is probably a combination of the social situations in which many people with epilepsy have to live, alcohol and the ready availability to anyone with epilepsy of powerful anti-convulsant drugs which can be taken in deliberate overdosage. In terms of the management of depression and epilepsy, the possibility of attempted suicide should always be borne in mind, and all patients who have depressive symptoms should be specifically asked if they have intended to harm themselves. If suicidal intent is clear, then admission to hospital (on a compulsory basis if necessary) should be arranged. Most patients who successfully kill themselves have given a warning to somebody before they do so, and therefore talk or threats of suicide should always be taken seriously.

ANXIETY

Of the other non-psychotic mental illnesses, hysteria (reviewed by Dr Trimble in Chapter 9) is almost certainly more common in people with epilepsy than would be expected by chance. Obsessional illness, on the other hand, is probably not. Although I have encountered a few patients with both conditions, the association has almost certainly been fortuitous. The number of people with epilepsy who also have an obsessional illness (not the same thing as obsessional personality) is small, and the content of the obsessional acts or ruminations, when such an association does occur, bears no relation to the epilepsy, nor is there a convincing

Table 6.3 Anxiety and epilepsy

1. Anxiety reaction to acquiring the label of epilepsy
2. Anxiety reaction to the social or family problems of epilepsy
3. Prodromal anxiety before a fit
4. Anxiety as an aura
5. Anxiety as an ictal experience
6. Anxiety (or agitation) occurring in association with an epileptic psychosis
7. Anxiety occurring in association with epilepsy-related brain damage
8. True phobic axiety related to seizures

time relationship: the two conditions seem completely independent.

Anxiety, however, does have a complex relationship with epilepsy: study of this is made difficult by the fact that in many reports anxiety is but loosely defined, is difficult to measure, and the differentiation of normal from abnormal anxiety is not easy. Many studies, also, fail to distinguish between 'state' anxiety (i.e. what the person is feeling at this moment) from 'trait' anxiety (the level of anxiety that a particular subject usually feels). The two are not necessarily the same, as some people normally have a higher degree of everyday anxiety than others, and people respond to the same stressful situation with differing degress of anxiety. Certainly in considering anxiety the context in which it is occurring has to be understood, as one cannot say that a particular degree of anxiety is pathological or not unless one does. This is more so than in depression, where often consideration of the person's symptoms would be enough to make this distinction.

We do not look at anxiety in the same way as depression, and the concept of 'endogenous' anxiety is not usually employed (although one could argue that it exists). Depressive and anxiety symptoms can also occur side by side. As in depression there are two components to anxiety, a psychic one of a felt unpleasant emotion of fear or dread or apprehension (though anticipatory feelings, the start of apprehension, can be pleasant), and a somatic component of physical symptoms (like nausea, diarrhoea, trembling, tachycardia, sweating etc), which can usually be interpreted as the components of a 'flight or fight' reaction. One of the problems of anxiety is that such physical symptoms can become self reinforcing — one becomes afraid of being afraid — and a particular anxiety response, that of overbreathing, can trigger off other somatic symptoms of peripheral tingling, tetany and eventual unconsciousness which can be mistaken for an epileptic attack. This problem is made more complex by the fact that there is now good evidence that involuntary overbreathing can trigger off epileptic attacks in the predisposed.

As anxiety occurs commonly in people under stress it is to be expected that anxiety symptoms will occur in people recently given the diagnosis of epilepsy and attempting to come to terms with it, or in people struggling with the problems of epilepsy. Both depressive and anxiety reactions, or a mixture, are common.

Anxiety, or agitation, can also occur as a regular prodromal phenomenon before a tonic–clonic seizure. This usually takes the form of restlessness, irritability and agitation for several days before a fit, or a mounting level of apprehension: one patient known to me also breaks out in an urticarial rash for two days before his clonic–tonic seizure as well as feeling anxious.

In a manner similar to depression, anxiety or fear can occur before, during or after other epileptic phenomena. Rarely fear can occur on its own as the sole ictal experience. Williams (1956) describes ictal fear as being both commoner and shorter lasting than ictal depression: ictal depression tends to carry on after the fit is over. Ictal fear often has an 'unnatural' quality—it does not feel like remembered fear but like, say, the fear of the supernatural. Very rarely the fear may have a pleasurable quality: I have one patient who was troubled from three to 12 years of age with fleeting feelings of pleasant anticipation (like the feeling before going to the circus'); at 12 the attacks continued but the feeling of pleasant anticipation was replaced by a feeling of fearful anticipation 'like going to the dentist'. Examination of the patient during the feelings shows clouding of consciousness, tachypnoea and a right anterior temporal spike wave discharge on electroencephalography.

Ictal fear can be accompanied by terrifying visual hallucinations (occasionally auditory) or by automatisms (sometimes relating to the fear) or by visceral sensations (tachycardia, palpitations, tachypnoea, 'gooseflesh', pallor, flushing, sweating, borborygmi, belching, flatus, vomiting, diarrhoea and micturition have been described). Sometimes automatisms occur which suggest fear, but the patient cannot recall the feeling afterwards (like cowering and shouting 'no, no,' or running with a look of terror from the room); sometimes the patient has the visceral accompaniments of fear without the psychological feeling (i.e. pallor, gooseflesh and sweating).

Sometimes the ictal nature of the patient's fear is not recognised, particularly when the brief ictal anxiety is mistaken for a panic attack or misidentified as some other phenomenon. In Betts (1981) I describe several examples of this, including a woman whose brief ictal anxiety was misinterpreted as evidence of occult powers. Of particular diagnostic difficulty is the patient who has both ictal anxiety and who has also become afraid of his experiences so that he also has true anxiety attacks. Panic attacks are particularly likely to be mistaken for ictal anxiety if the patient has evidence of temporal lobe dysfunction on electroencephalography as is not uncommon in phobic anxiety states. Only careful observation will reliably distinguish between the two (Betts 1981).

Williams (1956) felt ictal fear to be confined mainly to the anterior half of the temporal lobe with left-sided or bilateral discharges predominating.

Anxiety (agitation) is often seen as part of a depressive or schizophrenic psychosis: agitated depression is common and the perplexed unfocused anxiety of schizophrenia is characteristic. Both may be seen in epileptic psychoses. Likewise 'organic anxiety' exists: agitation may be a response to failing intellectual powers, or may be seen in states of clouded consciousness related to ictal activity. Anxiety can occur in patients who fail with academic tasks with which they can no longer cope—students with left temporal epileptic lesions seem particularly prone to it in my experience.

Many patients become fearful of their attacks; some develop a true phobic anxiety state related to them so that they are panic-stricken at the thought of going into a public place lest they have an attack (such patients, usually but not invariably, have made an imagined 'spectacle' of themselves in front of others). The patient then becomes housebound. The problem with such phobic anxiety is that, with epilepsy in particular, it tends to be self-reinforcing. The more anxious a person (particularly the more he overbreathes) the more likely he is to have a fit. The more fits he has the more anxious he will be about going out and the more likely he will be to have a fit. In my experience true phobic anxiety, related to a fear of going out or making a spectacle of oneself, is not at all uncommon in people with epilepsy; much more common, however, is the patient who does not have a true phobic anxiety state, but who, nevertheless, is frightened of his fits and has a general level of anxiety and stress which makes his fits more likely. If both types of patient can be helped to feel more relaxed about the fits and not care about them so much, fit frequency will decline and anxiety levels will reduce further. Such patients benefit enormously from experimenting with the self-control techniques that Fenwick describes in Chapter 22, as the more they feel in control of their illness, the less anxious they become and the fewer fits they have.

It is therefore very important to treat anxiety occurring in people with epilepsy well, because of the effect it will have on their fits. For some patients, as with depression, techniques of counselling, psychotherapy, social work intervention, and careful explanation about the illness work well, and diminish fear. In general terms one should try to avoid using medication to treat anxiety; this is particularly important in epilepsy as most benzodiazepine tranquillisers and hypnotic drugs are also anticonvulsants, so that withdrawal of the drug, after it has corrected the anxiety, is particularly difficult.

Behavioural methods of treatment of anxiety are becoming increasingly important, particularly as the dangers of the indiscriminant use of benzo-diazepines are becoming increasingly recognised. Behavioural treatment of anxiety implies the teaching to the patient of some mechanism which the patient can utilise to control or abolish the anxiety feelings.

General anxiety-reducing techniques include relaxation training and biofeedback. Once the patient has learnt control of his tension symptoms using such techniques he can learn to use them in previously anxiety-provoking situations. Generalised anxiety ('free floating' as opposed to phobic anxiety) can be treated in the same way. Once maintained, control skills also raise the patient's morale as he feels he has some control of his own illness, and has a technique that will last a lifetime. Relaxation skills need to be carefully taught and practised if they are to be successful; biofeedback needs to be used as a particular element in relaxation training and not as an end in itself. A demonstration of the methods taught patients with epilepsy in the Department of Psychiatry at the Queen Elizabeth Hospital is found in Betts, Pidd & Harvey (1976).

Relaxation or behavioural methods of anxiety reduction have been applied to patients whose epileptic attacks seem to be associated with or precipitated by anxiety (Pinto 1972, Standage 1972, Mostofsky & Balaschak 1977, Betts 1981) and lead to better control of the patient's epilepsy. In some patients coming to terms with one's fits by actually seeing them on videotape or seeing other patients with similar fits can be valuable in reducing the fear of the unknown which pervades some people with epilepsy: the videotape experiment of Feldman & Paul (1976) needs replication. I have no doubt that specific relaxation training is good for all people with epilepsy and may give some of them a control skill for the epilepsy itself; there are intriguing hints in the literature (Mostofsky & Balaschak

1977, Fenwick, Chapter 22) that behavioural techniques work in some non-anxiety related epilepsies.

It will be seen from this general review that both depression and anxiety pervade epilepsy and understanding the management of both is probably necessary for the good management of epilepsy. What we don't know for sure is how common they are, what particular phenomena they have, what special treatments they need and how much successful treatment of both would lead to reduction in epilepsy itself. To learn this would need a large epidemiological survey based on a general unselected population of people with epilepsy. Because depression and anxiety are often brief it would need to be longitudinal as well as cross-sectional and with a control population. The cost would be high, but the rewards might be great. It should at least answer one question: is there more depression and anxiety in people with epilepsy than in a comparative population of chronically sick people? Standage & Fenton (1975) suggest in their small number of patients that in terms of emotional response to their illness people with epilepsy may not be unique. It's a pity that a century on from Gowers we can't be more certain than that.

References

Betts T A 1974 A follow-up study of a cohort of patients with epilepsy admitted to psychiatric care in an English city. In: Harris P, Mawdsley C (eds) Epilepsy: proceedings of the Hans Berger centenary symposium. Churchill Livingstone, Edinburgh, p 326–336

Betts T A , Pidd S A, Harvey P G 1976 Relaxation and biofeedback. Videotape No. 0463. University of Birmingham Television and Film Service, Birmingham, England

Betts T A 1980 Three people with epilepsy. Videotape No. 0643 University of Birmingham Television and Film Service, Birmingham, England

Betts T A, Raffle A E 1980a Its only a fit—nothing to worry about: a film about becoming a person with epilepsy. Videotape No. 0637. University of Birmingham Television and Film Service, Birmingham, England

Betts T A, Raffle A E 1980b Temporal lobe epilepsy—an explanation. Videotape No. 0630. University of Birmingham Television and Film Service, Birmingham, England

Betts T A 1981 Psychiatry and epilepsy. In: Laidlaw J, Richens A (eds) A textbook of epilepsy, 2nd edn. Churchill Livingstone, Edinburgh

Feldman B G, Paul N G 1976 Identity of emotional triggers in epilepsy. Journal of Nervous and Mental Disease 162:345–353

Flor-Henry P 1969 Psychosis and temporal lobe epilepsy. Epilepsia 10:363–395

Gudmundsson D 1966 Epilepsy in Iceland. Acta neurologica scandinavica 43:Supplement 25.1–128

Gunn J 1969 Epileptics in prison. MD thesis, University of Birmingham, England

Hawton K, Fagg J, Marsack P 1980 Association between epilepsy and attempted suicide. Journal of Neurology, Neurosurgery and Psychiatry 43:168–170

Mackay A 1979 Self poisoning—a complication of epilepsy. British Journal of Psychiatry 134:277–282

Mellor D H, Lowitt I, Hall D I 1974 Are epileptic children behaviourally different from other children? In: Harris P, Mawdsley C (eds) Epilepsy: proceedings of the Hans Berger centenary symposium. Churchill Livingstone, Edinburgh, p 313–316

Mostofsky D I, Balaschak B A 1977 Psychobiological control of seizures. Psychological Bulletin 84:4 p 723–750

Perez M, Trimble M 1980 Epileptic psychosis—diagnostic comparison with process schizophrenia. British Journal of Psychiatry 137:245–249

Pinto R 1972 A case of movement epilepsy with agoraphobia treated successfully by flooding. British Journal of Psychiatry 121:287–288

Pond D A, Bidwell B H 1959 A survey of epilepsy in 14 general practices. II Social and psychological aspects. Epilepsia 1:285–299

Sanson-Fisher R, Maguire P 1980 Should skills in communicating with patients be taught in medical schools? Lancet 2:523–526

Shukla G D, Katiyar B C 1980 Psychiatric disorders in temporal lobe epilepsy: the laterality effect. British Journal of Psychiatry 137:181–182

Standage K F 1972 Treatment of epilepsy by reciprocal inhibition of anxiety. Guys Hospital Report 021:217–219

Standage K F, Fenton G W 1975 Psychiatric symptom profiles of patients with epilepsy: a controlled investigation. Psychological Medicine 5:152–160

Toone B K, Driver M V 1980 Psychosis and epilepsy. Research and Clinical Forums. 2:121–127

Trimble M R 1980 Psychotropic drugs in epilepsy. Research and Clinical Forums 2:113–120

Williams D 1956 The structure of emotions reflected in epileptic experiences. Brain 79:29–67

Suicide and epilepsy

INTRODUCTION

'Suicide although not a certainty is often a probable indication of a morbid family tendency and some weight must be given to it as an indication of a disposition to disease of which epilepsy may be a result even when it has an immediate exciting cause.' W. Gowers (1901)

Leaving aside progressive fatal brain disease, the excess mortality of epilepsy is attributed to death from status epilepticus and accidents associated with fits. The epilepsy literature has no systematic review that I have found reporting the association between epilepsy and suicide. The purpose of my enquiry is to fill this gap.

I searched the epilepsy literature from 1966–1979 using Medlars under the terms Suicide and secondly Epilepsy/Follow-up/Mortality. I included a paper if the number of suicides was given and the expected number or enough information to make an estimate. I calculated an expected number by multiplying together the number of persons in the cohort, the mean years of follow-up and the suicide rate of that country. The difference between observed and expected numbers is minimised by this method because cohorts of epileptics are on average younger than the general population to whom national suicide rates apply.

I found 11 papers from which it was possible to derive some evidence about the incidence of suicide in epileptics. Their dates of publication ranged from 1940–1979. The papers can be grouped broadly into: four papers about temporal lobe epilepsy, two papers on epileptic patients who resided in institutions, six papers about people with epilepsy who had been referred for diagnosis and treatment to general hospitals as in-patients or as out-patients, and lastly a paper based on life insurance statistics (Tables 7.1 and 7.2).

Temporal lobe epilepsy

In a sample of 666 patients diagnosed as having temporal lobe epilepsy at the London Hospital between 1949–1967 there were 54 deaths (Currie et al 1971). Of these 54, 42 were epilepsy-related and 12 were not, and of these 12, three or 25 per cent were suicides; the expected value was approximately 0.3. None of the suicides had been surgically treated.

Table 7.1 Follow-up studies of patients with epilepsy, reporting mortality from suicide

Author	Country	No. of suicides		No. of dead	% of deaths from suicide	Sample size	Follow-up period (yrs)
		Obs.	Exp.				
Temporal lobe epilepsy							
Currie (1971)	England	3	0.3*	54	6	493††	1–25
Stepień (1969)	Poland	2	0.03	3	67	77	1–9
Lindsay (1979)	England	1	0.05	9	11	100	13
Taylor (1977)	England	9	0.2	37	24	193	5–24
Epileptic patients in institutions							
Prudhomme (1941)	USA	8	1.7	1100	0.7	several thousand	14
White (1979)	England	21	3.9	636	3	1980	6–27
General hospital patients							
Dalby (1969)	Denmark	2	0.2	10	20	346	4–16
Henriksen (1970)	Denmark	21	7	104	20	2763	25
Sillanpää (1973)	Finland	1	0.001**	18	6	245	10
Zielinski (1974)	Poland	16	2†	218	7	6710	3
Life insurance							
Society of Actuaries (1954)	USA	2	0.7	157	2	1000	1–15

* Expected number based on sample size and follow-up period applying national suicide rate; all other expected numbers calculated by the authors of the paper in question
** Because original sample were children
† Calculated from author's statement that suicide was five times commoner in men and ten times commoner in women
†† Patients aged 15 and over from sample of 666

Table 7.2   Summary of papers reporting suicide in patients with epilepsy

	No. of papers	Observed suicides	Expected suicides	O/E
Temporal lobe epilepsy	4	15	0.6	25
Institutions	2	29	5.6	5
General hospitals	4	40	9.2	4
Insurance	1	2	0.7	4
Total	11	86	16	5

77 patients treated for temporal lobe epilepsy in Warsaw between 1960–1968 were followed up for between one and nine years (Stepién et al 1969). Ignoring the post-operative deaths and those resulting from malignancy, there were three deaths, of which one was from epilepsy and two were from suicide; the expected value is extremely small.

A hundred cases of children with temporal lobe epilepsy from Oxford, Northampton and Swindon identified between 1948 and 1964 and followed until 1977 yielded 14 deaths, nine after 15 years of age (Lindsay et al 1979); one of these was a suicide. The expected value here is again very small, probably less than 0.05.

Another English study (Taylor & Marsh 1977) reported the outcome of Falconer's series, people with temporal lobe epilepsy who had been treated by surgery between 1952 and 1971. Taylor followed this group and discovered 37 deaths. Nine were suicides, and two in circumstances suspicious of suicide; expected value 0.2. Suicide was the largest single cause of death. The suicides were young, aged between 30 and 40, three of the nine were under 20; five had no fits post-operatively, an interesting comment on the relationship between fits and suicide.

These four studies concur that temporal lobe epilepsy, whether or not treated surgically, is associated with a greatly increased risk of suicide. It is permissible to sum the observed numbers of suicides and compare with the expected for an approximation to the increased risk. There are 15 suicides and an expected value of 0.6. Temporal lobe epilepsy therefore has an increased risk of suicide by about 25 times.

Epileptic patients in institutions
Two papers describe the mortality of those with epilepsy resident in institutions. The earliest study found (Prudhomme 1941) is of this kind. It describes a postal survey conducted in 1940 of institutions and private physicians in the USA, the author's aim being to find the suicide rate in epilepsy. This was the only paper which directed its aim primarily at this problem. Most private physicians reported no suicides on their returned questionnaires, a reply that the author was sceptical of. 22 institutions reported suicides, and of these Craig Colony in New York State, which cared for severely handicapped epileptic patients, provided enough information for the author to conclude that the suicide rate for in-patients was 46 per 100 000, five times higher than the general population rate of 9.7. There were eight suicides, 1.7 being expected. The raw data for this paper are not given, the method approximate, but the result convincing.

The most convincing study found was published two years ago (White et al 1979), and reported an enquiry into the mortality of patients treated at the Chalfont Centre for Epilepsy. The study was directed to find the association between anticonvulsant drugs and malignancy, but a useful by-product was mortality from other causes. 1980 patients were followed for between 6 and 27 years, and their mortality compared with expected values derived from English life tables. Of 425 deaths, 21 were from suicide; the expected value was 3.9. This result is unassailable on grounds of method.

General hospital patients

Four papers described the mortality of those with epilepsy who had been patients at general hospitals.

Patients with paroxysms of two to five per second spike wave or polyspike wave activity investigated at Aarhus Hospital, Denmark, between 1949 and 1959 were followed up for between 4 and 16 years (Dalby 1969). They were exceptionally young, only 111 were 15 years and over. At follow-up, 10 people had died, two from suicide, the expected value being 0.2.

Another Danish study (Henriksen et al 1970) compared the mortality of patients with epilepsy with the mortality of first class lives insured with Danish life insurance companies. The sample comprised all patients discharged from four neurological clinics between 1950 and 1964 with the diagnosis of epilepsy. Patients with intracranial tumours and handicaps were excluded. The sample comprised 2763 patients who had been 'exposed to the risk of death' for more than 25 years. There were 104 deaths. 21 were from suicide, three times the seven expected, the expected value being calculated by the authors from the mortality experience of insured lives. Suicide accounted for one third of the 29 deaths unrelated to epilepsy.

Of 245 children hospitalised for epilepsy in Finland and followed up for a mean period of nine years, 18 died (Sillanpää 1973). The only suicide accounted for one of the two deaths in the under-18 group. The expected number of suicides is near to zero because the mean age of the sample was 5 years, and none were over 25 at the end of the study period.

The records of the National Insurance Office in Warsaw and patients at the neurological or psychiatric in-patient or out-patients or in long-term institutions provided 6710 epileptics. These were followed up for approximately two years (Zielinski 1974), during which time there were 218 deaths, of which 16 were from suicide with an expected of only two, a value calculated by the authors from the mortality of the Warsaw population.

Comparing the observed and expected values indicates that in this group of patients suicide is four times greater than expected.

Life insurance

The last paper (Society of Actuaries 1954) is concerned with those with epilepsy who were well enough to have been accepted for a life insurance policy. Among the 625 000 policy holders with insurable disability or disease accepted by the United States and Canadian Life Insurance Companies between 1935 and 1950 and followed up for 1 to 15 years, there were 1000 policy holders with epilepsy.

Insurable patients were aged between 30 and 64 with a history of one or more fits, the most recent being three years or longer before the insurance application. The policy holders were the subject of a report sponsored by the life insurance industry in America called the Impairment Study 1951. The group of 1000 with epilepsy had, according to the report, a significantly higher suicide rate than healthy policy holders. Their mortality was 2.5 times higher. The result is based on two deaths giving approximately four times the expected value calculated from the experience of unimpaired lives, a value which must be a good deal less than that for the general population.

We can now see by summing the observed and expected values what increased risk epilepsy has for suicide. There were 86 suicides and 16 expected, which gives an increased risk of suicide of approximately five. The highest increased risk is associated with temporal lobe epilepsy, the lowest with those accepted for life insurance.

CONCLUSION

Patients with epilepsy have about five times the risk of dying from suicide as the general population.

Acknowledgements

Mr Paul Hockney, of the National Institute for Medical Research, Mill Hill, London, conducted the literature search.

References

Currie S, Heathfield K W G, Henson R A, Scott D F 1971 Clinical course and prognosis of temporal lobe epilepsy: a survey of 666 patients. Brain 94:173–190

Dalby M A 1969 Epilepsy and 3 per second spike and wave rhythms. Acta neurologica scandinavica 45:supplement 40

Gowers W R 1901 Epilepsy and other chronic convulsive diseases, 2nd edn. J & A Churchill, London

Henriksen B, Juul-Jensen P, Lund M 1970 Mortality of epileptics. In: Brackenridge R D C (ed) Life assurance medicine. Pitman, London, p 139–148

Lindsay J, Ounsted C, Richards P 1979 Long-term outcome in children with temporal lobe seizures. 1 Social outcome and childhood factors. Developmental Medicine and Child Neurology 21:285–298

Prudhomme C 1941 Epilepsy and suicide. Journal of Nervous and Mental Disease 94:722–731

Sillanpää M 1973 Medico-social prognosis of children with epilepsy. Epidemiological study and analysis of 245 patients. Acta paediatrica scandinavica supplement 237

Society of Actuaries 1954 Impairment study 1951. Society of Actuaries, New York

Stepién L, Bidzinski J, Mazurowski W 1969 The results of surgical treatment of temporal lobe epilepsy. Polish Medical Journal 8:1184–1190

Taylor D C, Marsh S M 1977 Implications of long-term follow-up studies in epilepsy: with a note on the cause of death. In: Penry J K (ed) Epilepsy: the 8th international symposium. Raven Press, New York, p 27–34

White S J, McLean A E M, Howland C 1979 Anticonvulsant drugs and cancer (a cohort study in patients with severe epilepsy). Lancet 2:458–461

Zielinski J J 1974 Epilepsy and mortality rate and cause of death. Epilepsia 15:191–201

Personality and behavioural disorders in adults with epilepsy

INTRODUCTION

For centuries people with epilepsy have been said to be abnormal in personality. Aretaeus (Guerrent et al 1962), in the second century AD, described epileptics as 'languid, spiritless, stupid, unsociable.... slow to learn from torpidity of the understanding and of the senses [and with] utterances indistinct and bewildered either from the nature of the disease or from the wounds during the attacks.' Thus, eighteen hundred years ago not only was it asserted that people with epilepsy were of abnormal personality but also the question was raised as to whether the abnormalities were an essential part of the disease process or a consequence of it. This question still awaits a definitive answer. The thinking on this subject has shown a number of clear trends over the past hundred years. Gowers in his textbook of epilepsy published in 1881, in common with other writers of that period, suggested that patients with epilepsy underwent personality deterioration and that this was directly related to their fits. The changes were thought to be mainly intellectual in nature, and the rate of progress in direct proportion to the number or severity of the seizures. Frank psychosis was regarded as rare and the physical appearance of people with epilepsy received little attention, any alterations being considered the result of damage caused by the seizures.

At the turn of the century opinions changed and the belief that epilepsy was a constitutional disorder with specific personality changes as well as seizures became prevalent. People with epilepsy were considered to be rarely, if ever, normal mentally. Profound disturbances of mood, attitudes and behaviour followed by inevitable intellectual deterioration were the rule. The character changes were so characteristic that a diagnosis of epilepsy could be made in the absence of fits providing a family history was present. The whole syndrome was thought to have a congenital, constitutional basis rather like that of dementia praecox. The constitutional defect was also reflected in the physical characteristics of the face; an 'epileptic facies — characterised by a broad forehead, broad and flattened nose, prognathism, thick lips and staring eyes with wide pupils' (quoted from Kraepelin's textbook published in 1904). This concept evolved as a result of observations made on patients in institutions, where bromism was common and the reason for admission often disturbed behaviour. No doubt the teachings of

Kraepelin, which dominated psychiatry at that time, were highly influential. His main contribution was the description of clear-cut psychiatric syndromes such as dementia precox, genetically determined, with characteristic symptoms and a deteriorating progress to an inevitable end-state. The epileptic personality fits perfectly into this model and is described graphically in the works of Aldren Turner (1907), Kraepelin (1904), Bleuler (1924) and Pierce Clark (1931).

The development of more effective methods of neurological investigation and the consequent realisation that epilepsy is not a disease entity but a symptom of a variety of cerebral disorders, many of which may cause mental changes, led to a change in thinking about the middle of this century. Lennox (1944) reviewed the literature about the personality of epileptic patients. He commented that the majority of those he saw did not show the classical personality traits and pointed out the difficulties in distinguishing between the complex effects of heredity, brain damage, drug intoxication and the reactions to the psychological and social problems that the person with epilepsy has to face. It became recognised that many epileptic patients were well-adjusted people and that structural brain disease, chronic drug overdosage, uncontrolled seizures and the psychological problems associated with being an epileptic made a contribution to the genesis of psychiatric disorder in those who were mentally disturbed. As Lennox put it, much of the difficulty in assessing the mental state in epilepsy is due to the fact that 'the clear stream of essential epilepsy has been modified by a symptomatic tributary'. The change of climate in psychiatry with the development of a more dynamic approach may have also played an important role in this change in attitude.

In the late 1940s and early 1950s the intensive application of clinical electroencephalography to the study of the epilepsies, especially the work of Penfield and his colleagues in Montreal, led to the identification of the syndrome of temporal lobe epilepsy. Surveys of large numbers of patients with epilepsy by Gibbs and others reported an unduly high prevalence of functional psychiatric disorder in patients with temporal lobe epilepsy. The psychiatric symptomatology was not specific in any way, a wide spectrum of neurotic, psychotic and behavioural symptoms being present. In parallel with these clinical observations, the work of Papez, Maclean and others on the physiology of the limbic system and its possible role in the control of affect, the temporal lobe ablation studies of Kluver and Bucy, and the electrical stimulation studies carried out by Penfield and associates during operations for the relief of epilepsy, drew attention to the relation between temporal lobe function and emotion. No doubt these experimental observations have also had a profound influence on current thinking about psychological disorder and temporal lobe dysfunction. The view that temporal lobe dysfunction predisposes the epileptic patient to a high risk of psychiatric breakdown and personality change is currently the most popular one, though it is by no means universally accepted.

EPIDEMIOLOGICAL AND CLINICAL ASPECTS

Reliable estimates of the prevalence of personality and behaviour disorder in patients with epilepsy are difficult to obtain. Indeed, the same observation can be applied to the psychiatric morbidity of epileptics patients in general. Surveys have shown that between 4 per cent and 5 per cent of patients resident in mental hospitals have epilepsy (Liddell 1953, Betts 1974). The prevalence of chronic epilepsy in the general population can be assumed to be around 6 per 1000. Therefore the number of people with epilepsy under in-patient psychiatric care is around seven or eight times greater than the number expected by chance. Further, amongst epileptic patients living in the community, 7 per cent will have been admitted to a psychiatric hospital at some time in their lives (Pond & Bidwell 1960). The prevalence of overt psychiatric disorder in patients with seizures attending general hospital clinics or their general practitioners is surprisingly high, as many as 1 in 3; mainly conduct disorders in children and adolescents and mild affective disorders in adults (Pond & Bidwell 1960, Standage & Fenton 1975).

It is probable that the relatively high prevalence of psychiatric symptoms and conduct disorders in epileptic patients attending general hospitals reflects a tendency for patients with psychiatric complications to be referred for specialist investigation. Pond & Bidwell (1960) have shown that psychological difficulty is twice as common in patients referred to hospital by their GP than those who are not. Hence hospital-based studies will have an undue loading of subjects with psychological problems. In any event, only half of the general practice patients in the Pond & Bidwell survey were actually attending hospital for management of their seizure disorder. Hence community studies are necessary in order to obtain unbiased estimates of the distribution of psychiatric disorder in epileptics.

The findings of Rutter et al (1970) obtained by a survey of Isle of Wight schoolchildren are of special interest because of the careful sampling method and detailed psychiatric, physical and cognitive assessments carried out. The prevalence rate for psychiatric disorder in a random control group was 6.8 per cent. The rate was slightly higher (11.5 per cent) for children with physical handicaps not involving the brain, and about four times greater (28.6 per cent) for epilepsy uncomplicated by brain disease. The prevalence rates for psychiatric disorder rose to 37.5 per cent in children with lesions above the brain stem without fits. The maximum prevalence, more than eight times that of the controls, occurred in those children with epilepsy complicated by lesions above the brain stem (58.3 per cent).

Hence children with uncomplicated fits are much more likely to develop psychiatric complications than those with physical handicaps in the absence of epilepsy. Damage to the cerebral cortex and higher CNS areas further increases the risk. Factors significantly associated with psychiatric disorder were the presence of psychomotor attacks, and evidence of emotional disturbance in the mother and parental social class. Psychiatric disability was less common in children whose fathers had non-manual occupations. This study demonstrated clearly that multiple factors interact to produce psychiatric disorder in epilepsy as in other child psychiatric syndromes. Organic brain dysfunction, temporal lobe disorder as manifest by the psychomotor fits and adverse familial influences all predispose to psychiatric breakdown. The symptom cluster displayed by the epileptic children did not differ from the controls nor other patients. Antisocial and mixed neurotic/antisocial disorders were the most common.

However, when disturbed children with epilepsy are selected by EEG criteria, the site of origin of the epileptogenic process does appear to influence symptom profile. Nuffield (1961) demonstrated that children with temporal lobe spikes had high aggression and low neuroticism ratings while those with generalised spike-wave complexes showed the reverse trend, low aggression and high neurotic ratings.

Stores (1978), in a series of studies in which the behaviour of epileptic and non-epileptic children was compared, found that those with seizure disorders were significantly more anxious, inattentive, overactive and socially isolated as well as unduly dependent upon their mothers, mainly for emotional needs. However, the most important finding in these studies was that such characteristics did not apply generally. Boys with epilepsy and epileptic children of either sex with left temporal lobe abnormalities appeared to be specially vulnerable to this range of behaviour problems.

The surveys of adult epileptics are less satisfactory. Nevertheless, the study by Pond & Bidwell (1960) of epilepsy patients of 14 general practices specially selected to be representative of the population of the country (England and Wales) as a whole is worthy of note. 245 epileptic patients were identified. Nearly 1/3 (29 per cent) had psychiatric problems, mainly neuroses in adults and conduct disorders in children. Only 4 per cent showed features of the 'epileptic' personality. 7 per cent of the total sample had been patients in psychiatric hospitals; half of the latter having temporal lobe epilepsy. In fact, temporal lobe epilepsy, low intelligence and adverse environmental difficulties were the factors which seemed to predispose to psychiatric breakdown, especially behaviour and personality disorders. As in children, no specific symptom profiles could be identified.

These findings in both children and adults confirm the clinical impression that in epilepsy the phenomenology of the psychiatric syndrome the person presents with is essentially similar to that seen in non-epileptic patients. The clinical features the patient develops are also strongly influenced by the age of the subject. Children and adolescents tend to present with behaviour difficulties; usually antisocial or mixed antisocial/neurotic disorder. In contrast, adults tend to develop affective symptoms. This is especially so in those patients with late onset epilepsy. Personality disorder, unless a direct result of a focal brain lesion, is usually a reflection of a life-long disturbance with early onset of fits and a history of maladjustment with behaviour and/or neurotic problems during childhood and adolescence. The diagnosis of personality disorder can not be made with confidence until the early 20s since the time scale of the process of personality maturation must be allowed for. Hence personality disorder exclusively applies to adult patients.

Epilepsy and personality disorder

Amongst the prejudices which have surrounded epilepsy and coloured public attitudes towards the disorder is the concept that people share specific personality characteristics.

Descriptions of traits specific to the 'epileptic personality' include the adjectives 'pedantic', 'circumstantial', 'religiose', 'egocentric', 'suspicious', 'touchy' and 'quarrelsome'. Their speech is slow and perseverative and their thought processes stereotyped and concrete. In both thought and emotions, they were described as 'adhesive', 'sticky' or 'viscous'.

It does appear that a small number of epileptic patients, usually with a chronic disorder and sometimes institutionalised for many years, do display many of these traits (4 per cent in Pond & Bidwell's general practice survey). However their development almost certainly results from multiple handicaps, both personal and environmental. Brain damage, childhood deprivation, the chronic effects of heavy anticonvulsant therapy, and difficulties with schooling, employment, accommodation and interpersonal relationships may all contribute.

Assessment of personality disorders associated with epilepsy presents considerable methodological problems (Tizard 1962). First, there are selection factors; observations made on patients in institutions do not generalise to patients in the community. Secondly, allowance has to be made for the different types of epilepsy and for the presence, location and extent of brain lesions or damage. Tizard points out that most studies in which personality tests have been employed have not taken into consideration the intelligence of the patients or possible effects of medication. Like most recent authors (Betts et al 1976, Lishman 1978, Scott 1978a) she concludes that there is no specific personality disorder associated with epilepsy.

Apart from the observations of Pond & Bidwell (1960) on epileptic personality traits in epileptic patients living in the community, the prevalence of personality problems in people with epilepsy living in the community is unknown. As one would predict, personality difficulties are common in patients presenting at specialised epilepsy clinics and psychiatric units. For example, of 80 consecutive admissions to the Maudsley Hospital with epilepsy and psychiatric disorder, 60 per cent had a primary diagnosis of personality disorder. Though no specific category of abnormal personality predominated, immature and passive dependent traits were common. Clearly such a high prevalence of personality disorder reflects the specialised nature of the hospital. Also it is not known whether the categories of abnormal personality amongst the epileptic group differ from those of non-epileptic patients referred to the same hospital.

The hypothesis by Gibbs (1951), Gastaut (1954) and others that behaviour and personality disorder in epilepsy can be related to the presence of long-standing seizure discharge in the mesial temporal lobe/limbic structures has led to the view that a specific temporal lobe syndrome exists. The concept of a temporal lobe syndrome has been argued persuasively by Geschwind (1978), Blumer (1977), Bear & Fedio (1977) and others. According to this view, the syndrome consists of an excessive tendency to adhere to each thought, feeling and action (hypometamorphosis or viscosity); irritability and deepened emotionality (hyperemotionality); decreased sexual interest and arousal (hyposexuality). It is considered that this syndrome represents the opposite of the Kluver-Bucy syndrome. In the latter syndrome, bilateral temporal lobe ablation causes hypermetamorphosis, hypoemotionality and hypersexuality. Bear & Fedio (1977) have developed a questionnaire to rate 18 personality traits in patients with epilepsy. These were selected from descriptions of the personality and behaviour of epileptic patients published in the literature, though a few were used following pilot testing by the authors themselves. The traits were assessed in two equivalent questionnaires, one of which the subject answered about himself and the second completed about the subject by a close observer. The questions were answered on a 'true'/'false' basis. Each trait was sampled by five items composed by the two investigators and judged representative by three additional professionals. In addition to these 90 trait-derived items, 10 questions were modified from the lie scale of the MMPI. Two equivalent 100 item questionnaires were employed: a personal inventory that the subject completed about himself, and a personal behaviour survey, consisting of third-person versions of the same items that a long-time observer completed about the subject. The items were presented in random order, within the self-inventory, but grouped by trait for the rater survey. Each block of questions, in the latter, was introduced by a neutral description of the trait.

The authors found that compared to normal controls and patients with chronic neuromuscular disorders, the temporal lobe epileptic patients displayed a distinctive pattern of traits, namely humourless sobriety, dependence, circumstantiality, obsessionality, undue preoccupation with religious and philosophic concerns, emotionality and irritability. Bear & Fedio point out that there is now extensive evidence that destructive lesions within the temporal lobe of primates may act to disconnect emotion-mediating limbic structures such as the amygdaloid complex and hippocampus from the sensory association cortices of the visual and auditory system, resulting in the loss of learned emotional associations (Geschwind 1965). Surgical disconnection appears both to disrupt old emotional bonds and to inhibit formation of new stimulus-reinforcement (or sensory-limbic) linkages (Jones & Mishkin 1972). The authors speculate that in temporal lobe epilepsies, similar limbic system structures and adjacent cortex are electrically stimulated by the epileptic focus. This leads to enhanced affective association with previously neutral stimuli, events or concepts. Thus experiencing objects and events with an unduly intense affective colouring engenders a mystically religious view of the world. If the patient's immediate actions and thoughts are so coloured, the result is an augmented sense of personal destiny. Sensing emotional importance in even the smallest acts may lead to these being performed ritualistically and repetitively, with lengthy circumstantial speech or writing.

Further, Bear & Fedio showed that right temporal lobe patients differed from those with left-sided foci in displaying externally or overtly emotive traits such as periods of sadness, irritability, elation, emotionality, etc. In contrast, the left temporal lobe patients had a pattern of internal ideational (verbal) traits, for example a ruminative intellectual tendency, religiosity, philosophical interests and an augmented sense of personal destiny. Bear & Fedio tentatively interpret these results to mean that each hemisphere utilises its own characteristic style of cognitive processing in the development of limbic-sensory associations; the right hemisphere utilising non-verbal reactions (emotive, impulsive and dispositional), while the left hemisphere showed a predeliction for ideational, contemplative and perhaps verbal expressions of affect. Finally, the right temporal lobe patients tended to exaggerate socially acceptable traits and deny undesirable traits; the left temporal patients in contrast showed exactly the opposite pattern, tending to over-report traits that showed them up in a bad light. The authors again speculate that these contrasting styles of self-reporting reflect specialized right and left hemisphere modes of cognitive processing.

Though the patients were drawn from five general epilepsy clinics, the numbers in each sample were small (a total of 48 patients). The controls were healthy adults or patients with neuromuscular diseases. Epileptic patients without temporal lobe involvement were not studied. Hence their claim that these behavioural profiles are a specific feature of temporal lobe epilepsy is not valid. Indeed, the concept of a specific temporal lobe syndrome faces the same methodological problems as the 'epileptic personality'. The association with temporal lobe epilepsy may be a consequence of sample bias and lack of regard for the validity and reliability of behavioural assessment.

Nevertheless, I think that Geschwind's comments are very valid. He points out that research on the effects of temporal lobe epilepsy and behaviour have been held up by asking the wrong questions. We have kept putting the question 'What are the behaviour disorders associated with temporal lobe epilepsy?'. He feels that the proper question is 'What are the behavioural changes produced by temporal lobe epilepsy?'. He feels that we should beware of describing the behavioural changes by means of the standard nomenclature and classification of other psychiatric conditions. We should treat the behaviour change in temporal lobe epilepsy as a phenomenon in its own right. It is probably not valid to compare the mechanism of a disease of unknown pathophysiology to others of different or unknown pathophysiology. Certainly the quantitative approach introduced by Bear & Fedio to the study of behavioural profiles in epilepsy is a very interesting one. Providing the test-retest and inter-rater reliability of their questionnaires can be established, they could be readily applied to large numbers of patients identified during community prevalence surveys. The epidemiological approach is the only one capable of resolving the dispute over the relationship between temporal lobe epilepsy and behaviour, since it is only by total population surveys that one can get round the problem of sample bias introduced by studying hospital populations.

Aggression and epilepsy

The possibility that dangerous violence can occur during a period of epileptic automatism has been known for many years. Delasiauve (1854) in his textbook on epilepsy devoted a chapter to the legal responsibility of the epileptic and cited a number of instances in which an individual had committed a crime of violence during or after an attack. Maudsley (1874) stated: "Whenever we meet with isolated acts of violence, outrages on persons, homicide, suicide, arson, which nothing seems to have instigated, and when, upon attentive examination and thorough enquiry, we find a loss of memory after the perpetration of the act with a periodicity in the recurrence of the same act, and, a brief duration, we may diagnose 'larval' epilepsy." Nevertheless violent behaviour in relation to seizures is rare, the evidence in favour of such an association being confined to occasional case reports (Gunn 1979; Chapter 13).

Knox (1968), in the first systematic study of the relationship between epileptic automatism and violence, found only one patient who had acted in an extremely aggressive and violent fashion during an epileptic automatism out of a total of 434 epileptic out-patients. Surveys of more deviant populations have confirmed these findings. Although a survey of epileptic offenders in prisons and borstal institutions in England and Wales has indicated that the prevalence of epilepsy in these institutions is significantly higher than in the general population, there were only two persons out of a total of 158 whose crime was probably committed during or following a seizure: one during the postictal phase and the other in a possible ictal automatism. A parallel electroclinical study of the epileptic population of Broadmoor Hospital, one of the special hospitals in England and Wales for psychiatric offenders and patients displaying dangerously antisocial behaviour, revealed a prevalence of epilepsy similar to that of a conventional mental hospital. Of the 29 male patients who had committed offences, in only two could a definite relationship be established between their crimes and the occurrence of seizures: both behaved violently during a postictal confusional state (Gunn 1979, Gunn & Fenton 1969, 1971).

Explosive aggressiveness, moodiness and irritability unrelated in time to the occurrence of fits have long been considered features of the 'epileptic' personality. During the last few decades, interictal aggressive behaviour has come to be regarded as a specific manifestation of temporal lobe epilepsy. The published studies on the relation between aggression and temporal lobe epilepsy have used a variety of definitions. Some authors have restricted their attention to outright physical assault, while others have included verbal abuse, bullying, stubbornness and assertiveness.

Kligman & Goldberg (1975) have carried out a comprehensive review of the possible connections between temporal lobe epilepsy (TLE) and aggression. They critically reviewed the eight published controlled studies. All the studies were open to question because of sampling bias and only two produced definite evidence of a positive association between TLE and aggression. Only the study by Nuffield (1961) on children was regarded as being methodologically sound. Though this study did offer some support for the association in children, Kligman & Goldberg feel that it will be necessary to have Nuffield's study replicated and applied to adults before a conclusion can be reached. They conclude that TLE is too heterogeneous and ill-defined and human aggression too complex to allow definite interpretations of correlations between them at present.

Aggressiveness has been a not uncommon finding in those temporal lobe patients referred for anterior temporal lobectomy. About 1/3 of a large series of TLE patients operated on by Mr Murray Falconer were noted to have displayed overtly aggressive behaviour (Serafetinides 1965, Falconer 1973). This behaviour was much more common in males, especially those in their teens. It tended to be associated with left-sided lesions, a pathological diagnosis of mesial temporal sclerosis and a favourable outcome in terms of successful rehabilitation after the operation and a cessation of fits.

It may well be that temporal lobe epileptic patients with drug-resistant fits complicated by aggressive behaviour are more likely to be referred and selected for surgical treatment because the presence of the aggressiveness undoubtedly causes greater management and social adjustment problems. Indeed comparison of temporal lobe epileptic patients treated medically with those treated surgically indicates that the latter have an early age of onset (the majority within the first 15 years) and a much higher prevalence of disturbances of personality and behaviour

(Currie et al 1971). This early age of onset within the first decade of life tends to be associated with mesial temporal sclerosis (MTS) and may account for the relation between TLE, aggression and MTS in the surgically treated patients.

As discussed previously, the occurrence of frequent fits throughout childhood may have adverse effects on parental and peer group attitudes, the processes of social learning and personality maturation. A cluster of other environmental factors that may produce a coincidental correlation between TLE and aggression by leading to a high incidence of both in the same people include low socio-economic status, parental psychopathology and child abuse. Antisocial children are more likely to have a low socio-economic background than neurotic children. The same background may expose children to poor parental and medical care with greater risks of acquiring brain damage due to poor obstetric care, head injuries due to parental neglect or abuse and infections which may provoke febrile convulsions and consequent mesial temporal lobe sclerosis. Unfortunately, little attention has been paid to controlling for socio-economic status in many of the studies on TLE and aggression. Indeed such criticisms can be applied to most investigations of the relation between epilepsy and behaviour.

Sexual dysfunction in epilepsy
The same problems arise in the relationship between sexual behaviour and temporal lobe epilepsy as exist between TLE and aggression. This subject is reviewed by Scott (1978b). There is no doubt that partial seizures with a focal onset on the medial surface of a hemisphere in the central region can have contralateral genital sensations as part of the initial seizure phenomena. The patient's behaviour both during and after epileptic automatism may simulate rather crudely sexual behaviour (Currier et al 1971, Hooshmand & Brawley 1969). Hooshmand & Brawley described three patients who showed exhibitionist behaviour as a result of undressing during epileptic automatisms. In at least one patient (Hoenig & Hamilton 1960) with temporal lobe epilepsy, partial seizures were triggered by orgasm. Occasionally seizures occur early during coitus and terminate the act, usually occurring in the female partner. In such cases their occurrence seems to reflect difficulties in the relationship between the two partners (Scott 1978b). The temporal lobe has been implicated in those cases where an association between sexual deviation and epilepsy has been reported. Fetishism and transvestism have been described. The abnormal sexual behaviour in both cases was abolished by successful temporal lobectomy. The case of fetishism is particularly interesting, being a 38 year old man who derived sexual satisfaction from staring at a safety pin, following which activity he would have a partial seizure. An active left temporal lobe focus was seen in the EEG and an attack, while viewing a safety pin, was monitored. A temporal lobectomy was performed and this resulted in control of both his seizures and his fetish. In the second patient transvestism was abolished following operation. It is tempting to speculate a relationship between the sexual abnormalities and limbic system dysfunction although it is difficult to draw any firm conclusions from such a small number of patients. In any event temporal lobe dysfunction is rare among sexual deviants.

Much more common in patients with epilepsy are complaints of reduced libido and impotence. As with other associations between epilepsy and behaviour, the relationships are complex. In many cases, the poor sexual skills are a reflection of poor social skills in persons of immature and dependent personality. However, there is no doubt that the chronic effects of anticonvulsant medication play an important role. Toone et al (1980) have recently carried out a pilot study of the relationship between sexual function, sex hormone levels and medication. Estimates of free testosterone circulating in the serum were low in a group of chronic epileptic patients. There was a positive correlation between low free testosterone levels and increased serum gamma-glutamic-transaminase concentrations. The latter is a measure of increased liver enzyme induction. Hence it would seem that the chronic medication leads to rapid metabolism of testosterone by liver enzymes induced by anticonvulsant drug action. Further, a low serum-free testosterone level correlated with ratings of low sex drive and activity. If these findings are replicated in a larger series of patients, the case for sex hormone replacement therapy in patients on chronic anticonvulsant medication will have to be considered. Whether the reduced sex drive and impotence can also be related to limbic system dysfunction in patients with temporal lobe epilepsy, as is often claimed, remains an open question and awaits further controlled studies of less biased samples of patients.

PATHOGENESIS OF PERSONALITY AND BEHAVIOUR DISORDER IN PATIENTS WITH EPILEPSY

As discussed above, epilepsy with onset in early childhood and frequent fits throughout the growing-up period is quite likely to have adverse effects on parental and peer group attitudes, the learning of social skills and academic achievement and to put severe restrictions on the patient's activities and life-style. These influences may interfere with personality maturation and the development of personal competence. Taylor (1972) presents an interesting model to explain the effect of seizures on the various stages of personality maturation based on a modified version of Erikson's schematic view of personality development.

These factors are likely to be further aggravated by the existence of parental psychopathology and poor socio-economic conditions, which indeed may have created the milieu for the development of both the epilepsy and behaviour problems. It has been demonstrated clearly by Gruneberg & Pond (1957) and Rutter et al (1970) that adverse family and environmental factors play a major role in the genesis of psychiatric disorder in epileptic children.

Temporal lobe dysfunction acquired at an early age is likely to have a particularly serious effect on personality development because of the role of the temporal lobes in the processes of learning, memory and ego development. Early, acquired diffuse cortical damage will have similar adverse effects on the individual's potential for personal growth. As well as its influence on general intelligence and learning capacity, the irritability, impulsiveness and psycho-motor slowing associated with diffuse loss of cortical neurones will accentuate the difficulties.

The depressant effects of anticonvulsant drugs on cognitive function and emotional control are a further complication in both patients with and without acquired cerebral lesions. In particular, phenobarbitone may have a paradoxical exciting effect with a consequent increase in irritability and hyperkinetic behaviour. Phenytoin-induced hirsuitism and soft tissue hypertrophy are special problems for the female patient.

Increased fit frequency often leads to a temporary exacerbation of the behaviour difficulties. The increase in seizure activity presumably causes a global disruption of cortical function with consequent disinhibition of behaviour. An inverse relation between behaviour and fits is rare, except as a reflection of an adverse reaction to medication. The influence of seizure pattern on psychiatric morbidity has not been examined in detail. In common sense terms, the experience of complex, frightening auras might be expected to arouse anxiety. Frequent major convulsions with threat to life and limb will lead to greater restriction of activity and dislocation of social and vocational opportunities. The potential risk of loss of consciousness and self-control during automatisms would seem to be an especially potent threat on the individual's wellbeing. Yet, one's clinical impression is that such factors do not play a significant role in the onset of psychiatric morbidity.

Finally, the potentially precarious adjustment of the person with epilepsy may be undermined by difficulties in obtaining work because of the inevitable restrictions of choice applied due to having fits, often reinforced by the prejudices of both employers and employees. The inability to have a driving licence is particularly frustrating for the male adolescent, who sees his friends happily riding motor-cycles at the age of 16 years. The loss of a licence in an adult with late onset epilepsy may also have serious consequences both in terms of employment prospects and leisure pursuits.

Personality difficulties acquired by having epilepsy, especially the dependency, general lack of social skills and low self-esteem, combined with parental overprotectiveness and popular prejudice, will cause problems in finding friends of both sexes as well as work. This, in turn, will lead to social isolation, feelings of rejection, frustration and despondency.

Hence, the personality and behaviour difficulties in people with epilepsy are caused by an interaction of many factors, both organic, psychological and social. The relative importance of any particular causative factor will vary from individual to individual. It is a general rule that the early onset of epilepsy in the developing child especially in the presence of either temporal lobe dysfunction or diffuse cortical damage is particularly likely to result in psychiatric morbidity; conduct disorder being the most common manifestation. In the adult, where the personality maturation is complete and the person's life style stable, the onset of fits has less serious psychological consequences and the prospects of successful adjustment are much better. In this situation, personality change or behaviour disorder is rarely seen, unless as the result of focal brain disease causing the fits or overmedication. Nevertheless mild depressive or anxiety symptoms with lowered self-esteem are common, though no more so than in other chronic illnesses. It would seem that these affective symptoms are a response to the stresses induced by living with a chronic illness and its social consequences, possibly complicated in some people by the effects of long-term drug treatment on mental or bodily function.

MANAGEMENT

It is necessary to establish the type of epilepsy (whether generalized, partial or unclassifiable) and to attempt to identify the nature of the underlying pathology, if any. This requires careful history taking, clinical, EEG and radiological investigation. The efficacy of the anticonvulsant medication must also be assessed and careful enquiry for toxic effects conducted. Serum vitamin B_{12} and folate estimations need to be done as well as a full blood picture, in order to exclude a drug-induced megaloblastic change. Similarly serum calcium and alkaline phosphatase levels should be checked because of the risk of anticonvulsant-induced osteomalacia. Serum anticonvulsant concentrations require to be measured, to make sure that the levels are not toxic on the one hand nor below the therapeutic range on the other.

A conventional psychiatric diagnostic formulation must be carried out. This will include diagnosis of the presenting psychiatric syndrome and an evaluation of the relative importance of genetic, organic, environmental, personality factors and current situational problems in the genesis of the behaviour and personality difficulties. The respective aetiological roles of the following epileptic variables must be considered:

1. the influence of the underlying epileptogenic lesion on the patient's cognitive function, behaviour and emotional state because of its extent (diffuse), location (temporal lobe) or occurrence of frequent subclinical seizure discharges.

2. the relation between seizure type and frequency (increased/decreased) and mental state disturbance.

3. the respective effects of the medication on the individual's behaviour, mental processes, neurological, metabolic and haematological status.

4. the effects of having fits and being labelled epileptic on the person's emotional development, acquisition of social, academic and vocational skills. The impact of all these personal and social factors on the development of the individual's social competence and capacity to cope with current life events should be evaluated. The person's individual style of reacting to the problems of living with a chronic handicap should also be noted e.g. the use of the sick role, aggressive acting out behaviour etc.

After the neuropsychiatric assessment is complete, a satisfactory anticonvulsant drug regime should be established, care being taken not to further impair the patient's level of functioning by overmedication with consequent psychomotor slowing, lack of alertness, ataxia and perhaps irritability. Hence phenobarbitone should be avoided. Polytherapy with the prescription of multiple drugs must also be avoided, not more than two anticonvulsant drugs, preferably one, with adequate serum levels being used at any one time. If necessary, the drug treatment should be adjusted by gradual withdrawal of the unnecessary extra drugs. This more careful use of drugs will reduce the risk of toxic effects, drug interactions, improve compliance and often the patient's level of alertness and behaviour (Chapter 23).

The management of the mental state and behaviour follows the same principles applied to psychiatric patients without fits. A psychotherapeutic approach is necessary. During the initial few interviews devoted to detailed history taking, rapport will be established with the patient. This will facilitate the processes of clarification and non-directive discussion of the patient's symptoms, emotional difficulties, current life problems and their interrelationship. Providing the patient's intelligence level is appropriate and motivation for self-examination present, the exploratory psychotherapy can progress to an in-depth examination of the psychological meaning for the patient of the illness and the person's habitual defence mechanisms against anxiety. Such an approach will tend to focus on an examination between therapist and patient and how this reflects relationships in his formative years and problems in his current life. The number of sessions of such focal psychotherapy will depend on the amount of available therapeutic time and the therapist's assessment of the patient's capacity to benefit. The aggressive patient will often benefit by active encouragement to verbalize his aggressive feelings as an alternative to 'acting' them out. Such a process may be facilitated, in suitable patients, by role play methods. If this dynamic approach is inappropriate, a more supportive psychotherapeutic role is likely to help by permitting abreaction, reducing emotional distress, providing encouragement and guidance, support of the necessary neurotic defences and manipulations of the current life situation. In the adolescent or child with behaviour problems associated with epilepsy, work with the parents will be necessary. This will include simple explanation, provision of support, encouragement to ventilate anxiety and other feelings about the patient and his behaviour, discussion and exploration of parental attitudes towards the epilepsy and attempts at modification of those that are abnormal such as overprotectiveness, unduly high or low expectations of the patient's academic or vocational achievement, etc. Family or marital psychotherapy may occasionally be indicated if serious family or marital problems are evident. It should be stressed that the selection criteria for admission to psychotherapy of the person with epilepsy should not differ from those applied to nonepileptic patients with neurotic, personality or psychosomatic disorders.

Because of their very socially restricted and overprotected upbringing, many young people with epilepsy are grossly deficient not only in social skills but also in the basic skills of looking after themselves, e.g. basic cooking, washing clothes, shopping and the general aspects of self-care necessary for an independent existence. A ward milieu and occupational therapy programme to improve basic self-care skills and capacity for social interaction can do much to enhance the person's self-esteem and ability to function independently. Formal social skills training can also be helpful. Participation in a ward or out-patient group can help those with deficient interpersonal skills. Such group involvement may be encouraged by participation in the local Action for Epilepsy branch organised by the British Epilepsy Association, a voluntary organisation devoted to the welfare of people with epilepsy and their relatives. Active involvement in the local activities of the association will provide a source of advice and guidance about the problems of living with epilepsy, cater for the needs of those who are socially isolated and add to the restricted range of their leisure activities. For some, it will provide the setting for the development of hidden talents in organisation, administration, persuasion and in the practice of various types of handicraft.

Concerning vocational guidance and occupational rehabilitation, collaboration between the social worker and Disablement Resettlement Officer is vital. Skilled counselling may help someone with epilepsy who is looking for a job to take a realistic view of his prospects and to present his disability to a prospective employer in an acceptable way. Admission for assessment to an industrial rehabilitation unit can be arranged with consequent training in a skilled occupation in suitable cases at a Government Training Centre or residential training college. People with epilepsy should be encouraged to enter skilled trades and professions. Such skills, as well as making them more viable in the open employment market, will help to dispel some of the stigma which attaches to people with the disease by associating them only with poorly paid or unskilled work.

One hiatus in the system exists between the protected atmosphere of home or school, in which an adolescent with epilepsy may grow up and socially mature, and the vocational and industrial rehabilitation services which are intended to prepare for employment of people who have already achieved social maturity. There is a need for much more hostel and other residential accommodation where the immature, dependent person with epilepsy can be encouraged to develop independent attitudes under a degree of supervision which can be tailored to meet his needs.

If significant depressive symptoms are present, antidepressant drug therapy should be given. Nomifensine, 50 to 150 mg daily, is the drug of choice as it does not alter seizure threshold. Should anxiety symptoms be troublesome, the benzodiazepine group, especially diazepam, is useful; particularly because of their anticonvulsant action. However, care must be taken to make sure that the benzodiazepine drugs do not increase irritability or aggressiveness as sometimes happens. For seriously aggressive behaviour haloperidol or phenothiazine drugs in appropriate doses can be used. The potentially epileptogenic action of the latter drugs can be avoided by the addition of a small dose of diazepam, if necessary, or readjustment of the anticonvulsant regime. This is rarely a problem.

Finally, unilateral anterior temporal lobectomy is indicated in young patients with intractible partial epilepsy due to a unilateral temporal lobe lesion (usually mesial temporal sclerosis), and seriously aggressive behaviour. Providing the seizures are controlled following the surgery, there is a high probability that the behaviour will also improve.

The sexual dysfunctions in epileptic patients require independent assessement. The adverse effects of overmedication must be considered and, if present, dealt with by readjustment of drug dosage. Sex hormone serum assays need to be carried out and any deficiency in hormone concentration corrected. After such organic factors are excluded or treated, a behavioural approach using the Masters and Johnson technique is worth trying. This may have to be followed by formal social skills training, if there is evidence of lack of social as well as sexual skills.

References

Bear D, Fedio P 1977 Quantitative analysis of interictal behaviour in temporal lobe epilepsy. Archives of Neurology 34:454–467

Betts T A 1974 A follow-up study of a cohort of patients with epilepsy admitted to psychiatric care in an English city. In: Harris P, Mawdsley, C (eds) Epilepsy: proceedings of the Hans Berger centenary symposium. Churchill Livingstone, Edinburgh, 326–333

Betts T A, Merskey H, Pond D A 1976 Psychiatry. In: Laidlaw J, Richens A (eds) A textbook of epilepsy. Churchill Livingstone, Edinburgh

Bleuler E 1924 Textbook of psychiatry (translated by Brill A A). Macmillan, New York Reissued by Dover Publications 1951

Blumer D 1977 Treatment of patients with seizure disorder referred because of psychiatric complications. In: Blumer D, Levin K (eds) Psychiatric complication in the epilepsies: current research and treatment. McLean Hospital Journal, special issue, p. 53–73

Clark L P 1931 The psychobiologic concept of epilepsy. In: Epilepsy and the convulsive state, Vol 2. Association for research in nervous and mental disease, Williams and Wilkins, Baltimore

Currie S, Heathfield K W C, Henson R A, Scott D F 1971 Clinical course and prognosis of temporal lobe epilepsy. Brain 94:173–190

Currier R D, Jackson M, Little S C, Suess J F, Andy O J 1971 Sexual seizures. Archives of Neurology 25:260–264

Delasiauve L J F 1854 Traité de l'épilepsie: histoire: traitement: médecine légale. Masson, Paris

Falconer M A 1973 Reversibility by temporal lobe resection of the behavioural abnormalities of temporal lobe epilepsy. New England Journal of Medicine 289:451–455

Gastaut H 1954 Interpretation des symptomes de l'épilepsie 'psychomotrice' en fonction des données de la physiologie rhinencephalique. Presse Medicale 62:1535–1537

Geschwind N 1965 Disconnexion syndromes in animals and man. Brain 88:237–294

Geschwind N 1978 Behavioural changes in temporal lobe epilepsy. Psychol. Med. 9:217–219

Gibbs F A 1951 Ictal and non-ictal psychiatric disorders in temporal lobe epilepsy. Journal of Nervous and Mental Diseases 11:522–528

Grunberg F, Pond D A 1957 Conduct disorders in epileptic children. Journal of Neurology, Neurosurgery and Psychiatry 20:65–68

Guerrant J, Anderson W W, Fischer A, Weinstein M R, Jaros R M, Deskins A 1962 Personality in epilepsy. Thomas, Springfield, Illinois

Gunn J 1979 Forensic psychiatry. In: Granville-Grossman K (ed) Recent advances in clinical psychiatry. Churchill Livingstone, Edinburgh

Gunn J, Fenton G W 1969 Epilepsy in prisons: a diagnostic survey. Br. med J 4:326–328

Gunn J, Fenton G W 1971 Epilepsy, automatism and crime. Lancet 1:1173–1176

Hoenig J, Hamilton C 1960 Epilepsy and sexual orgasm. Acta psychiatrica et neurologica scandinavica 35:448–457

Hooshmand J, Brawley B W 1969 Temporal lobe seizures and exhibitionism. Neurol 19:1119–24

Jones B, Mishkin M 1972 Limbic lesions and the problems of stimulus-reinforcement associations. Experimental Neurology 36:362–377

Kligman D, Goldberg D A 1975 Temporal lobe epilepsy and aggression. Journal of Nervous and Mental Disease 160:324–341

Knox S J 1968 Epileptic automatisms and violence. Medicine, Science and the Law 8:96–104

Kraepelin E 1904 Lectures on clinical psychiatry (trans. Johnstone T). W Wood, New York

Lennox W G 1944 Epilepsy. In: Hunt J (ed) Handbook of personality and behaviour problems. Ronald Press, New York

Liddell D W 1953 Observations on epileptic automation in a mental hospital population. Journal of Mental Science 99:732–748

Lishman W A 1978 Organic psychiatry. Blackwell Scientific Publications, Oxford

Maudsley H 1974 Responsibility in mental disease. Appleton, New York

Nuffield E J A 1961 Neurophysiology and behaviour disorders in epileptic children. Journal of Mental Science 107:438–458

Pond D A, Bidwell B H 1960 A survey of epilepsy in 14 general practices. II Social and psychological aspects. Epilepsia 1:285–299

Rutter M, Graham P J, Yule W 1970 A neuropsychiatric study in childhood. Clinics in Developmental Medicine, Heinemann, London

Scott D F 1978a Psychiatric aspects of epilepsy. British Journal of Psychiatry. 132:417–430

Scott D F 1978b Psychiatric aspects of sexual medicine. In: Epilepsy '78. British Epilepsy Association, Workingham, England

Serafetinides E A 1965 Aggressiveness in temporal lobe epileptics. Epilepsia 6:33–42

Stores G 1978 School children with epilepsy at risk for learning and behaviour problems. Developmental Medicine and Child Neurology 20:502–508

Standage K F, Fenton G W 1975 Psychiatric symptom profiles of patients with epilepsy. Psychological Medicine 15:152–160

Stevens J F 1966 Psychiatric implications of temporal lobe epilepsy. Archives of General Psychiatry 14:461–471

Taylor D C 1972 Psychiatry and sociology in the understanding of epilepsy. In: Mandelbrote, B M, Gelder M G (eds) Psychiatric aspects of medical practice. Staples Press, London

Tizard B 1962 The personality of epileptics. Psychological Bulletin 59:196–210

Toone B K, Wheeler M, Fenwick P B C 1980 Sex hormone changes in male epileptics. Clin. Endocrinol. 12:391–395

Turner W A 1907 Epilepsy—a study of the idiopathic disease. Macmillan & Co., London

Hysteria and other non-epileptic convulsions

"Note that an epileptic, lunatic and demoniac have certain things in common, as Constantine says, *Practica* Book 9, Chapter 5 'On Epilepsy'. Therefore to discern whether the one who falls to the ground be a lunatic or an epileptic, make this test. Utter these words into the ear of the suspect: 'Depart demon, and go forth, because Effimolei commands thee.' If he be a lunatic or a demoniac, he immediately becomes [?]dead, for nearly an hour. When he arises ask him any question whatever, and he will give the answer. If he does not fall when he hears these words, then you know that he is an epileptic." (Lennox 1939)

Hysteria, as everybody knows, has a long history, with original descriptions going back to the Egyptian *Kahun papyrus*. In this text a variety of behaviour disorders are listed under the heading of 'Disorders of the Uterus', and from that time it has been suggested that there exists a group of disorders with diverse symptoms which are associated with the generative organs (Veith 1965). These ideas found their way into the Greek literature where the term 'hysteria' was first applied in the Hippocratic writings, and when a number of techniques were devised for the correct replacement of an errant womb. The association between convulsions and hysteria was recognised at this time, in particular by Hippocrates who stated in *Diseases of women*: "If a woman suddenly becomes voiceless you will find her legs cold, as well as the knees and the hands. And if you then palpate the uterus, it is not in the proper place; her heart palpitates, she gnashes her teeth, there is copious sweat, and all the other features characteristic of those who suffer from the 'sacred disease', and they do all sorts of unheard-of things" (Simon 1978).

Aretaeus classified epilepsy into two varieties, the ordinary and the hysterical. The latter was due to movement of the uterus, which he compared to an animal on account of its ability to move around of its own accord. His recommended treatment was logical, suggesting that foetid-smelling substances or old urine were given which would drive the uterus downwards, at the same time fragrant oils being rubbed into the female genitalia in order to attract the uterus back to its correct position (Whitwell 1936).

The first person to suggest that the uterus was not the seat of hysteria was probably Willis. Not only did he suggest that the brain was the organ most likely to be involved, he also discussed the origin of hysterical fits: 'The distemper named from the womb is chiefly and primarily convulsive, and chiefly depends on the brain and the nervous stock being affected . . .' Hysterical fits were caused by 'spirits inhabiting the brain, being now prepared for explosions.' (Willis 1684).

He suggested that men also could be subject to hysterical illness, and following post-mortem examinations in which patients who had suffered from hysteria were shown to have an intact uterus he concluded: 'Having weighed these and other reasons, we doubt not to assert the passions, commonly called hysterical, to arise most often for that the animal spirits possessing the beginning of the nerves within the head are infected with some taint.' Since, in further studies, he came to the conclusion that it was the animal spirits in the middle part of the brain which were finally disturbed in epilepsy, it seems that for Willis both epileptic and non-epileptic convulsions had a similar neuropathological basis (Brain 1963).

The association between hysteria and epilepsy continued throughout the 18th and 19th centuries. Boerhaave and Swieten both felt that hysteria could degenerate into epilepsy (Tempkin 1971), and Cheyne, in his book *The English Malady or a Treatise of Nervous Diseases of all kinds as Spleen, Vapours, Lowness of Spirits, Hypochondriacal and Hysterical Distempers* noted few differences between epilepsy and hysteria, saying that the former 'differs very little or not at all, or at most in a few circumstances only, from Hypochondrical and Hysteric Fits: which last, when violent, terminate always in these Epileptick Fits, as they, on the other hand, when they become weak, dwindle into the Hysterick Kind. (Cheyne 1733).

The mid- and late-19th century saw a further blending of these phenomena with the introduction by the French physicians of the term 'hystero-epilepsy'. This implied an association of the two disorders, and while most accepted that there were *accès-distincts*, where a clear differential diagnosis between an epileptic attack and a hysterical seizure was possible, others claimed the existence of *accès-complexes* in which both epileptic and hysterical symptoms were combined so as to make a distinction between these two impossible (Tempkin 1971). At the same time the concept of epilepsy was expanded to include a wide range of clinical phenomena. Todd used the word 'epileptiform' to describe fits in which consciousness was not impaired, and in which unilateral convulsive movements were noted, which may 'pass into the true epileptic fit' (Todd 1856). A number of authors recognised behavioural changes associated with epilepsy, especially acute changes. Griesinger introduced the term 'psychomotor' to refer to symptoms in 'epileptoid' conditions, and Hughlings Jackson discussed at length the associated phenomena of epilepsy which led him to his broad definition that it was 'an occasional, sudden, excessive, rapid and local discharge of grey matter'. There were for him many epilepsies, as opposed to one discrete disease, and the borderlands involved 'all conditions in which there is a transient impairment of voluntary motor power, sensation or consciousness' including migraine and the sneeze.

It was Briquet, and later Charcot, who were most influential in developing the concept of hysteria, and discussing the relationship to epilepsy. Briquet felt that hysteria with mixed attacks was in reality a particular form of hysteria, namely very intense hysteria, and the prognosis was that of this condition, not that of epilepsy. Charcot too delineated epilepsy from hysteria, and noted in particular alterations of temperature which were different following repeated attacks in the two disorders. As an alternative to hystero-epilepsy, he used the term 'hysteria major' to describe hysteria that presented with convulsive patterns. By careful clinical observation the Salpêtrière school outlined several stages of the convulsive episode, called respectively the prodromal stage, the epileptoid stage, the period of clownism, the period of emotional attitudes, and the period of delirium. In the third stage, the characteristic 'arc de cercle' was seen, in which the trunk is raised, and the body rests on the feet and occiput only (see Fig. 9.1). However, not all attacks were deemed to be typical, and often only small portions of the total pattern were recorded.

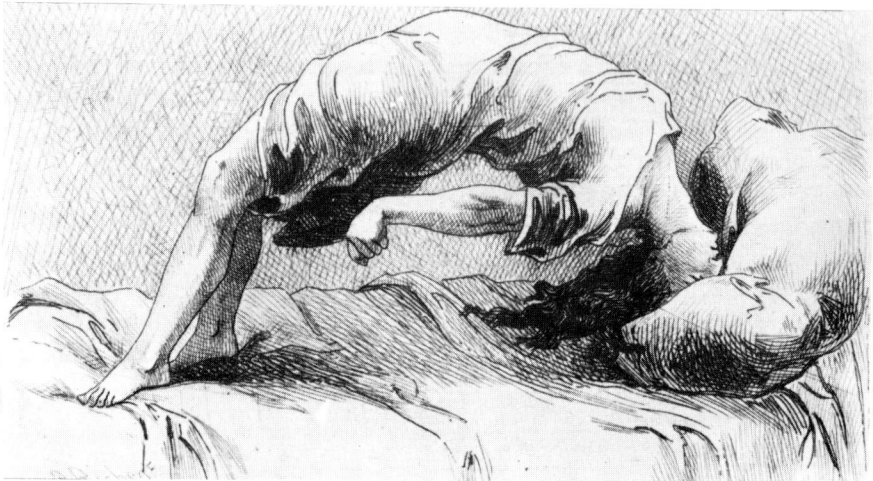

Fig. 9.1 Phase des contorsions (Arc de cercle).

Charcot in particular dwelt on other clinical phenomena noted in hysteria which could help the differential diagnosis. These included narrowing of the visual field, monocular polyopia, and sensory disturbances such as the anaesthesias. The latter could be complete or incomplete (hemianaesthesia), and the demarcation line of the abnormality was often perfect, and corresponded to the median line. Such anaesthesias, Charcot felt, were rarely seen in diseases other than hysteria, commenting: 'Its well-established existence is, therefore, a valuable indication, one which will often reveal the real nature of many symptoms, which would otherwise remain doubtful.' (Charcot 1877).

It was the end of the 19th century and the beginning of the 20th which led to a fundamental change in ideas regarding both epilepsy and hysteria. The growing ability of clinical neurologists to identify from clinical signs localised lesions within the brain, and the rapidly expanding field of neuropathology resulted in the clear identification of a number of disease states, amongst which were some forms of epilepsy. Although Charcot and his school had been instrumental in first describing many of these, he was also, albeit briefly, involved in educating the Viennese neurologist, Freud. The latter came to Paris and met Janet, with whom he must have discussed neuropsychiatric problems, and was led not only to a great interest in hysteria, but also towards new psychological explanations for disease which Janet and others had been developing. Reaffirming Briquet and Charcot, Janet felt that convulsive attacks were extremely frequent in hysteria, although did not give them the pride of place that Charcot had done. Janet felt that the convulsive episodes were a variety of somnambulism, and that the actions of the patient during them had psychological meaning. For example, he states: 'They begin, like somnambulisms, on the occasion of particularly affecting events, genital perturbations, sorrows, fears, etc. A man begins to have a crisis of hysteria because he has seen his son fall from a scaffolding and die before him; many girls or women begin to have attacks on the occasion of the death of a beloved person; in about ten observations the cause of the first fit is a conflagration, a petroleum lamp setting the subject's dress on fire; in others it is a fall from a tram-car or from a bicycle, a fight with comrades, heart-grief, reverses of fortune etc.' (Janet 1907). He also discussed 'associations of ideas' in which 'the dreaded perception and the remembrances which bring on the fit' are linked in the mind of the patient. The actual pattern of the fits were thus an 'ensemble' of emotional manifestations, and he could identify the emotions such as anger, and eroticism in the activity of patients.

Freud also regarded the motor phenomena of hysterical attacks as appropriate to the affect which accompanied the memory of some past trauma which was of importance in bringing about the hysteria. However, there were clearly relationships between epileptic and hysterical convulsions which he explained as follows: 'In infants, apart from the respiratory action of screaming, affects only produce and find expression in uncoordinated contractions of the muscles of this primitive kind — in arching the body and kicking about. As development proceeds the musculature passes more and more under the control of the power of coordination and the will, but the opisthotonus, which represents the maximum of motor effort of the total somatic musculature, and the clonic movements of kicking and thrashing about persist throughout life as a form of reaction for the maximal excitation of the brain — for the purely physical excitation in epileptic attacks, as well as for the discharge of maximal affects in the shape of more or less epileptoid convulsions (viz. the purely motor part of hysterical attacks).' Freud also considered the possibility that there existed 'purely motor convulsive attacks which are independent of any psychical factor, and in which all that happens is that the mass of excitation accumulated by summation is discharged, in just the same way as the mass of stimuli caused by anatomical modifications is discharged in an epileptic fit' (Freud & Breuer 1893–5).

A similar association between epilepsy and hysteria was observed and explained by other physicians. Pierce Clark (1923) attempted to present a psychobiological theory of epilepsy, which used later Freudian ideas in attempting to explain certain types of epilepsy. He pointed out that in many cases of epilepsy no neuropathological disorder could be demonstrated, and from his own studies of epileptic patients he was able to discern certain patterns of developmental traits prior to the onset of the epilepsy. He suggested that the fit itself served as an unconscious gratification for the libido. Thus, in both epilepsy, and in the neuroses, infantile motives, and the inadequate development of the individual's affects and instincts led to the later development of symptoms. Lehrman (1925) made a similar point, noting: 'The symptoms of psychoneuroses, psychoses, and essential (psychogenic) epilepsy, indicate not only the intensity of the unconscious strivings, but the necessity of the manner and degree of the withdrawal from reality. Thus a partial withdrawal is seen in the psychoneuroses, a complete withdrawal is seen in the psychoses, and a sudden withdrawal is seen in epilepsy.'

Jelliffe & White (1929) also considered this relationship by discussing energy and its flow within the nervous system. This could be blocked at any level, psychic, sensorimotor or physicochemical, and in the classical epileptic attack all levels were involved. However, different 'levels' could be so involved in other varieties of attack. 'The hysterical convulsion offers an example of a high level convulsive type of reaction ... next lower in the scale of levels are the psychaesthenic convulsions of Oppenheim (compulsion neurosis type) which are expressions of a more severe grade of neurosis ... then come the very interesting affect epilepsies ... distinctly epileptoid types of reaction conditioned by purely psychological situations.' The epileptic seizure itself was considered as a 'flight into unconsciousness', when occurring at times of stress. The fit was '... therefore a break in the life demand for adaptation or an attempt at escape from an intolerable stimulus whether from within (toxin, tumour) or from without (life situation).'

This association between hysteria and epilepsy at a pathophysiological level has been discussed more recently in the writings of Krapf (1957) and Rabe (1966, 1970). The former author felt that a complete dualism between epilepsy and hysteria was unacceptable, as was a return to Charcot's ideas. Krapf noted that the electroencephalogram was often normal in epilepsy, and that dysrhythmias were a frequent finding in neurotics, psychopathic personalities, and children with behaviour problems. In addition he commented on the relationship between age and the EEG pattern, pointing out that "the abnormal EEG does not indicate in the first place the predisposition of the brain to 'explosive discharges of neuronal energy', but rather the degree of functional maturity of the central organ." He suggested therefore that psychologically meaningful seizures could appear in somatically predisposed individuals, and that 'physiogenesis and psychogenesis could be integrated together such that heredity, external stimuli and psychological factors are involved in all convulsive states, although, in different degrees and working in different ways through different predispositions.'

Rabe discussed the relationship at length, and himself described a number of cases in which both epileptic and hysterical attacks appeared in the same patient, suggesting common underlying causative factors based primarily on immaturity of physiological and psychological mechanisms. He noted the relative paucity of work on the differential diagnosis of the two disorders, partly because it was thought that hysterical fits were declining in frequency and partly because *grande hystérie* became concealed under the diagnosis of epilepsy, and treated with anticonvulsants. He made the point that the EEG was often used to make a diagnosis of epilepsy with neglect of clinical findings, when in reality only dysrhythmias were recorded. The reason for this 'shift away from the fit description to the EEG' was that, in practice, seizures were rarely observed first-hand. Fit-provoking EEG techniques, he felt, provided contradictory evidence, since in patients prone to hysteria the metrazole threshold is lower anyway, and there is a danger of provoking a first epileptic seizure in the predisposed.

This brief historical view indicates first, that an association between epilepsy and hysteria was founded in Egyptian and Greek medicine, and still finds expression today in the writings of several authors. Secondly, that of the two trends particularly noted, namely the one being an attempt to isolate and separate hysterical from epileptic attacks, and the other to seek a common pathogenesis for at least some cases, the latter held sway until the late 19th century when the former took the dominant role, and is still the trend today, but with notable exceptions. Thirdly, the idea of a dichotomy in the two disorders reflects to some extent the growing separation between psychiatry and neurology which became apparent at that time, based mainly on the clear identification of a number of organic lesions, particularly cortical, in relation to neurological disorders. Before going on to consider some more recent experimental work in relation to non-epileptic, in particular hysterical, attacks, it is germane to consider some recent ideas in the development of the concept of hysteria.

HYSTERIA—THE LAST 30 YEARS

Chodoff & Lyons (1958) drew attention to the semantic difficulties in the literature that hysteria presented, and clearly emphasised the separation between *hysteria*, a particular kind of psychosomatic symptomatology often referred to as conversion hysteria or conversion reaction, and the *hysterical personality*, a pattern of behaviour habitually exhibited by certain individuals. In addition to these two separate meanings, they noted other uses of the word including 'mass hysteria', in which there was an epidemic spread of symptoms in the absence of well-defined somatic pathology; 'anxiety hysteria', which was used by Freud to describe a psychoneurotic disorder manifesting principally with phobias in which 'repression' was the principal defence mechanism, a use now no longer employed; and its use as a pejorative term, which should be confined to the lay public.

The essential features of the hysterical personality include egocentric attitudes, exhibitionism and dramatism, labile affects with excitability, emotional shallowness, flirtatiousness associated with sexual frigidity, dependency, and suggestibility. In its florid form this personality style is easily recognised, and experimentally, by use of standardised questionnaires, a number of authors have identified these trait patterns using factor analysis, and clearly distinguished them from, for example, obsessional personality traits (Lazarre et al 1970). Its distinction from hysteria was a decisive step forward in understanding, vindicated by further work which has attempted to delineate the relationship of the personality style to hysteria. Chodoff & Lyons in their study reported 17 patients with conversion phenomena, uncontaminated by known neurological disease, and noted three with the hysterical personality, the others having a variety of personality disturbances, the main one being passive-aggressive. Ljungberg (1957), in a study of 381 patients, found 43 per cent of the men and 47 per cent of the women to have deviant personalities, 20.7 per cent of the total having hysterical personalities. Merskey & Trimble (1979), using a control group of patients with psychiatric illness, reported that the personality types of 89 patients with conversion symptoms included 17 with hysterical personalities, 17 with passive-immature-dependent personalities and seven with obsessional personalities. In contrast, control psychiatric patients had a lower frequency of hysterical personalities, and a greater frequency of obsessional personalities. These data thus suggest that there is an increased prevalence of patients with the hysterical personality in those who present with conversion hysteria. However, it is also clear that the majority of patients do not conform to this particular style. While assessment of the personality is therefore of importance clinically, the presence of the hysterical personality does not lead to a diagnosis of hysteria, and hysteria can occur in patients with clinically normal personalities.

The relationship of hysteria to organic neurological disease has also received much attention, and is responsible for several misunderstandings in this field. Gowers himself (1893) pointed out that hysterical symptoms frequently accompany diseases of the nervous system, and reported that there was hardly a single neurological disease that did not sometimes cause hysterical phenomena.

More recently Whitlock (1967) reported that 62.5 per cent of patients with hysterical symptoms had significant coexistent or preceding histories of organic disorder, compared to 5 per cent of a control group, and Merskey & Buhrich (1975) reported that 61 of 89 patients with conversion symptoms also had organic disease, epilepsy being the commonest. Merskey (1979) has accumulated the evidence that temporal lobe abnormalities, epileptic and otherwise, may be related to the hysterias, and that modification of epileptic discharge with anticonvulsant drugs may lead to brief episodes of loss of consciousness associated with hysterical behaviour.

It was however Slater (1965) who emphasised the relationship most strongly, using his evidence to suggest that a diagnosis of hysteria was 'a disguise for ignorance and a fertile source of clinical error'. In a survey of 85 patients with such a diagnosis he found 19 that initially had a combined diagnosis of hysteria and organic pathology, but at follow-up 12 of the total had died, and 22 went on to develop neurological illness not detected at the initial assessment. However, these results, far from devaluing the diagnosis of hysteria, lead to the conclusion that, with an understanding of the subtle interplay between personality factors and somatic disease, and the acknowledgement that a diagnosis of hysteria carries an uncertain prognosis, these patients need to be followed up by physicians aware of the progression of both psychiatric and neurological disease, and not discharged from the clinic with an appellation that 'nothing is wrong'.

The confusion over the validity of hysteria as a diagnosis led Pilowsky (1977) to introduce the concept of *Abnormal Illness Behaviour*. The term 'illness behaviour' was introduced by Mechanic (1968) to refer in patients to 'the way in which given symptoms may be differently perceived, evaluated and acted upon or not acted upon by different kinds of people and in different social situations'. He pointed out how ethnic variations, cultural and developmental experiences determine a patient's reaction to threatening circumstances, and the great variety of responses among different patients to the same illness condition. He says: 'Illness behaviour and the decision to seek medical advice frequently involve, from the patient's point of view, a rational attempt to make sense of his problem and cope with it within the limits of his intelligence and his social and cultural understandings, but this does not make it rational from a medical perspective'. Pilowsky, taking this concept further, defined 'abnormal illness behaviour' as 'the persistence of an inappropriate mode of perceiving, evaluating and acting in relation to one's state of health'. This concept allows for further understanding of a number of overlapping clinical phenomena including hysteria, hypochondriasis, Munchausen's syndrome, and factitious illness. As such, all these names have provided conceptual difficulties for many physicians confronted with the clinical problems they present, but as Pilowsky pointed out, these diagnoses are initially usually made by physicians without psychiatric training on the basis of a perceived discrepancy between the objective somatic pathology noted and the patient's reaction to it.

Pilowsky classified abnormal illness behaviour either as 'illness affirming', in which the patient says that he has some illness that the physician is unable to document, or as 'illness denying' when there is denial of illness that has been diagnosed or is apparent to another observer. In each of these categories the behaviour may be consciously or unconsciously motivated. Thus consciously motivated somatically focused abnormal illness behaviour covers malingering and the Munchausen syndrome. Unconsciously motivated illness behaviour of this category refers to hysteria, hypochondriasis, and phenomena such as conversion. Psychologically focused abnormal illness behaviour may also include malingering, but in addition covers such syndromes as Ganser states, fugues and amnesias.

From this brief discussion it seems that the term abnormal illness behaviour has broad usage, yet fills satisfactorily the void left by those who suggest that for example hysteria or hypochondriasis do not exist. Whether or not patients with non-epileptic seizures are similar to patients with other varieties of unconsciously motivated abnormal illness behaviour however, has yet to be determined.

Finally, there is growing literature on *Briquet's hysteria*, an apparently specific psychopathological entity named after Briquet by the St Louis group (Guze & Perley 1963). The patients they described were all young females, polysymptomatic, and characteristically had a history of an excessive number of surgical operations and hospitalisations, numerous vague complaints, frigidity and often dyspareunia. They suggested that this disorder had a genetic basis, and was linked to sociopathic personality traits. While it has been implied that Briquet's syndrome is a synonym for hypochondriacal neurosis, a variant of the hysterical personality disorder, or represents one end of a spectrum of hysterical disorders, the possibility that it exists as an independent entity is seriously maintained. It is reported in 1–2 per cent of consecutive female patients attending hospital for investigation, and in 10 per cent of psychiatric in-patients. Fits are common in this group and, in that it is by definition an intractable disorder and extremely difficult to treat, recognition of such patients would seem to be of vital importance to avoid unnecessary surgical or medical intervention.

SOME RECENT WORK ON HYSTERICAL SEIZURES

Prevalence

The frequency with which conversion symptoms occur in medical practice varies from 5–25 per cent, depending on the population chosen. Some settings such as neurological clinics and wards attract a particularly high number of such patients. Although some writers have suggested that hysterical convulsions were rare, this was not supported by the comprehensive study of Ljungberg (1957) in which fits occurred in 25 per cent of the males and 41 per cent of the females, or in over one-third of the total sample of patients with conversion symptoms. Purtell et al (1951) recorded fits in 12 per cent of a group of 50 women with Briquet's syndrome, figures of 9.1 per cent and 25 per cent being given by Reed (1975) and Merskey & Buhrich (1975) respectively. Stefanis et al (1976), in a study of hysteria in Athens in three two-year periods between 1948 and 1971, noted that hysterical fits were the commonest presenting symptom but that the prevalence was declining, the percentage with each period being 37, 40 and 25 per cent respectively. Their suggestion was that with major social, economic and cultural changes that were taking place in Greece, not only was the overall incidence of hysteria declining, but some of its more florid manifestations, in particular the epileptiform variety, was diminishing. Different evidence comes from the work of Trimble (1981), who reviewed patients with a diagnosis of hysteria at the National Hospitals for Nervous Diseases for three years selected from three decades. Whereas a decline in frequency was seen in the late 1950s, this was not manifested in the 1960s. The actual symptoms are shown in Table 9.1 which indicates no fall in the frequency of convulsions over the decades, suggesting that, in certain centres at least, hysteria

Table 9.1 Symptom distribution of patients with 'hysteria' over three decades

	1951, '53, '55	1961, '63, '65	1971, '73, '75
Total for all patients	166	144	159
Motor	51 (32.7%)	53 (36.8%)	40 (25.1%)
Tremors	2 (1.1%)	5 (3.4%)	7 (4.4%)
Convulsions	19 (11.1%)	19 (13.2%)	22 (13.8%)
Anaesthesias	10 (5.8%)	8 (5.5%)	11 (6.9%)
Visual	10 (5.8%)	12 (8.3%)	16 (10.0%)
Pain	43 (25.1%)	23 (16.0%)	36 (22.6%)
Amnesia, etc.	6 (3.5%)	8 (5.5%)	7 (4.4%)
Dizziness, etc.	16 (9.3%)	12 (8.3%)	15 (9.4%)
Other	9 (5.3%)	4 (2.8%)	5 (3.4%)

Note decline in frequency of motor symptoms in the 1970s

presenting as fits remains a common diagnostic problem. It is important to note that often these symptoms occur in non-epileptic patients, although their frequency occurrence in patients with epilepsy confirms the historical trend discussed above.

Differential diagnosis
In spite of all that has been written on this subject, few studies have actually been carried out to determine what differences may exist between hysterical and epileptic seizures, and most offer only clinical impressions. An early attempt was that of Laurés & Gascard (1920) who examined the urea content of the cerebrospinal fluid during various convulsions and were able to conclude: 'le taux de l'urée dans le liquide céphalorachidien, quel qu'il soit en dehors des crises est diminué pendent la crise histérique et augmenté pendent la crise épileptique'. Roy (1977, 1979) examined 22 patients who had been investigated for seizures with a final diagnosis of hysterical seizures, and compared them to a control group of patients with well-defined epilepsy. Clinical history was obtained, and both groups were given rating scales of psychopathology, including the General Health Questionnaire, the Wakefield Self-Assessment Depression Inventory, and the

Morbid Anxiety Inventory. Significant differences included, for the experimental group, a family history of psychiatric disorder, a personal history of psychiatric disorder, attempted suicide, sexual maladjustment and increased scores on the anxiety and depression inventories. A clinical diagnosis of a current affective disorder was made in 19 at the time of the investigation. He suggested that five factors, namely family history and past history of psychiatric disorder, attempted suicide, sexual maladjustment and a current affective syndrome helped differentiate hysterical fits from epilepsy.

Henry & Woodruff (1978) have recently described a physical sign which provides a positive basis for diagnosis of non-epileptic seizures during an attack based on variation of ocular deviation with the patient's posture. When the patient is on the ground and is turned from one side to another, the eyes are always deviated towards the ground, thus changing their position with posture. This sign was absent in 20 cases of coma where there was a clear 'organic' diagnosis.

More recently the use of EEG telemetry has been advocated for the elucidation of the aetiology of fits, and the differential diagnosis of epileptic from non-epileptic seizures (Bowden et al 1975). Porter et al (1977) described the use of 6-hour telemetered EEG and video records in 23 patients with a long history of uncontrolled epilepsy. One was eventually diagnosed as hysteria. Rowan et al (1980) noted that in 52 patients in which the most frequent clinical problem was differentiation of epileptic from non-epileptic seizures, the technique gave answers to the clinical questions in 52 per cent of the cases. The same authors examined six patients with 'psychogenic seizures' using 6–24 hour telemetered recordings. 42 seizures were monitored, all of which showed absence of epileptiform EEG activity during the seizure, and no post-fit slowing. Improvement in seizure frequency occurred in five on withdrawal of anticonvulsant medication.

Another approach which has been used recently is the investigation of anterior pituitary hormone output following seizures. Trimble(1978) measured prolactin levels in patients diagnosed as hysteria who presented with seizures that resembled major generalised epilepsy, and compared them with levels in patients with that form of epilepsy, and with a group of patients undergoing modified non-dominant unilateral ECT. Changes in serum prolactin were seen in the epilepsy and ECT groups, maximum increase above baseline occurring 15–20 minutes following a fit. In the majority of patients with epilepsy postictal levels were greater than $1000 \mu U/ml$. In contrast, the hysteria group showed no changes in prolactin levels and the conclusion was that 'when the prolactin concentration is above $1000 \mu U/ml$, in the absence of other causes such as a high baseline level or medication, the attack is epileptic rather than hysterical'. Some experimental support for these findings comes from the work of Meldrum et al (1979) who estimated a number of hormones in the plasma of the photosensitive baboon *Papio papio* following major generalised epileptic seizures. Prolactin showed marked rises postictally compatible with the findings in patients. More recently Abbott et al (1980) have repeated the clinical findings. They examined prolactin release following generalised tonic-clonic seizures, and in healthy male volunteers who were asked to simulate seizures. The mean prolactin level in post-ictal patients was $1195 \mu U/ml$, which was significantly higher than in control subjects. They also measured cortisol levels and noted no difference between the two groups.

In further studies, Oxley et al (1980) have compared prolactin changes, clinical impressions and EEG ambulatory monitoring in the differential diagnosis of seizure states. Eighteen subjects were assigned to one of three clinical groups, namely epileptic, non-epileptic or mixed, and 57 fits were recorded using the Medilog-4 recorder with on-head pre-amplification for prolonged EEG recordings. Following tonic-clonic fits with epileptic activity recorded on the EEG, large increases in prolactin were noted in contrast to the non-epileptic group in whom no changes were seen, confirming the earlier results. In general there was a high concordance between clinical diagnosis, based on positive criteria for a diagnosis of either epilepsy or hysteria, and the EEG findings, and the 4-channel ambulatory monitoring was found useful in helping with the clinical evaluation of both epileptic and non-epileptic fits.

Prognosis

Little information is available on the prognosis of hysterical fits. As noted above in the more general discussion on hysteria, prognosis is generally varied, although the later development of organic disease is well-described. In one study, Barham Carter (1949) noted that two out of four patients with a diagnosis of hysterical fits were unchanged or worse at follow-up 4–6 years later. Ljungberg (1957) noted that after one year 66 per cent of patients still had symptoms, and after five years 42 per cent. When comparing this prognosis with patients suffering from astasia-abasia, he noted that the fit group had a far less favourable outlook. Hafeiz (1980) followed up six patients with hysterical convulsions, three of whom relapsed, a higher rate than patients presenting with motor disturbances and aphonia.

On the diagnosis of hysterical fits

From the above, certain features regarding the diagnosis of hysterical as opposed to epileptic fits are apparent. As with other hysterical symptoms diagnosis should include not only negative neurological criteria, but also positive psychiatric evidence, and where they can be demonstrated, positive neurological signs. The initial feature is the discrepancy between the observed pathology and the patient's complaints. The history may reveal other episodes suggestive of conversion phenomena, and a personality disorder with a propensity to seek medical help. Illness experiences in childhood need to be explored, especially illnesses that may have occurred in significant other persons in a patient's life. A number of patients may be found who have a long history of operations, investigations and complaints which, when carefully probed, all seem to indicate early episodes of 'abnormal illness behaviour'. Psychopathology in the form of current affective illness may be quite clear and must always be looked for. However, often on account of the way the patient is presenting, it may easily be overlooked. Some authors write of 'la belle indifférence' — a tendency to deny problems and to show unconcern regarding apparently serious symptoms. Although this is not regularly present, it may lead to masking of psychiatric disturbance and be easily missed by the inexperienced physician. So-called secondary gain may be clear at the outset, or only be discovered later in the course of the patient's illness. However, secondary gain is often based on value judgements by physicians rather than necessarily reflecting reality for the patient, and the danger of hinging a diagnosis of hysteria on evidence of secondary gain cannot be over-emphasised. Stress in itself is often a necessary, but not a sufficient, criterion for the emergence of conversion symptoms.

Among positive neurological criteria, the presence of hemianaesthesia or other clearly defined anaesthetic patches, not conforming to anaesthesias seen following neurological illness, is perhaps the most important. Unfortunately, since the time of Charcot this fact has been forgotten, their presence often being attributed purely to suggestion. However, even today the eliciting of unusual anaesthetic patches on examination in patients at the first consultation is not at all uncommon, but is often ignored, or referred to as 'functional'. While to-date there is no evidence that they are pathognomonic for hysteria, in view of their frequent occurrence in that disorder it should be taken as a positive sign, lending weight to the diagnosis. Often all modalities of sensation are altered, and in hemianaesthesia the body and face of one side, most often the left, are affected to the midline. An interesting feature of the anaesthesia is its lateralisation. Briquet, in his series, noted that it occurred in 93 cases out of 400, and that in 70 the left side alone was affected. Gowers also commented on its common occurrence in hysteria, noted that patients seldom complain of it and were often unaware of its existence, and that it was commoner on the left side (Gowers 1893). Purves-Stewart (1920) also commented on this distribution, making the additional observation that in left-handed patients it is usually right-sided. That this lateralisation is not only confined to anaesthesia was noted by Janet (1931), who found similar results for a variety of hysterical symptoms, and Merskey & Boyd (1978) who noted an increased incidence of left-sided presentation for chronic pain. More recently Stern (1977) investigated the distribution of hysterical symptoms in 191 patients, taking specific note of handedness. 45 of these had sensory loss, 37 of whom had unilateral symptoms. Of these, both right- and left-handed patients experienced the anaesthesia more on the left side. The importance of these observations is that the asymmetry suggests mechanisms other than straightforward suggestion for their production. The growing interest in laterality differences between the two hemispheres raises the possibility that these phenomena are a reflection of non-dominant hemisphere activity, and that exploration of such findings will lead to further understanding of the pathophysiology of hysteria.

The clinical features of the attack itself clearly are important, as are any preceding subjective phenomena, or post-paroxysmal behaviour abnormalities. Precipitating events should be sought, and if necessary an attempt to produce an attack with hypnosis be made. During and after the attack reflex changes should be looked for, eye movements examined and, in major tonic seizures, a 20-minute prolactin level taken to assess against baseline values. A further sample at 40 minutes is useful additional information to see if any fall in levels is occurring post-paroxysmally.

Telemetry may need to be arranged, and of growing usefulness is prolonged 24-hour or longer ambulatory monitoring, which can continue if necessary until an attack occurs.

It is clear that full understanding of the patient's symptoms requires elaborate assessment of personality, past illness behaviour history, present mental state, and the patient's current environmental and interpersonal stresses. As Pilowsky pointed out this does not, and should not, require two separate examinations, and most relevant data can be obtained at a single interview if the appropriate technique is adopted. Often the initial examination of a patient, even when there is an early suggestion of abnormal illness behaviour, is entirely symptom and somatically focused. This is followed by a number of investigations all of which turn out to be negative, at which stage the approach is suddenly 'switched' to a probing of the psychiatric status of the patient. This sudden turnabout may upset the patient, who then becomes indignant when asked to see a psychiatrist since the implication must be that as 'nothing has been found' the symptoms are 'all in the mind' and thus imagined. It is better to make appropriate psychiatric and psychosocial enquiries at an early stage of the patient's investigation, pointing out to the patient that it is usual practice to ask a broad range of questions about themselves, their lives and their illness so that all aspects of their problem can be explored.

Even when all these possibilities are considered it is clear that the differential diagnosis in some patients remains obscure, more especially where complex partial seizures are considered as a cause of patients' symptoms. The follow-up studies (Harper — see below) suggest that the majority of these do not have epilepsy. In the first instance it is probably wiser to leave the diagnosis open since, with time, the history and prognosis will become clearer and to commit a patient to the label of epilepsy is serious, not only because it implies the taking of anticonvulsant drugs for many years, but also on account of the social stigma and restrictions that are attached to the disorder.

Management
Any associated psychopathology, in particular affective disorders, should receive prompt attention. Often patients in whom a diagnosis of hysterical fits is made have been receiving anticonvulsants and these should be reduced slowly and eventually stopped if there is no evidence of epileptic fits. Prompt cessation must be avoided as it may lead to withdrawal seizures and further complicate the diagnosis. Antidepressants should be substituted if necessary, but if depression is not a feature of the clinical picture small doses of minor tranquillisers, especially benzodiazepines, can be very helpful in arresting attacks. The life situation of the patient will need to be explored in often prolonged interviews, and help offered to solve conflicts, although formal psychoanalysis is nowadays rarely advocated. Relaxation and biofeedback have a part to play, especially in patients who are tense and describe muscle tightness before attacks. Patients should be introduced to the idea that their symptoms may reflect psychiatric disability early on in the course of their illness and intractable cases should be admitted to a psychiatric ward in order to assess and explore the patient's behaviour more thoroughly. While removal from the patient's life situation in itself can be therapeutic, the acceptance by the patient that it is to a psychiatric ward rather than to any other ward that they need to be admitted is an important therapeutic advance.

OTHER VARIETIES OF NON-EPILEPTIC FITS

There are a number of conditions which may lead patients without epilepsy to receive that diagnosis. In some, the patterns of the clinical activity observed resemble major tonic-clonic convulsions, and this has been particularly discussed under the heading of hysteria. However, many patients complain of a variety of subjective sensations, often associated with minor abnormalities of movement or loss of consciousness, which may lead to the possible diagnosis of epilepsy. Unfortunately, in many patients a diagnosis of epilepsy is given inappropriately, as is suggested by Jeavons (1977) who commented that 23 per cent of over 1000 patients seen at his epilepsy clinic did not actually have epilepsy. Common misdiagnoses included syncope and a variety of psychiatric disorders. It is appropriate to consider the differential diagnosis first in childhood and then in adults, following a brief discussion of the concept of 'borderlands of epilepsy'.

The borderlands of epilepsy

Although Hughlings Jackson, with his definition of epilepsy, expanded the concept to include a variety of phenomena in addition to motor convulsions and disturbance of consciousness, it was Gowers who first clearly formulated the idea of the 'borderland of epilepsy' (Gowers 1907). Under this heading were included faints, vasovagal attacks, tetanoid spasms, vertigo, migraine and some sleep disturbances. These he described clinically, and speculated on their pathogenesis. Some of them he felt were related to 'minor epilepsy' suggesting, for example, the possibility that 'its elements protracted with no tendency to be terminated by loss of consciousness, its features would be so different that its nature would not be suspected'. In addition, he put forward the idea that vertigo or syncopal faints may, with the correct predisposition, develop into minor epilepsy, similar to some of the suggestions about hysteria and epilepsy discussed above.

Williams (1975) has 'revisited' the borderlands of epilepsy. He noted that Gowers' interest in defining these conditions lay in those disorders of function where no structural changes could be described. He noted the large numbers of patients that were seen in neurological clinics whose problems were of emotional origin, and pointed out the multifactorial aetiology of many symptoms, which must include the setting in which they occur and the kind of person that they arise in. Obsessional personality styles were particularly frequent in patients presenting with borderland symptoms, and the latter developed in 'persistent homogeneous stress of a frustrating sort which deeply involves the self; being caught in a trap in life which cannot be sprung'. Williams recognised the borderlands as one casualty of the split between psychiatry and neurology which had occurred since Gowers' time, saying: 'In the study of patients with periodic disorder of function—the broad Borderland of Epilepsy—the attention to unitary aetiology with which we grew up, which is that of a specific disease due to a specific cause, must be changed to that of ecology—which is the study of the soil which encouraged the growth both of order and of disorder.'

Non-epileptic 'fits' in children

The main disorders requiring a differential diagnosis from epilepsy in children are syncopal attacks and breath-holding attacks. The former are extremely common, usually occurring in association with some emotional event, especially when indoors in a warm atmosphere. Adolescents, particularly those who are tall and thin, are likely to have such attacks following prolonged standing in an uncomfortable environment, or on rising from the sitting to the standing position. The episodes often begin with some anxiety sensations, often with epigastric discomfort, followed by palpitations, tremor and sweating. Light-headedness follows, sometimes with blurring of vision, following which consciousness is lost. Self-injury is not common, and the fall is more graceful than the sudden collapse in an epileptic seizure. Brief clonic movements may be noted by an observer, especially if attacks continue for any length of time.

The immediate cause of syncope is a diminution of cerebral blood flow associated with which there is bradycardia and peripheral vasodilatation. The attack is therefore usually terminated promptly when the patient lies down and cerebral blood flow is restored.

In breath-holding attacks children maintain the expiratory phase of breathing until they become cyanotic and lose consciousness. There may be brief stiffening or convulsive movements, thus resembling many of the features of epilepsy. In the majority of cases such attacks cease by the age of five (Lombroso & Lerman 1967) and mortality is extremely rare. Behaviour problems characterised by stubbornness, disobedience, aggression and enuresis occur with increased frequency in such children, and precipitating factors such as frustration and anger are commonly noted. It is of interest that a number of such patients go on to develop syncope in adult life, and some adults who suffer from syncope give a history of breath-holding in early childhood (Lombroso & Lerman 1967). A family history of breath-holding is often obtained, and although the mechanism of the episode is not understood, it is probably due to an acute reduction in cerebral blood flow in association with the Valsalva-like manoeuvre. Other disorders described in children include 'apparent fainting and sudden death', which occurs following strenuous exercise, and is associated with ECG abnormalities being similar to Stokes-Adams attacks in adults; benign paroxysmal vertigo; ritualistic movements, and night terrors (O'Donohue 1979). The latter occur in non-REM sleep, and are not to be confused with nightmares which occur in REM sleep, of which recall is vivid. Sleep-walking too is commonly seen in children, which also occurs in slow-wave sleep, in which purposeless behaviour, which may continue for up to 30 or 40 minutes, is observed for which there is usually an amnesia. Night terrors may be accompanied by sleep-walking.

Differential diagnosis in adults
The classification of syncope in adults as defined by Gilliatt (1977) is shown in Table 9.2. Vasovagal syncope is discussed above. Micturition syncope, which usually occurs in adult males who, at night, rise to micturate, may cause diagnostic difficulty since the loss of consciousness may be associated with incontinence.

Of particular importance are the cardiac causes of loss of consciousness including dysrhythmias. Not only may the latter lead to faints, dizzy spells and syncope, but they may also provoke an epileptic seizure, leading to diagnostic confusion. The more extensive use of simultaneous ambulatory elec-trocardiographic and electroencephalographic monitoring has led to a better definition of these phenomena. In such cases the inter-attack ECG is usually normal, the main abnormality being arrhythmias detected on prolonged monitoring. Schott et al (1977) reported that relevant cardiac arrhythmias may

Table 9.2 Classification of syncope (after Gilliatt 1977)

Reflex (vasovagal)
Haemorrhage
Upright posture
Anoxia
Emotion and pain
Micturition
Carotid sinus syndrome

Respiratory
Coughing
Trumpeting
Weight lifting

Cardiac
Arrhythmias
Aortic stenosis
Congenital heart disease

Areflexic or paralytic
Tabes
Diabetes
Polyneuropathy
Shy-Drager syndrome
Traumatic paraplegia
Alcoholism
Drug syndromes (hypotensive agents, phenothiazines, levodopa)
Old age (particularly with drugs)

Local brainstem
Migraine
Vertebrobasilar disease

---

occur in up to 20 per cent of patients with suspected idiopathic epilepsy, and suggest that, particularly when typically clinical features of epilepsy are absent and a routine EEG shows no abnormality, further cardiac investigations be pursued.

The carotid sinus syndrome is due to sensitivity of the sinus in elderly patients, in whom episodes of unconsciousness or vertigo occur on turning the head.

Other causes of abnormalities of sensation and consciousness, which need to be distinguished from epilepsy, include basilar-artery migraine; vertebrobasilar ischaemic attacks, especially in the elderly; transient ischaemic attacks which lead to brief episodes with neurological symptoms; hypoglycaemia, and sleep disorders such as narcolepsy and cataplexy. Migraine, particularly where there is brain-stem involvement, may lead to unconsciousness often associated with amnesia (Bickerstaff 1961). Rarely there may be transient neurological symptoms, such as hemiplegia, and associated unilateral EEG changes. Although some authors refer to an association between migraine and epilepsy (Williams 1975) the inter-attack EEG findings are usually normal in the former. Hypoglycaemia from a variety of causes can cause sweating, faintness, disturbances of behaviour and loss of consciousness, and is diagnosed by a prolonged glucose tolerance test. However, this test is not infallible, and it has been suggested that the only definitive way to establish the diagnosis is to obtain a blood sugar actually during an attack (Matthews 1970).

Gelineau's syndrome includes narcolepsy, cataplexy, sleep paralysis and hypnogogic or hypnopompic hallucinations. Narcolepsy itself consists of brief but unavoidable attacks of sleepiness which occur during waking hours. Cataplexy, during which loss of muscle tone and movement occur suddenly, usually in association with laughing or strong emotion, may be confused with epilepsy, particularly if the other elements of the tetrad are not clearly apparent. A number of patients with this syndrome have prolonged periods of automatic behaviour for which there is subsequent amnesia, which again may be confused with epilepsy. Narcolepsy responds to amphetamine-like compounds, and cataplexy to clomipramine, as opposed to anticonvulsant drugs.

Finally, there are a number of other psychiatric disorders which may be confused with epilepsy including panic attacks, anxiety states, rage attacks and fugues. Panic attacks are noted in patients with a prior history of anxiety neurosis, and often occur in the setting of stress. The onset is usually gradual with a growing dysphoria, and after the attack, which terminates slowly, feelings of apprehension may still continue.

Although patients complain of epigastric discomfort, there is never the clearly-defined sensation that rises to the back of the throat as noted in patients with complex partial seizures. In anxiety episodes, the feeling is more diffuse, and spreads to involve the whole body. Hyperventilation, tachycardia, sweating and other manifestations of anxiety will often be reported by the patient. Loss of consciousness may occur but careful attention to the time of onset, length and accompanying features will usually enable these attacks to be distinguished from epilepsy. There are a group of patients who hyperventilate and then, on account of this, have an epileptic seizure.

Harper, using clinical and electroencephalographic criteria, has systematically attempted to draw distinctions between temporal lobe epilepsy and the phobic anxiety-depersonalisation syndrome (PADS) (Harper & Roth 1962). The latter is a well-defined neurotic illness, in which a combination of phobias occur in association with depersonalisation. Often there are clear precipitating events for the onset, but the course may be protracted leading to considerable disability. In particular, the depersonalisation may suggest temporal lobe epilepsy, and other clinical features such as déjà vu experiences and perceptual disorders may further confuse the diagnosis. In their study, 30 cases of phobic anxiety-depersonalisation syndrome were compared to 30 patients with clearly defined epilepsy, which was probably the result of a focal lesion in the temporal lobes. A number of features clearly distinguished these two groups of patients which are outlined in Table 9.3. The phobic group had an older age of onset than the epileptic group, and in 28 of the former the disorder could be related to traumatic experiences immediately preceding onset, whereas the first epileptic attacks usually began out of the blue. Bereavement was a particularly common precursor of the neurotic illness, and only rarely was it impossible to identify precipitating factors from the history. The depersonalisation in the phobic patients was often associated with a sensation of fear, and some reported being drowsy; however in no case was it accompanied by aphasia, or clinical evidence of clouding of consciousness. Déjà vu and jamais vu were equally common in the two groups, although in the epileptic patients the experience was often extremely vivid and in PADS often continued for long

Table 9.3 Features distinguishing the phobic-anxiety-depersonalisation syndrome from temporal lobe epilepsy (after Harper & Roth 1962)

PADS	TLE
Family history of neurosis	*Severe birth trauma, prolonged anoxia, head injury with loss of consciousness, meningitis, encephalitis, mastoiditis
*Migraine Phobias in childhood *Episodic anxiety	
	Episodic speech disturbance Automatic behaviour Complete loss of consciousness
*No change of consciousness *Derealisation Loss of feeling of familiarity *Termination gradual	
	*Self-injury Incontinence Attacks followed by amnesia
*Phobias *Persistent anxiety *Depressive episodes *Feelings of unsteadiness *Irrational fears *Hypochondriacal symptoms Immaturity Dependence	
*One or more attacks a day	Epileptic EEG

* Highly significant

periods of time. The attacks themselves were experienced with greater frequency in the neurotic patients, often more than once a day, but in both groups they were preceded by a feeling of tension or anxiety, and began abruptly. However, the speed at which the attacks terminated was markedly different in the two groups, except where postictal confusion was noted. The EEG helped discriminate between the groups, although over one-third of the patients would fail to be classified by this index alone. Mild or non-specific abnormalities and in some cases sharp waves over the temporal regions were described in the neurotic patients, and were not of value in differentiation.

In further studies, Harper (1971) used both discriminant function analysis and principal component analysis to examine differences between the two groups. Items which had a strong relationship to neurotic disorder included sustained anxiety, phobias, and onset after stress, whereas phenomena such as the déjà vu and depersonalisation were relatively unimportant. An analysis of five items led to complete separation between the two groups, and these were the electroencephalogram, persistent anxiety, frequency of attacks, phobic anxiety symptoms, and stress at the onset of illness. 15 patients were noted in whom the diagnosis had been extremely difficult since they presented with clinical features of both neuroses and epilepsy. The mean age of this group was higher than the neurotic and the epileptic groups alone, as was the mean age of onset of illness. In nearly all of them the attacks began after stress, and a history of phobic anxiety, depression, or suicidal attempts were common, as were neurotic personality traits and a history of neurotic traits in childhood. On the five-item scale, only one case fell within the epileptic range, and on follow-up three to nine years later it was concluded that 12 of these 15 patients had neurotic illness without epilepsy.

In treatment, the PADS is best managed with MAOI antidepressants, while episodes of panic and anxiety respond well to minor tranquillisers, and poorly to conventional anticonvulsants. In particular, drugs of the benzodiazepine variety, as opposed to the barbiturate variety, are recommended.

Rage attacks, as ictal events, although described, are rare but aggression may occur postictally, especially in a confused patient who is forcibly contained. In these situations the aggression is poorly directed and there is usually more danger of the patient harming himself than others. However, recurrent outbursts of aggressive behaviour are almost never epileptic, often being related to a personality disorder, or to a lowered threshold for the release of aggression following brain damage. Mark & Ervin (1970) described the episodic dyscontrol syndrome. In this condition patients have repeated episodes of violence, often associated with abnormal EEG activity, especially temporal lobe disturbances, which may respond to anticonvulsant therapy.

Fugue states are prolonged episodes of amnesia associated with wandering that are associated with a variety of psychopathologies. The amnesia lasts hours, weeks, or occasionally years, and if related to psychiatric disability such as depression is usually seen in the setting of escape from difficult or intolerable circumstances (Stengel 1941). Unlike epileptic automatisms, which are briefer, the patient remains in contact with the environment and is able to manipulate it successfully, thus acting appropriately and failing to draw much attention to himself from others.

References

Abbott R J, Browning M C K, Davison D L W 1980 Serum prolactin and cortisol concentrations after grand mal seizures. J. Neurol. Neurosurg. & Psychiat. 43:163–167

Barham Carter A 1949 Prognosis of certain hysterical symptoms. Br. med. J. 1:1076–1078

Bickerstaff E R 1961 Basilar artery migraine. Lancet 1:15–17

Bowden A N, Gilliatt R W, Willison R G 1975 The place of EEG telemetry and closed-circuit television in the diagnosis and management of epileptic patients. Proc. R. Soc. Med. 68:246–248

Brain R 1963 The concept of hysteria in the time of William Harvey. Proc. R. Soc. Med. 61:321–323

Charcot J M 1877 Lectures on the diseases of the nervous system. (transl. Sigerson G) New Sydenham Society, London

Cheyne G 1733 The English malady. London

Chodoff P, Lyons H 1958 Hysteria, the hysterical personality and 'hysterical conversion'. Am. J. Psychiat. 114:734–740

Desai B T, Porter R J, Penry J K 1979 The psychogenic seizure by videotape analysis: a study of 42 attacks in six patients. Neurology 29:602

Fisher C M, Adams R D 1964 Transient global amnesia. Acta neurol. Scand. 40:suppl. 9 p 1–83

Freud S, Breuer J 1893–1895 Studies on hysteria. Penguin Books Ltd, Middlesex 1974

Gilliatt R W 1977 Syncope. Medicine 31:1999–2005

Gowers W R 1893 A manual of diseases of the nervous system. J & A Churchill, London

Gowers W R 1907 The borderland of epilepsy. Philadelphia, Maryland, USA

Guze S B, Perley M J 1963 Observations on the natural history of hysteria. Am. J. Psychiat. 119:960–965

Hafeiz H B 1980 Hysterical conversion: a prognostic study. Brit. J. Psychiat. 136:548–551

Harper M 1971 Temporal lobe epilepsy and neurosis. MD Thesis, University of Queensland

Harper M, Roth M 1962 Temporal lobe epilepsy and the phobic anxiety-depersonalisation syndrome. Comprehensive Psychiat. 3:129–151, 215–226

Henry J A, Woodruff G H A 1978 A diagnostic sign in states of apparent unconsciousness. Lancet 2:920–921

Jackson J H 1931–2 Selected writings of John Hughlings Jackson. Taylor J (ed) 2 volumes. Hodder & Stoughton, London

Janet P 1907 The major symptoms of hysteria. Macmillan Company, London

Janet P 1931 L'état mental des hystériques. Felix Alcon, Paris

Jeavons P M 1977 Choice of drug therapy in epilepsy. Practitioner 219:542–556

Jelliffe S E, White W A 1929 Diseases of the nervous system. H K Lewis, London

Krapf E E 1957 On the pathogenesis of epileptic and hysterical seizures. Bulletin of the World Health Organisation 16:749–762

Laurès G, Gascard E 1920 Variation du taux de l'urée dans le liquide céphalorachidien prévalé au moment et en dehors des crises convulsive épileptiques et hystériques. La Presse médicale 28:396–397

Lazare A, Klerman G L, Armor D J 1970 Oral, obsessive and hysterical personality patterns. J. psychiat. Res. 7:275–290

Lehrman P R 1925 In discussion. Some psychological data regarding the interpretation of essential epilepsy. J. Nerv. Ment. Dis. 51:55

Lennox W G 1939 John of Gaddesden on epilepsy. Ann. med. Hist. 3rd Series 1:No. 3, 283–307

Ljungberg L 1957 Hysteria. Acta psychiat. scand. Suppl. 112

Lombroso C T, Lerman P 1967 Breathholding spells. Paediatrics 39:563–581

Mark V H, Ervin E R 1970 Violence and the brain. Harper & Row, London

Matthews W B 1970 Practical neurology. Blackwells, Oxford

Mechanic D 1968 Medical sociology: a selective view. The Free Press, New York

Meldrum B S, Horton R W, Bloom S R, Butler J, Keenan J 1979 Endocrine factors and glucose metabolism during prolonged seizures in baboons. Epilepsia 20:527–534

Merskey H 1979 The analysis of hysteria. Ballière Tindall, London

Merskey H, Boyd D B 1978 Emotional adjustment and chronic pain. Bulletin of the London Psychiatric Hospital, Ontario. 1:111–125

Merskey H, Buhrich N A 1975 Hysteria and organic brain disease. Brit. J. med. Psychol. 48:359–366

Merskey H, Trimble M R 1979 Personality, sexual adjustment, and brain lesions in patients with conversion symptoms. Am. J. Psychiat. 136:2, 179–182

O'Donohue N V 1979 Epilepsies of childhood. Butterworths, Boston

Oxley J, Roberts M, Dana Haeri J, Trimble M 1980 Evaluation of prolonged 4-channel EEG taped recordings and serum prolactin levels in the diagnosis of epileptic and non-epileptic fits. In: Epilsepsy: proceedings of the 12th international symposium. Raven Press (in press)

Pierce Clark L 1923 The psychobiologic concept of essential epilepsy. J. Nerv. Ment. Dis. 57:433–444

Pilowsky I 1977 The classification of abnormal illness behaviour. Brit. J. med. Psychol. 51:131–137

Porter R J, Penry J K, Lacy J R 1977 Diagnostic and therapeutic re-evaluation of patients with intractable epilepsy. Neurology 27:1006–1011

Purtell J J, Robins E, Cohen M E 1951 Observations on clinical aspects of hysteria. J. Am. med. Ass. 146:902–910

Purves-Stewart J 1920 The diagnosis of nervous diseases. Butler & Tanner, London

Rabe F 1966 Hysterische Anfälle bei Epilepsie. Den Nervenarzt 37:141–147.

Rabe F 1970 Diagnostische probleme bei den unterscheidung von hysterischen und epileptischen anfällen. Der Nervenarzt. 41:426–429

Reed J L 1975 The diagnosis of hysteria. Psychol. Med. 5:13–17

Rowan A J, Binnie C D, Overweg J, Kamp T, de Vries J 1979 The value of prolonged EEG/video monitoring as a routine diagnostic procedure in epilepsy. In: Canger R et al (eds) Advances in epileptology. Raven Press, New York, p 139–142

Roy A 1977 Hysterical fits previously diagnosed as epilepsy. Psychol. Med. 7:271–273

Roy A 1979 Hysterical seizures. Arch. Neurol. 36:447

Schott G D, McLeod A A, Jewitt D E 1977 Cardiac arrhythmias that masquerade as epilepsy. Brit. med. J. 1:1454–1457

Simon B 1978 Mind and madness in Ancient Greece. Cornell University Press

Slater E 1965 Diagnosis of 'hysteria'. Brit. med. J. 1:1395–1399

Stefanis C, Markidis M, Christodoulou G 1976 Observations on the evolution of hysterical symptomatology. Brit. J. Psychiat. 128:269–275

Stengel E 1941 On the aetiology of fugue states. J. ment. Sci. 37:572–599

Stephenson J B P 1978 Reflex anoxic seizures. Archs Dis. Childh., 53:193–200

Stern D B 1977 Lateral distribution of conversion reactions. J. Nerv. ment. Dis. 164:122–128

Tempkin O 1971 The falling sickness. Johns Hopkins Press, Baltimore

Todd R B 1856 Clinical lectures on paralysis, certain diseases of the brain, and other affections of the nervous system. London

Trimble M R 1978 Serum prolactin in epilepsy and hysteria. Brit. med. J. 2:1682

Trimble M R 1981 Neuropsychiatry. John Wiley & Sons, Chichester
Veith I 1965 Hysteria: the history of a disease. University of Chicago Press
Whitlock F A 1967 The aetiology of hysteria. Acta psychiat. Scand. 43:144–162
Whitwell J R 1936 Historical notes on psychiatry. H K Lewis & Co., London
Williams D 1975 The borderland of epilepsy revisited. Brain 98:1–12
Willis T 1684 An essay of the pathology of the brain and nervous stock in which convulsive diseases are treated. (Transl. Pordage S) Dring, Leigh & Harper

Psychoses of epilepsy

According to conventional usage the term 'psychoses of epilepsy' applies to certain abnormal mental states and disorders associated with, or part of, seizure disorders. If there is a certain illogicality in subsuming under the same title heading conditions so diverse as minor status epilepticus, a neurological entity lasting often for a matter of hours only, and chronic psychotic states of unknown aetiology, it has the merit of widespread familiarity and general acceptance.

CLASSIFICATION

1. Psychoses directly related to the occurrence of seizure activity.
a. Abnormal mental states that are a direct and immediate consequence of underlying seizure activity and which may have some of the features of a psychotic state:
(i)   continuous auras
(ii) petit mal status
(iii) temporal lobe status
b. Postictal psychoses
2. Interictal psychoses
(a)   schizophrenia-like and paranoid psychoses
(b)   affective psychoses
The above description reflects, I think, fairly accurately prevailing views among British and American psychiatrists and has been stated in similar form elsewhere (Fenton 1978). It can readily be compared with the classification suggested by Betts et al (1976) (see Chapter 2) which divides the interictal psychoses into two principal categories and employs a third category termed 'organic psychosyndromes' to cover psychotic disorders directly related to epileptic activity. It takes no account of the brief periodic psychoses, including dysphoric states and alternating psychoses [a clinical entity that draws heavily on Landolt's (1958) theory of forced normalisation] and in this differs from the classification of Bruens (1974) which has wide currency among European psychiatrists. This is not to take an unduly partial view; the above classification may ultimately prove oversimplified, but in the present state of knowledge further subcategorisation seems unjustified.

PSYCHOSES DIRECTLY RELATED TO THE OCCURRENCE OF SEIZURE ACTIVITY

These range from organic confusional states, such as petit mal status, in which the classical features of psychosis may be completely lacking, to certain postictal psychoses in which typical psychotic phenomena may be observed in a setting of clear consciousness.

Continuous auras

Scott & Masland (1953) have described the appearance of prolonged auras following the successful institution of anticonvulsant therapy. 12 out of a consecutive series of 100 patients were so afflicted. Elementary sensory and motor auras were described, but visual and psychic auras were the most commonly encountered. The majority of patients had temporal lobe foci. The continuous aura usually represented a progression of the original aura but was occasionally a new development. It could be abolished either by increasing the drug dosage or, paradoxically, by drug withdrawal, thus permitting a major seizure to occur.

Petit mal status

This condition has reappeared under a number of descriptive terms since Lennox (1945) first reported it, e.g., 'epileptic twilight state' (Zappoli 1955), 'spike-wave stupor' (Niederemeyer & Khalifeh 1965). This probably reflects a growing recognition of the aetiological heterogeneity of what at first appeared a unitary condition.

The incidence of petit mal status among patients with primary generalised epilepsy is 6.2 per cent (Dalby 1969). Two-thirds of patients will already have experienced episodes of petit mal and most of the remainder will have grand mal seizures. Evidence of temporal lobe epilepsy is rare (Andermann & Robb 1972, Roger 1974) but is described (Jaffe 1962). Occasionally, and this is particularly so in the case of late onset, there is no previous history of epilepsy (Ellis & Lee 1978). In 75 per cent of cases the onset is before the age of 20 (Roger 1974) but there have been recent reports of first episodes in later life (Schwartz & Scott 1971). The onset may be gradual or abrupt and the duration variable, ranging from a few hours to a month or more. The salient clinical characteristic is an impairment of consciousness, which at its very least may be demonstrable only with the aid of sophisticated psychometric testing (Rennick et al 1969), but at its most profound results in a level of stupor resistant to all but intense and painful stimuli. In between, varying degrees of withdrawal, retardation, muteness and physical incoordination may be observed. Such attacks remit spontaneously but may be terminated by intravenous diazepam. Subsequently the extent of amnesia varies according to the degree of clouding and is by no means invariable.

Associated convulsive signs are found in approximately 50 per cent of cases. Fluttering of the eyelids is common and myoclonus of the upper limbs may also occur. Major seizures may develop during the episode and can terminate it. Brief automatisms may be observed particularly when true status with intervals of normal electric activity obtains rather than a single prolonged episode. The EEG may show generalised spike and wave activity with a frontal emphasis and a frequency of $1\frac{1}{2}$–$4\frac{1}{2}$ Hz (Roger 1974), but other authors have remarked on the predominance of multiple spike discharge (Andermann & Robb 1972).

Abnormal mental states other than clouding are distinctly uncommon and seem only to occur in atypical cases. Ellis & Lee (1978) have described six cases of late onset petit mal status in the absence of any previous history of epilepsy. Psychotic features including paranoid delusional ideation, visual and auditory hallucinations and thought blocking were described. However most of the cases had some kind of underlying metabolic disturbance. Wells (1975) has also reported on two middle-aged women in whom petit mal status presented as a depressive psychosis. One was receiving treatment for myxoedema and lacked any previous history of epilepsy. It seems possible therefore that metabolic disorders may in some way predispose towards the belated appearance of petit mal status.

In younger patients prolonged episodes, referred to by Lugaresi et al (1971) as 'absence status', may be associated with an abnormal EEG pattern and with mental dullness and lack of response to treatment. Such cases merge imperceptibly with the Lennox-Gastaut syndrome and some authors (Roger et al 1974) have argued that they should be classified separately. The appearance of mental confusion, clouding or stupor as a new and unexplained event should always prompt thoughts of petit mal status particularly in a child or young adult with primary generalised epilepsy. EEG examination will provide rapid confirmation and response to intravenous diazepam is usually prompt.

Psychomotor status

More than one author (Oller-Daurella 1970, Roger et al 1974) has remarked on the surprising rarity of temporal lobe status considering the frequency of temporal lobe epilepsy. Indeed it is only in the last decade that detailed reports of the condition have been published (Escueta et al 1974, Markand et al 1978). Such episodes may last from hours to days and may be ushered in or terminated by a major seizure. The patient is confused, withdrawn and retarded. Markand et al (1978) noted continuous movements of the hands, picking at clothes, and lip smacking, but Escueta et al (1974) were able to detect a recurring pattern in which for long periods the patient, although withdrawn, was able to respond to stimulation with simple but coordinated behaviour. These were interspersed with brief episodes of total unresponsiveness associated with spontaneous automatisms. The background EEG activity showed a unifocal, predominantly medial temporal lobe discharge, but during the latter episodes the discharge was bilateral and spread to involve the prefrontal and lateral temporal areas. In both studies periods of relatively normal EEG activity were interposed between attacks. The episodes were terminated by parenteral administration of anticonvulsants.

Postictal psychosis

This is probably the most commonly encountered ictus-related mental disturbance, although one of the least reported on. Dongier's (1959) extensive compilation of acute psychotic episodes may well contain a substantial number, if not a majority, of postictal states, but the temporal relationship of the psychotic state to seizure activity is nowhere made explicit. The most detailed account is provided by Levin (1952). In his series of 52 cases, males predominated (71 per cent). The average age was between 30 and 40 years. All but four of the cases were thought to have idiopathic epilepsy and in the majority the episodes began within 24 hours of a cluster of major seizures. All showed signs of confusion and half were aggressive and excited. Suicidal attempts were not uncommon and approximately one-quarter were either hallucinated or deluded. Hallucinations were usually in the auditory modality and delusions were almost always paranoid in content. Most had moderate to severe epilepsy and 20 per cent had had a similar episode before. Recovery was usually complete within one week. This description is entirely consistent with that of Clark & Lesko's earlier (1939) report. They also noted the marked tendency towards excitement and overactivity in contrast to the retardation and withdrawal characteristic of petit mal status. Treatment is symptomatic and best achieved by drugs of the butyrophenone group, e.g. haloperidol.

THE INTERICTAL PSYCHOSES

This term is used here to refer to certain chronic psychotic disorders, each of which has its counterpart among the functional psychoses. The schizophrenia-like, paranoid and affective psychoses that occur in association with epilepsy run a remitting and relapsing course with a tendency to chronicity. In contrast to the ictus-related psychotic states, the relationship between the interictal psychoses and the epileptic process is uncertain and controversial, and each disorder may run its course to a large extent independently of the other. Although there is some evidence that chronic psychotic states may occasionally develop after a series of confusional episodes (Slater et al 1963), ictus-related and interictal psychoses are best regarded as separate and, for the most part, unrelated groups of disorders.

Historical background
In a general sense epilepsy and schizophrenia may be related in one of three ways and this has given rise to three hypotheses: the theories of affinity, biological antagonism and coincidental association. Observations in support of each viewpoint can be encountered at an early date. Kraepelin (1910) refers to epileptiform attacks or attacks of dizziness and fainting spells in 16 per cent of patients with dementia praecox in his Munich clinic. For the next two decades there were frequent reports noting the prevalence of epileptic seizures among psychotic patients; the development of psychotic illness in epileptics was less commonly commented on. There was little general agreement. Some authors report a greater than expected prevalence of seizures (e.g. Vorkastner 1918), but interpretation is made more difficult by the obvious uncertainty in the writers' own minds in making a diagnostic distinction between epilepsy and giddiness (Kraepelin 1910), hysteria (Bleuler 1911) and catatonic manifestations (Urstein 1909). Later contributors took a more sceptical view. Krapf (1928), in a major review, dismissed the affinity hypothesis, but admitted that seizures occasionally occurred, a feature he regarded as part of the schizophrenic process. Esser (1938) noted a greater prevalence of epilepsy, but only after a considerable interval and was cautious in formulating any causal relationship.

In 1931 Muller (1931) reported on two catatonic patients who had partially recovered following spontaneous convulsions. Three years later Meduna introduced artificially induced convulsion therapy as a treatment for psychotic states. The 'antagonism' hypothesis gained support from fresh reports of low rates of association between epilepsy and schizophrenia (Wyrsch 1933, Kat 1937). The emerging era of EEG research offered a new means for investigating this relationship. Early studies failed to agree on the pathological nature of the EEG in schizophrenia although it was generally accepted that such abnormalities as did exist were less specific than in epilepsy. The EEG was considered essentially normal by several investigators (Berger 1931, Travis & Malamud 1937) or non-specifically abnormal (Jasper et al 1939, Davis 1940). One additional difficulty was the failure to establish distinct criteria for the EEG diagnosis of temporal lobe epilepsy, so that abnormalities in schizophrenia were often open to misinterpretation.

The next two decades witnessed a changing understanding of the temporal relationship between schizophrenia and epilepsy. Psychotic illness was seen to develop in the course of epilepsy rather than the reverse. This was first viewed as a symptomatic schizophrenia (Gruhle 1936). Later writers (Hill 1953, Pond 1957, Slater et al 1963) delineated a syndrome closely resembling schizophrenia but differing clinically in certain subtle but distinctive features and, perhaps more importantly, lacking evidence of a genetic predisposition. Temporal lobe epilepsy was implicated to a greater extent than other forms of epilepsy.

The most recent developments concerned a search for aetiological explanations. The role of lateralised cerebral dysfunction in relation to different phenomenological patterns of psychotic illness has been the subject of intensive investigation and has been paralleled by developments within epilepsy (Flor-Henry 1969). A growing interest in mechanisms underlying anticonvulsant action and the expansion of knowledge relating to central neurotransmitter function have resulted in biochemical hypotheses that seek to explain the observed increased association between epilepsy and psychosis as an artefact of complex drug side effects, and to assume a primary biological antagonism between the two disorders (Reynolds 1968).

By now it will be apparent that most of the reported work on interictal psychoses is concerned principally, or exclusively, with schizophrenia-like and paranoid states; cases of affective psychosis often form part of a mixed series (e.g. Flor-Henry 1969) but have yet to be dealt with in depth. As a diagnostic grouping they have not been given sufficient definition. For example, in Jensen & Larsen's (1979) series affective and schizo-affective psychoses were combined in the same category. It is likely that depressive symptoms, often of considerable severity, occur frequently among epileptics. In Betts' (1974) cohort of epileptic patients admitted in one single year into psychiatric care in the city of Birmingham, nearly a third were suffering from depressive symptoms; and depressive illness, endogenous type (17 per cent) and reactive type (14 per cent) were the two diagnoses most commonly made. However, it is not made clear what proportion, if any, of these patients were psychotically depressed. The same uncertainty applies to other studies. Pathological elevation of mood is probably uncommon. No cases were detected in two Maudsley Hospital series (Toone & Driver 1980, Pahla et al 1978). There are therefore no firm grounds at present for supposing the incidence of affective psychoses among epileptic patients to be greater than expected, nor does it appear that either of the two disorders, when they do occur together, have any distinguishing characteristics or are in any way atypical.

Prevalence

It is not easy to obtain a reliable and convincing estimate of the true prevalence of interictal psychotic states in association with epilepsy. There are a number of reasons for this. Persuasive arguments have been advanced that the effects of anticonvulsant drug therapy on folate metabolism (Reynolds 1968) and on central monoamine availability (Trimble 1977) may increase the risk of psychotic illness. It has also been suggested, on rather more slender grounds, that neuroleptic drugs may precipitate epilepsy. The possibility of an association between epilepsy and psychosis was recognised as early as 1854 (Falret) but there is little reliable information relating to prevalence statistics antedating the introduction of phenobarbitone in 1912. The prescription of anticonvulsant medication is virtually universal but Asuni & Pillutla (1967) have reported eleven schizophrenia-like psychotic states among a consecutive unselected series of 42 epileptic patients in Western Nigeria. Seven were untreated and four had received drugs only irregularly. Such a prevalence would of course be unusually high by Western standards and may be attributable to pathoplastic factors reflecting local cultural beliefs.

Ideally, estimates of prevalence should be ascertained in an unselected population. A number of community-based epidemiological studies of epilepsy have been carried out, e.g. Kurland (1969), but little account has been taken of psychiatric morbidity. Krohn (1960) examined 908 epileptics in northern Norway and identified 16 (2 per cent) patients who were, or had been, psychotic. In a study based on 14 general practices, Pond & Bidwell (1960) reported on 245 epileptic patients from a total population of 39 500. 29 per cent experienced psychological difficulties, but no cases of psychosis were noted.

Estimates drawn from selected populations are more plentiful but may be misleading. Studies based on neurology clinic attendance have reported the prevalence of psychotic illness among epileptics in general to be 4.4 per cent (Small & Small, 1967) and 2.4 per cent (Bruens 1974); and 2 per cent when only temporal lobe epileptics were considered (Currie et al 1971). However, Standage & Fenton (1975) examined 27 consecutive neurology outpatients and identified three (8 per cent) with a history of a previous psychotic episode, although none were receiving treatment at the time of the study.

Higher prevalence rates are encountered among series comprised of more intractible cases, or of patients undergoing intensive investigation. Thus Falconer (1973) found a pre-surgery psychosis rate of 16 per cent among those referred for temporal lobectomy, many of whom had come from a psychiatric hospital; while Lindsay et al (1979) followed up 87 children with limbic seizures for over a decade and found that nine (10.3 per cent) had developed a schizophreniform psychosis. As most of these subjects are still young adults this is almost certainly a substantial underestimate of lifetime risk.

Studies based on mental hospital populations reveal a different pattern. The proportion of epileptics may well remain constant: 4.3 per cent (Liddell

1953), 5.4 per cent (Betts 1974), and 5.3 per cent (Mann & Cree 1976). Rather surprisingly Liddell's detailed report makes no mention of any chronic psychotic states. Standage (1973) scrutinised a mental hospital population of 1835 patients. 53 were epileptic, 28 suitable for interview, and eight psychotic. Betts (1974) screened admissions to four mental hospitals over a six-year period. 72 patients received a diagnosis of epilepsy and of these 12 were endogenously depressed and three were considered to have a paranoid psychosis.

The admission rate to specialist referral centres is quite different. Slater et al (1963) ascertained 69 fresh cases of schizophrenia-like psychosis over an eleven year period at the National Hospital for Nervous Diseases and the Maudsley Hospital. The authors argued that this referral rate was so greatly in excess of that which would have been predicted on the basis of a coincidental combination of the two disorders that a positive association must be assumed. These findings were not confirmed by Bartlet (1957) and Slater's conclusions have been criticised on the grounds of selective referral (Stevens 1966). At the time of writing any attempt to arbitrate between these diverse explanations would be imprudent; nevertheless there remains a strong impression that in those studies in which follow-up has been comprehensive and painstaking (the work of Lindsay et al is a case in point) the prevalence of psychosis is greater than generally recognised. One caution should be emphasised. In any estimate of prevalence, the diagnostic criteria employed by the researcher merits consideration. Bleulerian concepts have to a considerable extent been replaced by more objectifiable operational definitions, e.g. Feighner's criteria (Feighner et al 1972). Even so a broader view of schizophrenia is still held in some European countries and in the United States in particular. Thus Ervin et al (1975) reported a diagnosis of schizophrenia in 81 per cent of 42 patients with unilateral or bilateral temporal spike foci.

Geographical Distribution

The vast majority of studies have come from Europe and North America but schizophrenia-like psychoses have been reported from India (Shukla et al 1979), West Africa (Asuna & Pillutla 1967) and Japan (Sawa 1963).

Clinical presentation

These disorders have acquired an extensive early literature particularly in German psychiatry. They are also the subject of numerous case reports. In the interests of brevity this review will place principal emphasis on recent publications comprising substantial series of subjects (Slater et al 1963, Flor-Henry 1969, Bruens 1971, Taylor 1972).

An association between epilepsy and schizophrenia was noted among others by Kraepelin (1910), but the more modern concept of a distinctive syndrome in which the clinical phenomenology resembles but is not identical to functional schizophrenia, a genetically determined predisposition is lacking and a particular association with temporal lobe epilepsy is apparent, owes its recognition to Hill (1953) who introduced the term 'chronic paranoid hallucinatory psychosis'. This view was endorsed in a review by Pond (1957), but a major descriptive analysis awaited the series of studies by Slater et al (1963). These authors ascertained those patients with a diagnosis of epilepsy and schizophrenia referred to two postgraduate hospitals (see above). Case selection was limited to those in whom epilepsy presented first. In terms of clinical presentation four groups of patients were identified; those in whom repeated, short-lived confusional episodes developed into a chronic psychosis (11 cases); two further groups, one closely resembling paranoid schizophrenia (46 cases), the other hebephrenic schizophrenia (eight cases); and finally a group of four patients whose epilepsy was of the petit mal type. This classification is, as Symonds has pointed out (Beard & Slater 1962), inconsistent in that the first three groups refer to the pattern of presentation of psychosis, the fourth to a particular type of epilepsy. No control group was used.

Two other British studies are of major importance. Flor-Henry (1969) compared 50 patients with temporal lobe epilepsy and psychosis (21 with a diagnosis of schizophrenia, 11 schizo-affective, nine manic depressive, and nine confusional states) with 50 epileptic non-psychotic controls, half of whom had been drawn from psychiatric referrals, half from referrals to a neurosurgical unit for consideration of lobectomy. The principal findings relating to laterality will be discussed later. Taylor (1972) has reported on the prevalence of psychosis among patients referred for temporal lobectomy and has related clinical features to histopathological findings.

Among recent European work the contribution of Bruens (1971) is outstanding. 19 cases were studied and categorized thus: those who experienced systematized paranoid delusions (nine cases); a group characterized by mental regression, bizarre behaviour and transient paranoid symptoms (5); schizophrenia-like psychoses (2) and confusional states of short duration (3), two of whom were diagnosed as primary subcortical epilepsy. The psychotic characteristics of the second group of patients are not particularly convincing, whilst it could be argued that the last group belong with the ictus-related psychoses. The complete absence of patients with affective psychosis is unexpected. However, Bruens observed that grandiose delusions formed the second most common type of delusion and it may be that some of these cases would be reclassified as manic-depressive psychotics by other authorities. Particular mention should also be made of work emanating from two neurosurgical centres for temporal lobectomy (Kristensen & Sindrup 1978a, 1978b, 1979, Jensen & Larsen 1979) as this affords the rare opportunity to relate clinical and pathological findings.

Certain clinical features and correlates will now be considered.

Sex distribution
The sex distribution of schizophrenia-like psychosis appears to be fairly even (Table 10.1), but the subject is of interest because, as Taylor (1971) has pointed out, in epilepsy males predominate in a ratio of 140:100. This observation is given added weight by the fact that between the ages of 15 and 35 (the period during which onset of psychosis in association with epilepsy is most likely to take place) admission rates for schizophrenia are substantially higher for males (Slater & Roth 1969). Taylor deduced that either females with epilepsy are more prone to psychosis, or that psychotic patients are drawn from a special sub-population of epileptics in which sex ratios are more equal. The latter explanation is more likely to be correct. A major study of unselected temporal lobe epileptics (Currie et al

Table 10.1 Salient characteristics of the interictal psychoses

Authors	n	Type of psychoses M = mixed S = schizophrenia-like P = paranoid	Male:Female	Age of onset epilepsy	Age of onset psychosis	interval	EEG % temporal lobe foci	% bilateral involvement
Bartlett (1957)	11	M					72	
Slater et al (1963)	69	S	46:33	15	30	15	80	25
Flor-Henry (1969)	50	M	26:24	13			*	44
Bruens (1971)	19	M	8:11	13	25	12	84	30
Taylor (1972)	13	M	5:8					20
Jensen & Larsen (1979)	20	M		14	28	14	*	
Kristensen & Sindrup (1978 a & b, 1980)	96	P	46:50	12	34	22	*	30
Perez & Trimble (1980)	23	M	15:8					
Toone & Driver (1980)	41	M						

* Selection limited to temporal lobe epilepsy

severely handicapped patients referred for special investigation with a view to surgery there is no sex difference (C. Polkey, personal communication).

Predisposition to psychosis

This may be judged on the basis of family history and on the presence or absence of characterological traits observed more commonly in those who ultimately develop schizophrenia.

Genetics

Earlier studies based on small case numbers reported a high incidence of psychosis among the relatives of psychotic epileptics (Krapf 1928, Glaus 1931). More recent work has been largely negative.

The most careful genetic study has been carried out by Slater et al (1963). In their series of 69 patients, one patient had a paranoid, two a schizophrenic, relative. These rates do not exceed the prevalence in the general population and are considerably less than in schizophrenia. This was confirmed by Flor-Henry (1969). Jensen & Larsen (1979) reported an excess of major psychiatric illness among the families of psychotic epileptic patients undergoing temporal lobe surgery compared with psychotic controls; however, they do not provide any information regarding psychiatric diagnosis.

Premorbid personality

An assessment of premorbid personality is always difficult, based as it must be to a large extent, on retrospective information. The problem here is compounded by the fact that the prepsychotic personality may well be influenced by the presence of epilepsy. Thus Slater et al (1963) found evidence of an 'epileptic personality', e.g., irritability, stubbornness, and aggressiveness, in 13 of their patients, but only two were described as schizoid and nine paranoid. All of these undesirable traits were associated with a relatively early onset of epilepsy. They considered that there were no grounds for suspecting personality abnormalities of a kind associated with vulnerability to schizophrenia. Bruens (1971) considered that normal premorbid personality was present in 16 of his 19 cases and reached a similar conclusion. In Jensen & Larsen's (1979) series psychotic epileptics were of higher intelligence and academic achievement than their epileptic non-psychotic controls. Flor-Henry (1969) found no excess of abnormal childhood experience in his psychotic group compared with controls, although within the psychotic group schizo-affective and affective psychotic patients fared better than schizophrenics.

Age of onset of schizophrenia

In most published series the age of onset occurs during the period spanning the middle of the third and fourth decades (Table 10.1). Slater & Moran (1969) have calculated the expected mean age of onset of psychosis, on the assumption that epileptic and psychotic processes are independent of one another. In each sex the onset was earlier than predicted, but significantly so only for women. Taylor (1971) confirmed that onset for women was earlier than for men (the opposite is the case in process schizophrenia) and that this was so in the case of onset of epilepsy also.

The relationship between the onset of epilepsy and schizophrenia

In their original publication Slater et al (1963) noted a correlation of 0.58 between the ages of onset and concluded that the development of psychosis was, to some extent, dependent on duration of epilepsy. It was later pointed out that, as their ascertainment criteria specifically excluded patients in whom the psychosis appeared first, such a statistical procedure was invalid, an observation the authors later acknowledged as correct (Slater & Moran 1969). Nevertheless, there is general agreement that psychosis usually follows the onset of epilepsy and that the interval may vary between 12 and 23 years (Table 10.1). This cannot be explained entirely in terms of the relative ages of onset of the two conditions when occurring independently of one another. Although temporal lobe epilepsy has a wider spread of age of onset, only a quarter of cases start before the age of 15 (Currie et al 1971), while the peak epoch is between 25 and 50. First admission for schizophrenia lies between 20 and 40 for two-thirds to three-quarters of subjects (Bleuler 1978).

If the two disorders occur independently one might expect a greater proportion of cases in which schizophrenia occurs first, particularly as Taylor (1971) has shown that, among cases referred for temporal lobe surgery, psychotic patients have a relatively late onset of epilepsy. On the other hand, if the development of a schizophrenia-like psychosis of epilepsy requires an interval of between one and two decades after the appearance of the epilepsy it is surprising that there are not more cases in which the psychosis develops in middle age. Only four of Slater's 69 cases had an onset after the age of 50. Part of the explanation may lie in the association between psychosis and certain types of pathology such as hamartomas (Taylor 1975) which are themselves linked with an early onset of epilepsy. Also it may be that in late onset cases the seizure frequency is less, although Currie et al (1971) found that success in control of seizures was independent of age of onset.

Phenomenology

The schizophrenia-like psychoses of epilepsy were first regarded as symptomatic schizophrenias (Gruhle 1936) and it was not thought that their clinical presentation differed in any significant way from functional schizophrenias. Hill (1953) first drew attention to the special relationship with temporal lobe epilepsy and described a paranoid hallucinatory psychotic state. Pond (1957), drawing on the same source of clinical material, emphasized the retention of warm and appropriate affect in contrast to 'true' schizophrenia. Slater & Beard's (1963) series confirmed these earlier findings. All but three of their cases were deluded, although primary delusions were uncommon. Paranoid, mystical, and grandiose delusions were frequently encountered as were feelings of passivity. Most of their patients experienced hallucinations, usually in the auditory modality and half exhibited thought disorder. Disturbances of mood were widespread. They were thought to differ from functional schizophrenics in their lack of catatonic features and the relative absence of affective flattening. Elsewhere Bruens (1971) reported that his largest psychotic group comprised patients with systematised paranoid delusions; Jensen & Larsen (1979) observed that 10 patients showed 'the chronic paranoid state described by Pond and by Slater & Beard'. Kristensen & Sindrup (1979) commented on their series that the 'majority of the patients tended to

1971) found an excess, though non-significant, of female patients. Among more remain in warm, affective contact'. Autistic and catatonic behaviour were exhibited by only one patient.

Thus a clinical syndrome has achieved widespread acceptance. However, it must be admitted that the very fact that the principal authors stem from the same institution and base their experience on an identical source of case referral constitutes something of a weakness. More serious is the absence of any psychiatric control group in any of these studies. Phenomenological description has been based on impression only. More recently Perez & Trimble (1980) have used the Present State Examination (Wing et al 1974) to demonstrate the diagnostic heterogeneity of psychotic states associated with epilepsy. Affective features were particularly prominent.

Mode of onset and subsequent course
In Slater et al's (1963) series just under half presented with an insidious onset, the majority of whom became chronically ill. A third presented acutely and had a better prognosis. The remainder followed an episodic course, half becoming chronic. This pattern is probably not untypical of functional schizophrenia in the absence of organic brain disease.

Outcome
This has been little studied. Slater et al (1963) followed up the majority of their cases until the end of a 10-year period of ascertainment. Approximately half still had psychotic symptoms; a further half, not necessarily the same, suffered psycho-organic sequelae, i.e. perseveration, retardation, pedantry and circumstantiality. In all, only five patients had made a full social recovery. Bruens (1971) also found that half of his patients remained psychotic after 10 years. However, formal cognitive assessment was not carried out in either of these studies and it cannot be assumed with any confidence that progressive intellectual deterioration had taken place.

Epileptic Variables

EEG focus
The development of EEG techniques has allowed more precise localisation of epileptic activity. Temporal lobe epilepsy appears to be more commonly associated with a wide spectrum of psychiatric illnesses than other forms of epilepsy (Gibbs 1951), but this view, though generally accepted, is not without its critics (Small et al 1962). This is not the place to discuss such wide issues. The majority of studies concerned with the schizophrenia-like psychoses of epilepsy have reported a preponderance of temporal lobe foci (Table 10.1). Only one author has reported contrary findings (Standage 1973). Stevens (1966) has criticised Slater's findings, noting that in her own series of unselected cases of epilepsy, 54 per cent had 'temporal-psychomotor seizures' compared with 65 per cent in Slater et al's (1963) series. Leaving aside the question of whether such a difference is significant, it will be noted (Table 10.1) that a computation of data from other available studies yields a figure of 71 per cent (this includes Standage's

finding in which he merely noted that none of his eight patients had psychomotor seizures and that there was no excess of temporal lobe foci). Small et al (1962) have considered this relationship further by taking 50 consecutive epileptic patients, 25 of whom had temporal lobe epilepsy, examining them clinically and submitting them to a battery of psychometric tests, some of which purport to evaluate the presence of psychotic traits. No differences were found between the temporal lobe epileptics and the remainder. However, the size of these groups was such that few if any psychotic patients could be expected; moreover, the authors do not appear to have taken anamnestic data into consideration and place too much importance on psychometric tests of dubious validity in the diagnosis of psychosis. The observation (Stevens 1966) that the association between temporal lobe epilepsy and schizophrenia merely reflects the age distribution of the two disorders is therefore spurious.

Type and frequency of seizures

In two series of psychotic patients unselected for epilepsy (Slater et al 1963, Bruens 1971) psychomotor seizures occurred in the majority of patients; in the third series (Standage 1973) they were absent. Slater et al (1963) based their assessment of seizure frequency on grand mal episodes only and, while admitting the difficulty in making retrospective judgements on observations of this kind, were unable to discriminate between their groups using this criterion and were of the impression that seizure control did not differ between psychotic and non-psychotic patients. Of greater interest are those studies that have compared temporal lobe epileptic and control groups. Kristensen & Sindrup (1978a) observed a reduction in frequency of complex partial seizures in psychotic patients; Flor-Henry (1969) also found less psychomotor and minor temporal attacks. However, Jensen & Larsen (1979) recorded a higher frequency of grand mal, petit mal, focal seizures and automatisms among psychotic patients while Taylor (1972) was unable to establish any relationship between fit frequency and any particular type of mental state.

Type of aura

Karagulla & Robertson (1955) were the first to draw a convincing parallel between the content of the epileptic aura and that of subjective psychotic experience. They did this by comparing the recorded experiences of patients undergoing cortical electrical stimulation immediately prior to surgery in Wilder Penfield's department at the Montreal Neurological Institute with a description of psychotic experiences obtained from psychotic patients in Edinburgh. Thought insertion, 'écho de la pensée', and auditory and visual hallucinations could be elicited during cortical stimulation, usually of the temporal cortex. Pond (Beard & Slater 1962) has raised the possibility that persistent psychotic states may have their basis in the abnormal experience encountered during the ictal and postictal state, but surprisingly little information has been gathered relating specific aura patterns to form and content of psychotic illness. Kristensen & Sindrup (1978a) found, using a classification according to Janz (1969), an excess of automatisms, epigastric and déjà vu auras over 'psychical seizures' among their psychotic group. Jensen & Larsen (1979) described more hallucinations and delusions, presumably in the form of auras, among their psychotic group, while the controls were more prone to visual symptoms. Hermann & Chabrias (1981) have noted an association between ictal fear auras and elevation in the pathological range on five Minnesota Multiphasic Personality Inventory scales including paranoia and schizophrenia.

Causes of Epilepsy

In most studies cause can only be deduced from anamnestic information and must be largely speculative; but in a few instances surgical intervention has made available histopathological confirmation. Slater et al (1963) reported that 28 of their cases gave a history suggestive of a significant cerebral insult. This was distinctly less common in the hebephrenic group. Kristensen & Sindrup (1978a) noted that a history of events liable to result in cerebral damage was more commonly obtainable from psychotic subjects than controls. The controls were more likely to have a family history of epilepsy. Jensen & Larsen (1979) found that psychotic patients had been more often exposed to perinatal complications. They also reported that the psychotic group were more likely to have a focal neuropathological lesion although unfortunately they do not specify the nature of such lesions. This finding was confirmed by Taylor (1975) who observed an association between psychosis and 'alien tissue', a term which was intended to cover small focal tumours, hamartomas, and focal dysplasia. Mesial temporal sclerosis was by contrast under-represented. These findings are not entirely consistent. On one hand the development of psychosis is associated with a history of cerebral insult implying more widespread brain damage; on the other, histological examination shows a predominance of discrete focal rather than diffuse lesions.

Age of onset

Ascertainment criteria for age of onset vary. Thus Slater et al (1963) excluded cases in which psychosis occurred first and ignored isolated seizures in early childhood. Kristensen & Sindrup (1978a) dated onset from the time of the first seizure. Despite this there is a fair measure of agreement. Epilepsy usually appears first in early adolescence (Table 10.1) and this is so whether the series is unselected (Slater et al 1963) or a temporal lobe series (Kristensen & Sindrup 1978a). Comparison with non-psychotic epileptic populations are few. In Kristensen & Sindrup's (1978a) series, the average age of onset for psychotic and non-psychotic groups was 12 and 10 years respectively. Jensen & Larsen (1979) reported a later age of onset for psychotics. In neither series was the difference significant. Taylor (1971) has analysed Slater et al's (1963) data and concluded that the age of onset was earlier in females than males.

Brain damage

As might be predicted, given the association between psychosis and temporal lobe epilepsy, evidence of brain damage is to be found in the majority of cases. Slater et al (1963) reported that air encephalography was abnormal in 70 per cent of their patients. Clinical findings regarded by the authors as indicative of organic change, e.g. perseveration, were usually present but formal psychometry was considered 'uninformative'.

Whether the degree and extent of brain damage contributes to the development of psychosis remains unclear. The majority of controlled studies have been comprised of temporal lobectomy series; conventional criteria for temporal lobe surgery would lead one to suppose that among these series, patients with bilateral brain damage would be under-represented. In any case there is no general agreement. Kristensen & Sindrup (1978a) found that a larger proportion (80 per cent) of their psychotic group had abnormal lumbar air encephalograms; however this was not significant.

Flor-Henry (1969) examined a number of indices of brain damage, but also reported negative findings. However, within the psychotic group, patients with schizophrenia-like psychoses showed more evidence of brain damage than those with manic depressive psychoses. Several authors have observed a comparative excess of bilateral EEG abnormalities among psychotics; others have not (see Table 10.1).

Laterality

Flor-Henry (1969) was the first to report an association between lateralisation of temporal lobe foci and any specific forms of psychosis. Hill (1953) and Pond (1957) had recognised the strength of the relationship between schizophrenia-like psychoses and temporal lobe epilepsy but had failed to comment on any laterality effect. Slater et al (1963) considered the possibility, but obtained negative findings. Flor-Henry reported an association between schizophrenia-like psychosis and left temporal lobe foci, and between manic depressive psychosis and right-sided foci, with schizo-affective psychosis occupying an intermediate position. Subsequent reports have provided confirmation (Gregoriades et al 1971, Sherwin 1977, Lindsay et al 1979, Toone & Driver 1980, Perez & Trimble 1981) and refutation (Kristensen & Sindrup 1978b, Jensen & Larsen 1979). Possible causes for such a diversity of opinion are not hard to discern. There is an excess of sinistrality among epileptics and this may be particularly marked among psychotic epileptics (Kristensen & Sindrup 1978a). In Taylor's (1975) series over half of the cases were left-handed. No immediate assumptions can be made regarding cerebral dominance among such subjects and when they form a sizeable proportion of the sample a confusing variable of some considerable importance is introduced. However, one study which analysed its sample before and after the exclusion of sinistrals still found an excess of left temporal epileptic activity in a ratio of 2:1 (Toone & Driver 1980). The diagnosis of psychosis is all too often poorly defined. Only in recent years have precise operational criteria been used (Toone & Driver 1980, Perez & Trimble 1980). Moreover, the extent to which either schizophrenic or affective features may predominate at varying times in a chronic remitting and relapsing illness is probably insufficiently appreciated by many of the contributors. Toone & Driver (1980) found that inconsistency of diagnosis in those cases who required readmission was such that only two-thirds received the same diagnosis as the first admission on subsequent readmissions.

The same reservations apply to any analysis of the relationship between psychosis and brain damage. Sherwin (1977) reported that, of 14 cases with temporal lobe abnormality on lumbar air encephalogram, 13 were left-sided and one bilateral. However, psychiatric criteria for inclusion in this lobectomy-based series was limited to 'psychotic-like reactions and aggressivity'. Toone & Driver (1980) performed CAT scans on 56 psychotic epileptic patients. Among those with a diagnosis of schizophrenia, left-sided abnormalities were three times as common as those on the right.

Relationship between seizure activity and psychotic symptomatology

Reference has already been made to the EEG phenomenon of 'forced normalisation' (Landolt 1958) and its clinical equivalent, the inverse relationship between symptoms of psychosis and frequency of epileptic seizures. It is likely that these may be more readily observed in association with brief ictus-related psychotic states. Slater et al (1963) reported that in six cases psychotic symptoms appeared at a time when fit frequency was falling. A further four cases showed a fluctuating course and an inverse relationship. Bruens (1971) reported that 12 of 19 cases showed a similar course, but Shukla & Katiyar (1980) noted that as many patients manifested an increase in fit frequency with the onset of psychosis as showed a decrease. Forced normalisation appears an altogether rarer phenomenon; Slater et al noted it in one case, and Bruens in three.

A development that may have implications for Landolt's hypothesis is the emergence reported in several neurosurgical series of psychosis following successful temporal lobectomy. In one study (Jensen & Larsen 1979) nine patients became psychotic in the post-operative follow-up period, six of these after apparent cure of their epileptic seizures. All had displayed severe behavioural disturbances prior to onset of psychosis. Taylor (1972) has also reported post-operative psychosis in three cases.

Aetiology

Any discussion of this topic must first take into account the uncomfortable observation that there is as yet no agreement as to whether chronic psychotic illness develops more commonly in the presence of epilepsy or the converse. Recent studies suggest a positive association (e.g. Slater & Beard 1963) but proponents of the theory of biological antagonism argue that this relationship is artefactual and due to the action of pharmacological agents (Reynolds 1968). Regrettably, little reliance can be placed on the epidemiological surveys dating from the pre-anticonvulsant era, although it is worth noting that an association beteen epilepsy and schizophrenia was reported as early as 1854 (Falret). The issue must therefore turn on less direct observation.

If epilepsy and psychosis are unrelated but occur together by coincidence, there is little reason why either disorder should possess particular characteristics that set it apart from the generality of epileptic or psychotic states. However, the schizophrenia-like psychoses associated with epilepsy have the following characteristics:

a family history of psychosis is lacking

the premorbid personality is normal

phenomenological distinctions, e.g. the preservation of normal affect, may be noted

there is a specific association with temporal lobe epilepsy.

These defining characteristics suggest that we are dealing with a specific syndrome, the emergence of which may reflect, at least in part, a disturbance in temporal lobe function.

If, on the other hand, there is a fundamental antagonism between the two conditions, certain predictions may be made. If seizure activity has some prophylactic value against psychosis it should also be of therapeutic benefit in the established case. In a minority of cases the onset of psychosis precedes the onset of epilepsy, but there is little evidence that the latter development has a beneficial effect on the course of the psychosis. Although ECT was first introduced for the treatment of schizophrenia, its usefulness is extremely questionable (Salzman 1980) and it is now used largely in the management of affective disorders. Other clinical observations support this hypothesis. Psychomotor seizure activity is less marked in psychotic patients (Flor-Henry 1969); the onset of psychosis not infrequently occurs at a time when the frequency and severity of epileptic activity is waning (Slater & Beard 1963). More strikingly a number of patients become psychotic for the first time years after a successful temporal lobectomy. Finally, the inverse relationship between epilepsy and schizophrenia which characterises the alternating psychoses may also occur intermittently during the more chronic course of the interictal psychoses.

It is, of course, more than probable that the schizophrenia-like psychoses of epilepsy are a heterogenous group. A patient in whom temporal lobe malfunction is a critical contributory factor may form one sizeable subgroup; another may be composed of those in whom an association between epilepsy and schizophrenia is quite coincidental. Nor are the hypotheses stated above incompatible. An increased susceptibility to psychosis may accompany some forms of epilepsy, but within the fluctuating course of two chronic conditions an inverse relationship may manifest itself.

A number of causal factors have been suggested in relationship to both the affinity and biological antagonism hypotheses:

Affinity hypothesis
Psychodynamic mechanisms
Subictal activity
Brain damage

Biological antagonism
Folate hypothesis
Monoamine hypothesis
Other biochemical hypotheses.

Psychodynamic mechanisms
Under this heading may be subsumed those arguments that propose a causal link between the bizarre nature of the epileptic experience and the subsequent development of a psychosis. Thus Pond (1957) has suggested that the complexity and misinterpretations arising out of a postictal confusional state may prepare the ground for a later psychotic development. Karagulla & Robertson (1955) have drawn a close parallel between the context of certain of the auras experienced by Penfield's patients and psychotic experience in non-epileptics. Certainly Slater &

Beard (1963) described a subgroup of patients in whom chronic psychosis had been preceded by the repeated occurrence of short-lived confusional episodes, but these constituted only a minority. Such theories would explain the greater prevalence of interictal psychosis in temporal lobe epileptics, but not the observation that temporal lobe seizures are, if anything, less common among psychotics (Flor-Henry 1969, Kristensen & Sindrup 1978a). Moreover, the present writer is not aware of any attempt to trace the evolution, in terms of actual content, of ictal and postictal experience into the psychotic state.

Subictal activity

The clinically observable epileptic seizure represents only the peak of abnormal electrical activity. Subictal discharges may result in abnormal behaviour, a view most cogently advanced by Sir Charles Symonds (Beard & Slater 1972). More recently mechanisms derived from the animal experimental model of kindling have been suggested as a possible explanation for such phenomena. Stevens & Livermore (1978) have reported the induction of fear, staring, searching and withdrawal responses as a result of electrical and pharmacological kindling of the mesolimbic dopamine system in the cat. However, a number of experiments that have focused on possible long-term effects of kindling show either no change or changes, particularly passive avoidance deficits, similar to those produced by lesions (Racine 1978).

Brain damage

The psychoses of epilepsy occur more commonly in association with temporal lobe foci. This implies the presence of underlying structural brain damage and it may well be that this is as significant a factor in the evolution of the psychotic process as ictal or subictal activities, if not more so. A paranoid hallucinatory psychosis has been described as a complication of brain damage in the absence of epilepsy (Hillbom 1960) and schizophrenia-like psychosis may appear in association with diverse cerebral pathologies, e.g. neoplasm, trauma and encephalitis (Davison & Bagley 1969).

Anatomical distribution

Numerous studies already mentioned attest to the possible relevance of left-sided or dominant temporal lobe pathology in the schizophrenia-like psychoses of epilepsy. This is in accordance with some psycho-physiological laboratory findings in process schizophrenia. Gruzelier & Venables (1974) have shown that electrodermal activity is diminished on the left side of the body and, assuming homolateral control by higher centres, have inferred damage to the dominant temporal lobe. However, their data is open to other interpretations, while Toone et al (1979) failed to demonstrate any asymmetry of electrodermal activity in patients who had undergone unilateral temporal lobectomy for epilepsy. Perceptual discrimination tasks involving tachistoscopically presented verbal material (Gur 1979) and dichotic listening techniques (Alpert et al 1976) claim to have demonstrated impaired dominant hemisphere processing in schizophrenia, but these findings have yet to be substantially confirmed.

The folate hypothesis

Reynolds (1968) has re-examined Meduna's theory of biological antagonism in the light of recent developments in neurochemistry and with particular reference to disturbances in folate metabolism. In his view the paradoxical coexistence of two antagonistic conditions may be resolved by postulating that a deficiency in body folate, a recognised complication of anticonvulsant treatment, may result in a range of mental disorders including psychosis. However, whether folate deficiency has a role in the production of psychotic symptoms, as a prime mover or as a contributory factor, or is merely a consequence of the altered physical state of the patient, due for example to associated dietary deficiency, polypharmacy, etc. remains unclear (see Chapter 19). Serial observations of the mental state during folate replenishment could go some way towards providing an answer, but unfortunately, although several such studies have been reported, methodological considerations have rendered interpretation difficult (Reynolds 1981).

The amine hypothesis

The 'antagonism' hypothesis has also been interpreted in terms of central neurotransmitter function. In this view (Trimble 1977) an increase in central monoamine activity may raise the threshold for seizures while having a deleterious effect on any propensity to psychosis.

There is a substantial body of experimental work dealing with the effect of manipulation of central monoamines on seizure thresholds. This has been reviewed recently by Maynert et al (1975) who concluded 'that almost any treatment that increases monoaminergic transmission will restore seizure thresholds'. However, in this respect a better case can be made for noradrenergic than for serotonergic or dopaminergic transmission, and release of the latter may actually facilitate seizures. Clinical observations in man fail to clarify the picture. Drugs that increase central monoamine levels e.g. the tricyclic antidepressants, may provoke seizures, but so also may monoamine depletors such as reserpine. Amphetamine is effective against minor seizures but may aggravate grand mal.

There is some evidence that anticonvulsant treatment may lead to an increase in monoamine metabolism, but less reason to believe that this is central to its therapeutic effects. Although some early studies produced conflicting findings (Bernheimer et al 1966) the small number of cases examined and the failure to report anticonvulsant effects make interpretation difficult. Shaywitz et al (1975) compared an epileptic group, most of whom were on drugs, with a control group with assorted neurological disorders. Levels of CSF 5-HIAA and HVA were lower in the first group; they did not correlate with serum anticonvulsant levels. In a larger study Reynolds et al (1975) found that CSF, HVA and 5-HIAA were increased in treated epileptics compared with both untreated epileptics and neurological controls. This was particularly true of those patients with toxic anticonvulsant levels. However, a recent study (Young et al 1980) reported CSF. 5-HIAA as unchanged in untreated epileptics and diminished after exhibition of anticonvulsant treatment.

One study (Peters 1979) has compared monoamine metabolism in psychotic and non-psychotic temporal lobe epileptics. CSF, homovanillic acid, as measured by the probenicid technique, was lower in the former group. Unfortunately the size of the groups was small and the presence of psychosis determined by scores on Minnesota Multiphasic Personality Inventory scales. The monoamine hypothesis therefore remains an attractive explanation but awaits a definitive investigation.

Other biochemical hypotheses
Platelet monoamine oxidase activity is reported both as raised (Kruk et al 1980) and lowered (Shohnori et al 1975) in epilepsy. The findings in schizophrenia are equally conflicting but one recent review (Wyatt et al 1979) has concluded that there is a strong likelihood of a subgroup in which monoamine oxidase activity is reduced.

Diagnosis
Taken as a class, the schizophrenia-like psychoses of epilepsy present certain distinctive characteristics, but at the level of individual case diagnosis that is no longer so. The presentation and course of a psychotic illness may be identical whether it occurs in association with epilepsy or is entirely functional. The problems of diagnosis therefore are those that appertain to psychosis in general and are beyond the scope of this chapter. The interictal psychoses may sometimes be confused with the ictus-related psychotic states or with confusional states due to anticonvulsant toxicity. Occasionally these conditions occur together in the same patient; otherwise the distinction should be easily made. The ictus-related psychoses are brief, self-terminating states characterised by clouding of consciousness, disorientation and subsequent amnesia, and accompanied by an abnormal EEG pattern. A close temporal relationship to seizure activity is usually apparent. These features, excepting the last, may be observed in confusional states due to anticonvulsants. In addition there is usually evidence of impaired cerebellar function. Plasma anticonvulsant levels are confirmatory.

Management
The treatment of epilepsy and of psychosis when they occur together does not differ in any important way from that which each should receive when they occur alone. The schizophrenia-like and paranoid psychoses will usually respond symptomatically to categories of drugs that produce dopaminergic receptor blockade. This is particularly the case when the clinical features are 'positive', e.g. delusions and hallucinations, as opposed to 'negative' features such as social withdrawal and poverty of speech. The acute symptoms are best treated with drugs of the phenothiazine or butyrophenone type administered orally to allow optimal dosage flexibility. Maintenance therapy may be achieved by use of a depot preparation such as flupenthixol or fluphenazine prescribed and administered through specialised outpatient clinics. In this way non compliance may be reduced to a minimum. Even so 40 per cent of patients will relapse in the first two years of treatment. Extrapyramidal side effects are not uncommon and usually indicate that the dosage is excessive and should be reduced. Anti-parkinsonian drugs of the anticholinergic type may be used to achieve symptomatic relief, but should not be employed as a substitute for reduction in dose of the antipsychotic agent, and should not be used prophylactically.

In the case of a first episode of psychotic illness, once symptoms are controlled and the mental state stable antipsychotic drugs should be cautiously withdrawn. Relapse will suggest the need for medium-term maintenance therapy, but further attempts to withdraw should be deferred rather than abandoned and the possibility of a spontaneous remission always borne in mind.

Manic symptoms respond to either phenothiazines or butyrophenones, the latter being sometimes preferred because of greater flexibility in the upper range of dosage. Lithium carbonate may also be effective but the delay in onset of action makes it unsuitable as a drug of first choice.

Depressive symptoms should be treated in the first instance by monoamine reuptake inhibiting drugs, the so-called tricyclic antidepressant drugs, along with certain newer non-tricyclic antidepressant compounds. Phenothiazines, particularly those with sedative characteristics such as thioridazine, may also be introduced when agitation is prominent. ECT should be considered when the patient has failed to respond to an adequate course of drugs or when delay constitutes a major threat to health, for example when there is a definite suicidal risk. In bipolar, that is manic depressive psychosis, and a unipolar depressive psychosis after two successive episodes, lithium carbonate should be used prophylactically and plasma levels monitored regularly.

The treatment of epilepsy should proceed in the usual manner; for a detailed account of drug management a recent review by Richens (1976) is recommended. It has been argued (see above) that anticonvulsant drugs may aggravate psychotic symptoms, but there is no clinical evidence of this effect and no reason to suppose any one drug would be particularly culpable. Diphenylhydantoin can cause dyskinesias and may possess dopamine antagonistic properties (Chadwick et al 1976), but it is not known whether this is of any benefit in the treatment of psychosis.

Many, if not most, psychotropic drugs are epileptogenic and this applies particularly to antipsychotic and antidepressant classes of drugs. Seizures may be provoked even in patients in whom any evidence of an epileptic diathesis is lacking (Toone & Fenton 1977), and this is especially prone to occur when more than one potentially epileptogenic drug is prescribed.

The effect of such drugs on seizure frequency in epileptics has not been properly evaluated, but it would seem prudent to take this fact into consideration when choosing drugs for the treatment of psychosis. Either maprotiline or nomifensine are to be preferred to the tricyclic antidepressants, and flupenthixol, an antipsychotic drug with some antidepressant properties, may lack the epileptogenicity of the phenothiazines (Trimble 1978). The possibility of anticonvulsant/psychotropic drug interactions should also be recognised. Plasma levels of antidepressants, in particular, may be low in the presence of anticonvulsants (Richens 1976) and lead to inadequate response to treatment.

References

Alpert M, Rubinstein H, Kesselman M 1976 Asymmetry of information processing in hallucinators and non-hallucinators. Journal of Nervous and Mental Disease 162:258–265

Andermann F, Robb J P 1972 Absence status. Epilepsia 13:177–187

Asuni T, Pillutla V S 1967 Schizophrenia-like psychoses in Nigerian epileptics. British Journal of Psychiatry 113:1375–1379

Bartlet J E A 1957 Chronic psychosis following epilepsy. American Journal of Psychiatry 114:338–343

Beard A W, Slater E 1962 The schizophrenic-like psychoses of epilepsy. Proceedings of the Royal Society of Medicine 55:311–316

Berger H 1931 Uber das elektrenkephalogramm des Menschen III. Archiv für Psychiatrie und Nervenkrankheiten 94:16–60

Bernheimer H, Birkmayer W, Hornykiewicz O 1966 Homovanillisäure im Liquor cerebrospinalis-Untersuchingen bein Parkinson-Syndrom und anderen Erkrankungen des ZNS. Wiener Klinische Wochenschrift 78:417–419

Betts T A 1974 A follow-up study of a cohort of patients with epilepsy admitted to psychiatric care in an English city. In: Harris P, Mawdsley C (eds) Epilepsy: proceedings of the Hans Berger centenary symposium. Churchill Livingstone, Edinburgh, p. 326

Betts T A, Merskey H, Pond D A 1976 Psychiatry. In: Laidlaw J, Richens A (eds) A textbook of epilepsy. Churchill Livingstone, Edinburgh

Bleuler E 1911 Dementia praecox. Deuticke, Leipzig-Wien

Bleuler M 1978 The schizophrenic disorders. Yale University Press, New Haven and London, p 195

Bruens J H 1971 Psychoses in epilepsy. Psychiatria, neurologia, neurochirurgia 74:174–192

Bruens J H 1974 Psychoses in epilepsy. In: Vinken P J, Bruyn G W (eds) Handbook of clinical neurology, vol 15. North-Holland Publishing Company, Amsterdam, American Elsevier Publishing Co., New York

Chadwick D, Reynolds E H, Marsden C D 1976 Anticonvulsant-induced dyskinesias: a comparison with dyskinesias induced by neuroleptics. Journal of Neurology, Neurosurgery and Psychiatry 39:1210–1218

Clark R A, Lesko J M 1939 Psychoses associated with epilepsy. The American Journal of Psychiatry 96:595–607

Currie S, Heathfield K W G, Henson R A, Scott D F 1971 Clinical course and prognosis of temporal lobe epilepsy. Brain 94:173–190

Dalby M A 1969 Epilepsy and 3 per second spike and wave rhythms. Acta neurologica scandinavica, supplement 40/45

Davis P A 1940 Evaluation of the electroencephalogram of schizophrenic patients. American Journal of Psychiatry 96:851–860

Davison K, Bagley C R 1969 Schizophrenia-like psychoses associated with organic disorders of the central nervous system: a review of the literature. In: Herrington R N (ed) Current problems in neuropsychiatry. British Journal of Psychiatry special publication no. 4, p 113

Dongier S 1959 Statistical study of clinical and electroencephalographic manifestations of 536 psychotic episodes occurring in 516 epileptics between clinical seizures. Epilepsia 1:117–142

Ellis J M, Lee S I 1978 Acute prolonged confusion in later life as an ictal state. Epilepsia 19:119–128

Ervin F, Epstein A W, King H E 1975 Behaviour of epileptic and non-epileptic patients with 'temporal spikes'. Archives of Neurology and Psychiatry 74:488–497

Escueta A V, Boxley J, Stubbs N, Waddell G, Wilson W A 1974 Prolonged twilight state and automatisms: a case report. Neurology 24:331–339

Esser P H 1938 Die epileptiformen anfalle der schizophrenen und die differentialdiagnostischen schwierigheiten im grenzgebit von epilepsie und schizophrenie. Zeitschrift für die Gesamte Neurologie und Psychiatrie 162:1–24

FalconerM A 1973 Reversibility by temporal-lobe resection of the behavioural abnormalities of temporal-lobe epilepsy. The New England Journal of Medicine 289:451–445

Falret J P 1854 Mémoire sur la folie circulaire. Bulletin de l'Académie Impériale de Médecine (Paris) 19: 382–400

Feighner J P, Robins E, Guze S B, Woodruff R A, Winokur G, Munoz R 1972 Diagnostic criteria for use in psychiatric research. Archives of General Psychiatry 26:57–63

Fenton G W 1978 Epilepsy and psychosis. Journal of the Irish Medical Association 71:315–324

Flor-Henry P 1969 Psychosis and temporal lobe epilepsy. Epilepsia 10:363–395

Gibbs F A 1951 Ictal and non-ictal psychiatric disorders in temporal lobe epilepsy. Journal of Nervous and Mental Disease 113:522–528

Glaus A 1931 Ueber kombinationen von schizophrenie und epilepsie. Zeitschrift für die Gesamte Neurologie und Psychiatrie 135:450–500

Gregoriades A, Fragos E, Kapslakis Z, Mandouvalos B 1971 A correlation between mental disorders and EEG and air encephalography findings in temporal lobe epilepsy. Fifth World Congress of Psychiatry, Mexico. Prensa Medica Mexicana, 325

Gruhle H W 1936 Ueber den wahn bei epilepsie. Zeitschrift für die Gesamte Neurologie und Psychiatrie 154:395–399

Gruzelier J H, Venables P H 1974 Bimodality and lateral asymmetry of skin conductance orienting activity in schizophrenics: replication and evidence of lateral asymmetry in patients with depression and disorders of personality. Biological Psychiatry 8:55–73

Gur R E 1979 Cognitive concomitants of hemispheric dysfunction in schizophrenia. Archives of General Psychiatry 36:269–274

Hermann B P, Chabrias S 1981 Interictal psychopathology in patients with ictal fear. Archives of Neurology (in press)

Hill D 1953 Psychiatric disorders of epilepsy. Medical Press 229:473–475

Hillbom E 1960 After-effects of brain injuries. Acta psychiatrica et neurologica scandinavica 35, Supplement 142

Jaffe R 1962 Ictal behaviour disturbance as the only manifestation of seizure disorder: case report. Journal of Nervous and Mental Disease 34:470–476

Janz D 1969 Die epilepsein. Georg Thieme Verlag, Stuttgart

Jasper H H, Fitzpatrick C P, Solomon P 1939 Analogies and opposites in schizophrenia and epilepsy. Lectures in electroencephalographic and clinical studies. American Journal of Psychiatry 95:835–851

Jensen I, Larsen J K 1979 Mental aspects of temporal lobe epilepsy. Journal of Neurology, Neurosurgery, and Psychiatry 42:256–265

Karagulla S, Robertson E E 1955 Psychical phenomena in temporal lobe epilepsy and the psychoses. British Medical Journal 1:748–752

Kat W 1937 Over de tegenstelling epilepsie-schizophrenie. Psychiatrische en Neurologische Bladen. Amsterdam. 41:733–745

Kraepelin E 1910 Psychiatrie 8th edn. Barth, Leipzig

Krapf E 1928 Epilepsie und schizophrenie. Archiv für Psychiatrie und Nervenkrankheiten 83:547–586

Kristensen O, Sindrup E H 1978a Psychomotor epilepsy and psychosis. I Physical aspects. Acta neurologica scandinavica 57:361–369

Kristensen O, Sindrup E H 1978b Psychomotor epilepsy and psychosis. II Electroencephalographic findings. Acta neurologica scandinavica 57:370–379

Kristensen O, Sindrup E H 1979 Psychomotor epilepsy and psychosis. III Social and psychological correlates. Acta neurologica scandinavica 59:1–9

Krohn W 1960 Study of epilepsy in Northern Norway; its frequency and character. Acta psychiatrica et neurologica scandinavica, supplement 150:215–225

Kruk Z L, Moffett A, Scott D F 1980 Platelet monoamine oxidase activity in epilepsy. Journal of Neurology, Neurosurgery, and Psychiatry 43:68–70

Kurland L T 1969 The incidence and prevalence of convulsive disorders in a small urban community. Epilepsia 1:143–161

Landolt H 1958 Serial electroencephalographic investigations during psychotic episodes in epileptic patients and during schizophrenic attacks. In: Lorentz de Haas A M (ed) Lectures in epilepsy. Elsevier Publishing Company, Amsterdam, p 91–133

Lennox W G 1945 The treatment of epilepsy. Medical Clinics of North America 29:1114–1128

Levin S 1952 Epileptic clouded states. Journal of Nervous and Mental Disease 116:214–225

Liddell D W 1953 Observations on epileptic automatisms in a mental hospital population. Journal of Mental Science 99:732–748

Lindsay J, Ounsted C, Richards P 1979 Long-term outcome in children with temporal lobe seizures. III Psychiatric aspects in childhood and adult life. Developmental Medicine and Child Neurology 21:630–636

Lugaresi E, Pazzaglia P, Tassinari C A 1971 Differentiation of 'absence status' and 'temporal lobe status'. Epilepsia 12:77–87

Mann S, Cree W 1976 'New' long-stay psychiatric patients: a national sample survey of 15 mental hospitals in England and Wales 1972/73. Psychological Medicine 6:603–616

Markand O N, Wheeler G, Pollak S 1978 Complex partial status epilepticus (psychomotor status). Neurology 28:189–196

Maynert E W, Marczynski T J, Browning R A 1975 The rôle of the neurotransmitters in the epilepsies. In: Friedlander W J (ed) Advances in neurology, volume 13. Raven Press, New York

Muller G 1931 Anfälle bei schizophrenen erkrankungen. Allgemeine Zeitschrift für Psychiatrie 93:235–240

Niedmeyer E, Khalifeh R 1965 Petit mal status ('spike-wave stupor'). Epilepsia 6:250–262

Oller-Daurella L 1970 Crises épileptiques psychiques de longue durée. Revue de neuropsychiatrie infantile et d'hygiene mentale de l'enfance 18:547–557

Pahla A, Fenton G W, Driver M V, Fenwick P C B 1978 Epilepsy and psychiatric disorder (in preparation)

Perez M M, Trimble M R 1980 Epileptic psychosis — diagnostic comparison with process schizophrenia. British Journal of Psychiatry 137:245–249

Perez M M, Trimble M R 1981 (in preparation)

Peters J G 1979 Dopamine, noradrenaline and serotonin spinal fluid metabolites in temporal lobe epileptic patients with schizophrenic symptomatology. European Neurology 18:15–18

Pond D A 1957 Psychiatric aspects of epilepsy. Journal of the Indian Medical Profession 3:1441–1451

Pond D A, Bidwell B H, Stein L 1960 A survey of epilepsy in 14 general practices. I demographic and medical data. Psychiatria, neurologia, neurochirurgia 63:217–236

Racine R 1978 Kindling: the first decade. Neurosurgery 3:234–252

Rennick M, Perez-Borja C, Rodin E A 1969 Transient mental deficits associated with recurrent prolonged epileptic clouded state. Epilepsia 10:397–405

Reynolds E H 1968 Epilepsy and schizophrenia: relationship and biochemistry. Lancet 1:398–401

Reynolds E H 1981 Anticonvulsant drugs, folate metabolism and mental symptoms. In: Proceedings of XII epilepsy international symposium. Raven Press, New York (in press).

Reynolds E H, Chadwick D, Jenner P, Chanarin I 1975 Folate and monoamine metabolism in epilepsy. Journal of the Neurological Sciences 26:605–615

Richens A 1976 Clinical pharmacology and medical treatment. In: Laidlaw J, Richens A (eds) A Textbook of epilepsy. Churchill Livingstone, Edinburgh

Roger J, Lob H, Tassinari C A 1974 Status epilepticus. In: Vinken P J, Bruyn G W (eds) Handbook of clinical neurology, volume 15. North-Holland Publishing Company, Amsterdam, American Elsevier Publishing Co., New York

Salzman C 1980 The use of ECT in the treatment of schizophrenia. American Journal of Psychiatry 137:1032–1041

Sawa M 1973 Epileptoid psychosis: a group of atypical endogenous psychoses. Folia psychiatrica et neurologica japonica 16:320–329

Schwartz M S, Scott D F 1971 Isolated petit mal status presenting de novo in middle age. The Lancet 2:1399–1401

Scott J S, Masland R L 1953 Occurrence of 'continuous symptoms' in epilepsy patients. Neurology 3:297–301

Shaywitz B A, Cohen D J, Bowers M B 1975 Reduced cerebrospinal fluid 5-hydroxy-indoleacetic acid and homovanillic acid in children with epilepsy. Neurology 25:72–79

Sherwin I 1977 Clinical and e.e.g. aspects of temporal lobe epilepsy with behaviour disorder, the role of cerebral dominance. In: Blumer D, Levin K (eds) McLean Hospital Journal, special issue, p 40

Shohnori T, Kaneyuki T, Kobayashi K, Mori A, Kohsaka M 1975 Reduced blood platelet monoamine oxidase activity in epileptic patients. IRCS Medical Science: Clinical Pharmacology and Therapeutics 3:558

Shukla G D, Srivastava O N, Katiyar B C, Joshi V, Mohan P K 1979 Psychiatric manifestations in temporal lobe epilepsy: a controlled study. British Journal of Psychiatry 135:411–417

Slater E, Moran P 1969 The schizophrenia-like psychoses of epilepsy: relation between ages of onset. British Journal of Psychiatry 115:599–600

Slater E, Roth M 1969 Clinical Psychiatry, third edition. Baillière, Tindal and Cassell, London, p 239

Slater E, Beard A W, Glitheroe E 1963 The schizophrenia-like psychoses of epilepsy. British Journal of Psychiatry 109:95–150

Small J G, Small I F 1967 A controlled study of mental disorders associated with epilepsy. Recent Advances in Biological Psychiatry 9:171–181

Small J G, Milstein V, Stevens J R 1962 Are psychomotor Epileptics different? Archives of Neurology 7:187–194

Standage K F 1973 Schizophreniform psychosis among epileptics in a mental hospital. British Journal of Psychiatry 123:231–232

Standage K F, Fenton G W 1975 Psychiatric symptom profiles of patients with epilepsy: a controlled investigation. Psychological Medicine 5:152–160

Stevens J R 1966 Psychiatric implications of psychomotor epilepsy. Archives of General Psychiatry 14:461–471

Stevens J R, Livermore A 1978 Kindling of the mesolimbic dopamine system: animal model of psychosis. Neurology 28:36–46

Taylor D C 1971 Ontogenesis of chronic epileptic psychoses: a re-analysis. Psychological Medicine 1:247–253

Taylor D C 1972 Mental state and temporal lobe epilepsy. Epilepsia 13:727–765

Taylor D C 1975 Factors influencing the occurrence of schizophrenia-like psychoses in patients with temporal lobe epilepsy. Psychological Medicine 5:249–254

Toone B K, Driver M V 1980 Psychosis and epilepsy. Research and Clinical Forums 2, No 2:121–127

Toone B K, Driver M V 1980 Psychosis, epilepsy and laterality (in preparation)

Toone B K, Fenton G W 1977 Epileptic seizures induced by psychotropic drugs. Psychological Medicine 7:265–270

Toone B K, Cooke E, Lader M H 1979 The effect of temporal lobe surgery on electrodermal activity: implications for an organic hypothesis in the aetiology of schizophrenia. Psychological Medicine 9:281–285

Travis L E, Malamud W 1937 Brain potentials from normal subjects, stutterers, and schizophrenic patients. American Journal of Psychiatry 93:929–937

Trimble M 1977 The relationship between epilepsy and schizophrenia: a biochemical hypothesis. Biological Psychiatry 12:299–304

Trimble M 1978 Non-monoamineoxidase inhibitor antidepressants and epilepsy: a review. Epilepsia 19:241–250

Urstein A 1909 Die dementia praecox und ihre stellung zum manisch-depressiven irresein. Urban und Schwarzenburg, Berlin

Vorkastner W 1918 Epilepsie und dementia praecox. Karger, Berlin

Wells C E 1975 Transient ictal psychosis. Archives of General Psychiatry 32:1201–1203

Wing J K, Cooper J E, Sartorius N 1974 The measurement and classification of psychiatric symptoms. London. Cambridge University Press

Wyatt R J, Potkin S G, Murphy D L 1979 Platelet monoamineoxidase activity in schizophrenia: a review of the data. American Journal of Psychiatry 136:377–385

Wyrsch J 1933 Ueber schizophrenie bei epileptikern. Schweizer Archiv für Neurologie und Psychiatrie 31:113–132

Young S N, Gauthier S, Anderson G M, Purdy W C 1980 Tryptophan, 5-hydroxy-indoleacetic acid and indoleacetic acid in human cerebrospinal fluid: interrelationships and the influence of age, sex, epilepsy and anticonvulsant drugs. Journal of Neurology, Neurosurgery, and Psychiatry 43:438–445

Zappoli R 1955 Two cases of prolonged epileptic twilight state with almost continuous 'wave-spikes'. Electroencephalography and Clinical Neurophysiology 7:421–423

Epilepsy and mental retardation

INTRODUCTION

Gowers succinctly and correctly identified the two main issues concerning the relationship between epilepsy and mental retardation (1881). Firstly that mental deterioration occurs in some people who have suffered from seizures. His conclusion that we often do not know the cause of this association, except insofar as it relates to a subtle interaction between underlying brain damage, cerebral dysrhythmia, drugs and other factors is equally true today. The relative contribution of each of these factors remains a matter for active investigation and has been discused in other contributions to this volume. As those suffering from such deterioration not infrequently come under the care of the mental retardation services, particularly if it arises early in life, it will be further considered later in this chapter.

Gowers' second main conclusion was that epilepsy is particularly common in people with mental retardation, and that it was 'the expression of a cerebral imperfection of which epilepsy is another manifestation'. It is therefore relevant to review our present knowledge of this association.

Prevalence of epilepsy in the mentally retarded

Epidemiological studies suggest that 3–6 per cent of children with an IQ between 50 and 70 suffer from epilepsy (Peckham 1974, Rutter et al 1970). This figure depends upon whether uncomplicated seizures or cases associated with other handicaps are considered, and compares with a frequency of seizures in the past year in school age children of 0.7 per cent (Cooper 1965, Graham & Rutter 1968, Pond & Bidwell 1960, Ross et al 1980). Until recently most studies have been of institutionalised populations and this accounts for the higher figure of 19.5 per cent given by Margerison (1962) in high grade institutionalised patients.

In an epidemiological study of severely retarded children under the age of 14 years, from the Camberwell district of South East London, it was found that 32 per cent had had a seizure at some time during life but, although many of these continued to be labelled as having epilepsy and received anticonvulsant drugs for long periods of their childhood, only 19 per cent had suffered a seizure in the year prior to the study (Corbett et al 1975) (Table 11.1).

Table 11.1 Epilepsy and degree of mental retardation (Corbett et al 1975)

	n	Lifelong seizures %	Seizures in past year (%)
IQ 35–49	65	23	15
IQ 20–34	35	28	26
IQ <20	41	50	27
Total	141		

This increase in seizures in the severely retarded and those in contact with services for the mentally handicapped persists into adult life in the Camberwell study, and, with increasing age, more of those with epilepsy tend to be institutionalised (Corbett 1974) (Fig. 11.1).

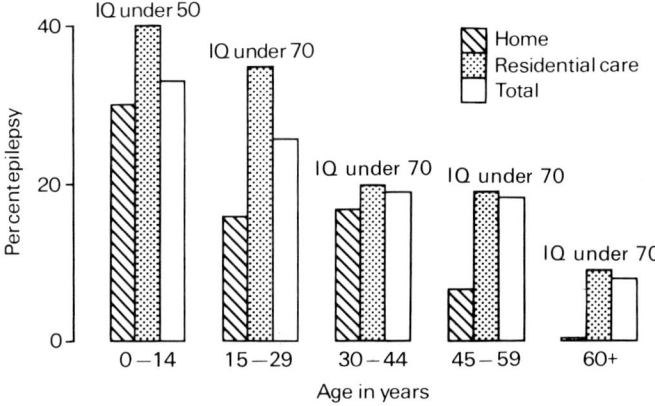

Fig. 11.1 Lifelong history of seizures in mentally retarded people from Camberwell (n = 540) (Corbett, 1974)

Richardson and his co-workers (1979, 1981) reporting recently on mentally retarded people from the Aberdeen case register who were followed up until the age of 22 years found an even higher frequency of epilepsy. Nearly half the subjects with an IQ of less than 50 had suffered a seizure by that age: a third with IQs. between 50–59 and a quarter of those with an IQ over 60, who had been in contact with services for the mentally retarded by the time of school leaving age 16. The impression from the 10-year follow-up of the Camberwell children bears out the finding that the mentally retarded suffer from an increased incidence of seizures in late adolescence.

This very marked increase in seizures in the severely retarded is understandable as most children with an IQ of under 50 have overt signs of brain damage and the normal distribution of intelligence in the population is skewed for this reason at the extreme lower end. The relationship between epilepsy and severe mental retardation is strongly age-related and children with profound retardation and the severest brain damage have the highest frequency of life-long seizures, the damage occurring in the perinatal period or the first five years of life. In the Camberwell study 25 per cent of children under the age of 5 years had had a seizure in the previous year compared with only 5 per cent between the ages of 10 and 15 years (Table 11.2).

Table 11.2 Frequency of seizures in severely retarded children related to age (Corbett et al 1975)

Age in years	n	% children having seizures
0–5	56	25
5–10	61	18
10–14	38	5
Total	155	

Boys are more vulnerable to brain damage and hence to seizures, and in the Camberwell study 39 per cent of the boys had suffered from seizures compared with only 26 per cent of the girls.

Apart from this biological vulnerability of boys to early brain damage it is possible to distinguish three common periods during early infancy when brain damage associated with epilepsy is particularly likely to occur.

1. Seizures and brain damage in the perinatal period

The causes of neonatal seizures are very varied and it is convenient to classify them according to the times at which the cause first operated, whether prenatal, perinatal or postnatal (Table 11.3).

Postnatally the most important distinction seems to be between seizures associated with pre- or perinatal brain damage or with hypoglycaemia and other biochemical changes, and seizures of late onset, occurring for the first time between the fifth and eighth days of life associated with hypocalcaemia or hypomagnesaemia. The latter are probably due to bottle feeding with cow's milk preparations high in phosphorous which lower the serum calcium. As this practice has declined with greater awareness, the prognosis of the latter is improving and for this reason it seems unlikely that the fits themselves cause brain damage (Brown et al 1972).

Table 11.3 Causes of neonatal seizures

Factors present or operating before birth
   Cerebral malformations
   Intra-uterine infections e.g. rubella

Factors operating during labour or at delivery
   Birth trauma
   Perinatal hypoxia

Factors operating after birth
   Transient biochemical disturbances
     Hypoglycaemia
     Hypocalcaemia
     Hypomagnesaemia
   Infection-meningitis
   Inborn errors of metabolism
   Intracranial haemorrhage
   Drug withdrawal

2. Infantile spasms

The onset of infantile spasms tends to be commonly between the ages of three and eight months. In about half the cases they are idiopathic while the rest are associated with brain damage of various kinds ranging from tuberose sclerosis to inborn errors of metabolism (Jeavons & Bower 1964). The control of seizures by steroids in some studies has suggested a better outcome in the cryptogenic cases and adds support to the idea that the seizures themselves may be damaging (Jeavons et al 1973). Infantile spasms are, like many seizures associated with severe encephalopathy in early childhood, followed by severe regression in behaviour and cognitive development. In some cases, language development and social relationships are particularly affected in a way similar to that seen in early infantile autism (Taft & Cohen 1971). In cryptogenic cases there has usually been a period of apparently normal development and the condition is probably more appropriately entitled non-progressive disintegrative psychosis of childhood (Corbett 1979).

3. Prolonged febrile convulsions

Febrile convulsions which proceed to status epilepticus, seizures associated with meningitis or encephalitis in early infancy in which there has been a delay in initiating treatment, or non-accidental head injury in childhood are amongst the most important preventable causes of mental retardation associated with subsequent epilepsy. The most important measures, in addition to effective treatment of the underlying cause, are effective prophylaxis and early energetic treatment to terminate the seizures.

In addition to generalised retardation occurring as a result of prolonged status epilepticus, focal neurological damage may also occur which is often more extensive in one hemisphere than the other. This may cause temporary hemiplegia and late focal epilepsy may supervene months or years later. The studies of Ounsted and his colleagues showed that one third of their cases of psychomotor epilepsy followed prolonged status in early childhood, and that when temporal lobe epilepsy was associated with an acute or chronic anatomical cerebral insult the prognosis for mental development was poor (Ounsted et al 1966, Lindsay et al 1979) (Chapter 15).

EPILEPSY IN PARTICULAR MENTAL RETARDATION SYNDROMES (Table 11.4)

There have been very many accounts of the association of mental retardation with epilepsy in isolated case reports of particular conditions. While epilepsy is reportedly rare in Down's syndrome, kernicterus and cretinism (Crome 1965) it is much commoner in conditions associated with evidence of more extensive or localised brain damage affecting the cerebral hemisphere, such as spastic cerebral palsy, and almost universal in those where extensive cortical involvement is associated with severe mental retardation. For example, in the Sturge-Weber syndrome or epiloia, if the subject is severely mentally retarded, that is with an IQ of less than 50, then seizures seem almost inevitable. Similarly in biochemical disorders such as phenylketonuria or homocysteinuria, if the condition is untreated, epilepsy is common, and again there is an association in treated cases between the intellectual level and frequency of seizures.

Table 11.4 Frequency of epilepsy in severely retarded children and diagnosis (Corbett et al 1975)

	n	Lifelong history of seizures (%)
Infections	23	34
Trauma	9	33
Metabolic	6	51
Gross brain disease	8	100
Other perinatal causes	16	41
Chromosomal abnormalities	35	16
Others with family history	13	23
Others with family history	30	30
Total	140	

Epilepsy and Down's syndrome

In looking at trends in the relationship between epilepsy and mental retardation it is helpful to examine the situation in Down's syndrome which is now the commonest single known cause of retardation accounting for a quarter of all severely affected children. The prevalence of severe mental retardation has not changed dramatically over the past fifty years, since reliable epidemiological studies were first carried out in this country (Lewis 1929) and the age-specific prevalence rate remains in the order of 3.5–4/1000 for school children (Wing 1972). In early studies less than 10 per cent of children with Down's syndrome survived until school age, but increased survival has led to improved insights into the prevalence of epilepsy in this condition. It used to be said (see above) that epilepsy was very uncommon in cases of Down's syndrome, but it is now clear that this is not so. Young children suffer from febrile convulsions at least as frequently as non-retarded children. Young Down's children also suffer from a form of myoclonic epilepsy which seems to be pyridoxine dependent, and may be related to abnormalities in cerebral neurotransmitters in this condition (Wolcutt & Chun 1973).

Veall (1974) has shown that patients with Down's syndrome also have an increasing tendency to epilepsy as they get older. It is not yet clear whether this is related to intellectual deterioration which tends also to be more apparent as more people with this condition survive into middle age.

Epilepsy and cerebral palsy

Children with cerebral palsy, usually resulting from pre- or perinatal brain injury, frequently suffer from epilepsy and in the Camberwell study seizures were reported in 60 per cent of such children compared with only 20 per cent of severely retarded children without cerebral palsy. Now that these children have been followed up for ten years it is apparent that epilepsy is the commonest cause of death in this population in childhood.

The rate is highest in spastic children and lowest in those with athetoid cerebral palsy. Infantile hemiplegia, which is more frequently post-natal in origin, has a particularly high incidence of seizures and the resulting HHE syndrome ('hémiconvulsions, hémiplegie, épilepsie') described by Gastaut et al (1960) presents particular problems in management, as to this triad of symptoms may be added disabling hyperkinetic behaviour. Occasionally where the seizure disorder proves resistant to anticonvulsant treatment, neurosurgical intervention is indicated if the degree of retardation is not too severe.

TYPES OF SEIZURE DISORDER IN THE MENTALLY RETARDED

Every type of seizure pattern occurs in people with mental retardation but a number of issues need to be considered. First, seizures are often mixed in type and the pattern may change from time to time so that, even in older mentally retarded subjects, it may be similar to that seen in normal younger subjects. Secondly, among partial seizures, temporal lobe epilepsy is not, as was previously thought, uncommon. It may give rise to particular difficulties in diagnosis in people who have insufficient language to describe their subjective experience, particularly in those who show apparently unpredictable behaviour changes for other reasons. Even more important may be the behavioural change resulting from prolonged postictal confusion, as the mentally retarded person has more difficulty in reorientating himself following a fit.

Minor status epilepticus may mimic mental retardation or childhood psychosis and cause an organic confusional state. This may be more difficult to recognise in the mentally retarded subject, and for this reason an EEG should be part of routine screening in people with mental retardation, where the cause of the intellectual impairment or disturbed behaviour is not immediately apparent.

A particularly difficult problem is presented in the mentally retarded child with the Lennox–Gastaut syndrome or petit mal variant in which seizures begin for the first time, usually after infancy, with disabling myoclonic or astatic fits or other forms of complex partial seizures. The diagnosis is confirmed by the EEG which is said to show a typical pattern of high voltage slow spike and wave which is more regular than the hypsarrhythmia of infantile spasms (Gastaut et al 1966, Chevrie & Aicardi 1972). This condition is difficult to treat, and may be associated with progressive intellectual deterioration. Sodium valproate and nitrazepam may be helpful in the management of the myoclonic attacks, and occasionally a trial of ACTH or a ketogenic diet using medium chain triglyceride oil is indicated.

EPILEPSY AND BEHAVIOUR DISORDERS IN THE MENTALLY RETARDED

People with epilepsy and mental retardation have an increased risk of psychiatric disorder, although in children this is offset to some extent by the fact that epilepsy is more common in those with cerebral palsy, where, with the exception of the HHE syndrome, behaviour disorders are less frequent. All types of psychiatric disorder are seen, although in children hyperkinetic behaviour disorders are more frequent, especially in association with complex partial seizures. Children with Kanner's syndrome or classical infantile autism less frequently suffer from epilepsy in early childhood, although approximately one third develop seizures for the first time in adolescence or early adult life (Rutter et al 1967).

Even without accepting the idea of there being a specific epileptic personality, many authors have considered that mentally retarded people with epilepsy, like epileptic people of normal intelligence, are particularly liable to certain symptoms such as aggressive behaviour and either hyperactivity or hypoactivity. The latter refers to the slowness or 'stickiness' of response seen in some chronic adult epileptic patients. Eyman et al (1969), in a study of three large hospitals for the mentally retarded, found that hyperactivity was more common in mentally retarded patients with seizures than those without. Aggressive behaviour, speech problems and difficulties in eating and dressing were also more common, but this may well have been a reflection of the more severe degree of retardation of the patients with epilepsy. In this study, however, all the patients were institutionalised, and drugs were thought to play an important part in causing behaviour disturbance.

In the Camberwell study, 40 per cent of adults with a history of epilepsy were free from psychiatric disorder compared with 60 per cent of those who had never had a seizure. Epilepsy was not frequent in those with schizophrenia, depression or manic depressive psychosis but more frequent in those with a history of childhood psychosis or behaviour and personality disorders (Corbett 1979).

Treatment
The additional handicap of epilepsy causes particular problems for families and others caring for the mentally retarded. Anxiety and fear for the life of the child, engendered by the seizures themselves, frequently compound the sense of partial bereavement caused by the presence of the handicapped child in the family. Also, because the epilepsy tends to be regarded as a strictly medical problem, it may lead to exclusion of the child from residential care facilities in the community and special schooling leading to long-term hospital care.

It follows that there is a particular need to facilitate access of people with epilepsy and mental retardation to outpatient services for epilepsy. Special investigations such as EEGs and neuroradiology will need to be carried out at hospital. However, ongoing supervision and monitoring of serum anticonvulsant levels may be best carried out by the same team of specialists visiting special schools, adult training centres or residential facilities in which the handicapped person works or lives. This also provides the opportunity for staff counselling and support.

Little is known about the effects of anticonvulsant drugs on the behaviour or intellectual performance of people with mental retardation but a number of facts stand out. First, patients tend to be maintained on medication over long periods of time, often in combination, and there is often a reluctance, because of the existence of brain damage, to reduce or discontinue this once the seizures have ceased. There is also evidence that the mentally retarded are more prone to become intoxicated with anticonvulsant drugs, and may show side effects such as intellectual deterioration and psychomotor slowing with anticonvulsant serum levels, for example of phenobarbitone and phenytoin, within the conventionally accepted normal range (Reynolds & Travers 1974, Trimble & Corbett 1980). Whether this is due to the difficulty in eliciting neurological signs of intoxication in people who are already likely to show evidence of neurological disorders, or because the damaged brain is more vulnerable to the effects of anticonvulsants is not clear, although the former seems most likely.

Among the other chronic disturbances in metabolism which are likely to remain undetected in people with mental retardation are those involving folic acid and calcium. Both require monitoring, and although there have been no specific studies of folate metabolism in mentally retarded populations, it is clear that children on long-term anticonvulsant therapy, particularly with phenytoin, who show intellectual deterioration, tend to suffer from folate depletion (Trimble et al 1980). There have been a number of reports of calcium deficiency in patients receiving long-term anticonvulsants and this has been confirmed in mentally retarded patients with epilepsy (Viukara et al 1972).

The indications for the use of different anticonvulsants are similar in retarded patients to those of normal intelligence, although there is much to be said for a determined attempt, where possible, to restrict their use to a minimum number of drugs of proven low toxicity, bearing in mind the additional burdens placed on those caring for the retarded.

Particular attention needs to be given to the practical aspects of administration. For example, anticonvulsants often have to be given to the retarded child in liquid form, and it is important to bear in mind that some anticonvulsants, such as phenytoin, do not stay in suspension easily and unless the bottle is shaken vigorously variation in drug dose is likely to occur. Similarly many retarded patients have difficulty in chewing food and cleaning their teeth, so that the associated gum hypertrophy due to the drug causes them to be prone to develop gingivitis.

In summary, when epilepsy occurs with mental retardation, because of its association with other handicaps, it presents particular problems in management, and presents an important challenge to all those working in the multidisciplinary team caring for retarded people.

References

Brown J K, Cockburn F, Forfar J A 1972 Clinical and chemical correlates in convulsions in the newborn. Lancet 1:135–139

Chevrie T J, Aicardi J 1972 Childhood epileptic encephalopathy with slow spike and wave. A statistical study of 80 cases. Epilepsia 13:259–271

Cooper J E 1965 Epilepsy in a longitudinal study of 5000 children. Br. Med. J. 1:1020–1022

Corbett J A 1974 Epilepsy and mental retardation. In: Parsonage M J (ed) Total care in severe epilepsy. Proceedings of 6th international symposium on epilepsy, Belgium 1974. International Bureau for Epilepsy, London

Corbett J A, Harris R, Robinson R 1975 Epilepsy. In: Wortis J (ed) Mental retardation & developmental disabilities, vol VII. Bruner Mazel, New York

Corbett J A 1979 Psychiatric morbidity and mental retardation. In: James F E, Snaith R P (eds) Psychiatric illness and mental handicap. Gaskell Press, London

Crome L 1965 In: Hilliard L T, Kirman B H (eds) Mental deficiency. Churchill, London

Eyman R K, Capes L, Moore B C, Zachofsky T 1969 Retardates with seizures. Am J Ment Defic 74:651–9

Gastaut H, Roger J, Soulayrol R, Tassinari C A, Regis H, Dravet C 1966 Childhood epileptic encephalopathy with diffuse slow spike waves (otherwise known as petit mal variant) or Lennox Syndrome. Annales de Pédiatrie (Paris) 13:489–99

Gowers W 1881 Epilepsy and other chronic convulsive diseases. Their causes, symptoms and treatment. Churchill, London

Graham P, Rutter M 1968 Organic brain dysfunction and child psychiatric disorder. Br Med J 13:695–700

Jeavons P M, Bower B D 1964 Infantile spasms. Spastics Society, Heineman, London

Jeavons P M, Bower B D, Dimitrihoudi M C 1973 Long-term prognosis in 150 cases of West's syndrome. Epilepsia 14:153–164

Lewis E O 1929 Report of an investigation into the incidence of mental defect in sex areas 1925–27. Report of the Mental Deficiency Committee, part IV. HMSO, London

Lindsay J, Ounsted, D C, Richards P 1979 Long-term outcome in children with temporal lobe seizures. 1. Social outcome and childhood factors. Devel Med & Child Neurol 21:285–298

Margerison J H 1962 In: Proceedings of the London conference on the scientific study of mental deficiency. I.A.S.S.M.D. London

Ounsted C, Lindsay J, Norman R 1966 Biological factors in temporal lobe epilepsy. Clinics in Dev Med 22. London Spastics Society MEIU, Heinemann Medical

Peckham C 1974. National child development study (1958 cohort). Personal communication.

Pond D A, Bidwell B H 1960 A survey of epilepsy in fourteen general practices. II Social psychological aspects. Epilepsia 1:283–299

Reynolds E H, Travers R D 1974 Serum anticonvulsant concentrations in epileptic patients with mental symptoms. Br J Psychiat 124:440–5

Richardson S A, Katz M, Koller H, McLaren J, Rubenstine B 1979 Some characteristics of a population of mentally retarded young adults in a British city. Jour Ment Defic Res 23:275–287

Richardson S A, Kolle R H, Katz M, McLaren J 1981 Seizures and epilepsy in a mentally retarded population over the first 22 years of life. (in press)

Ross E M, Peckham C S, West P B, Butler N R 1980 Epilepsy in childhood: findings from the national child development study. Br Med J 1:207–211

Rutter M, Graham P, Yule W 1970 A neuropsychiatric study in childhood spastics. Int Med Pub. Heinemann, London

Rutter M, Greenfield D, Lockyer L 1967 A five to fifteen year follow-up study of infantile psychosis. II Social and behavioural outcome. Br J Psychiat 118:1183–99

Taft L T, Cohen M J 1971 Hypsarrhythmia and infantile autism: a clinical report. J Autism & Childhood Schiz 1:27–36

Trimble M, Corbett J A 1980 Behaviour and cognitive disturbances in epileptic children. Irish Medical Journal Supplement 73:21–28

Trimble M R, Corbett J A, Donaldson D 1980 Folic acid and mental symptoms in children with epilepsy. Journal of Neurology, Neurosurgery & Psychiatry 43:1030–1034

Veall R M 1974 Survey of epilepsy among mongols in subnormality hospitals. J Ment Defic Res 18:99–106

Viukara N M A, Tannisto P, Kauho K 1972 Low serum calcium levels in forty mentally retarded subnormal epileptics. J Ment Defic Res 16:192–195

Wing L, Corbett J A, Pool D, Woollen W, Yeates S 1972 Services for mentally retarded children and adults. In: Wing J K, Hailey A (eds) Evaluating a community psychiatric service. The Camberwell Register 1964–71. Oxford University Press, London

Wolcott G, Chunn R W M 1973 Myoclonic seizures in Down's syndrome. Devel Med Child Neurol 15:809–821

Cognitive impairment in epileptic patients

INTRODUCTION

In the nineteenth century it was widely believed, especially by psychiatrists, that intellectual, moral and social deterioration was the frequent or inevitable outcome of epilepsy on an hereditary basis. In Chapter 1 Hill traces the origins of this view in large measure to the degeneracy theory of B-A. Morel (1857), the pervasive influence of which was to last for nearly a century, reinforced by studies of unrepresentative groups of patients in psychiatric and other institutions. As Hill points out, not all neurologists of this period shared this gloomy concept of ultimate mental deterioration, based on their own experience of a rather different, often private practice, population of epileptic patients. Nevertheless Gowers in his (1881) classic book which is based on a study of the idiopathic or, as he put it, the 'functional' form of epilepsy (as far as could be ascertained with the clinical methods of that time) wrote as follows:

'The mental state of epileptics, as is well known, frequently presents deterioration and this constitutes one of the consequences of the disease which is much dreaded, and is often most serious. In the slighter form there is merely defective memory especially for recent acquisitions. In more severe degree there is greater impairment of mental power, weakened capacity for attention and often defective moral control. Mischievous restlessness and irritability in childhood may develop to vicious and even criminal tendencies in adult life. Every grade of intellectual defect may be met with, down to actual imbecility.'

Gowers recognised however that deterioration was not necessarily the effect of the epilepsy itself. 'It is certainly, in some, the expression of a cerebral imperfection of which the epilepsy is another manifestation. In such instances mental defect exists before the occurrence of the first fit'. Nevertheless he went on 'in other cases, however, which constitute a majority of the whole, the failure must be regarded as a consequence of the disease. It distinctly succeeds the fits in point of time, and may lessen very much when the fits are arrested by treatment. It is not surprising, therefore, that in cases in which a mental defect exists before the fits commenced, this should be greatly intensified by the subsequent attacks. It is among these cases that many of the worst forms of mental failure are met with'.

It is not clear how commonly deterioration, at least of the milder kind, occurred in Gowers series because in his analysis of the factors leading to dementia he compares 64 patients with 'conspicious' mental failure with some 1000 patients in whom mental failure was 'mild or absent'. Factors associated with conspicious failure included early age of onset of epilepsy, the duration of the disorder, and, to only a slight extent, the frequency of seizures. He was unable to discern an influence of sex, character of attacks, or interestingly, heredity ('it may certainly be inferred that heredity does not increase the probability of mental failure'). He concluded that 'mental failure is determined less by single conditions than by their combinations, and that it is probable that a more potent cause than the attacks themselves consists in a predisposition to suffer from fits—a predisposition which is related to the ultimate cause of the disease rather than to its developed characters'.

The reversal of the older idea of frequent and inevitable deterioration, which was clearly not shared in its fullest extent by Gowers, has been a slow process which received its main impetus from the studies of Lennox (1942) (see Lennox & Lennox 1960), who showed that some two-thirds of epileptic patients are mentally normal, a view confirmed by more modern epidemiological studies (e.g. Pond & Bidwell 1960, Graham & Rutter 1968). It has become clearer that the commonest cause of mental handicap in epileptic patients is the cerebral pathology which is associated with many types of seizure disorders, especially those with partial (focal) attacks. Nevertheless the impression has remained that deterioration in cognitive function does occur with time in a proportion of patients, and varying views have been expressed about the relative importance of heredity, brain damage, seizures, chronic anticonvulsant therapy and psycho-social factors (e.g. Lennox 1942, Pond 1961, Rodin 1968, Lishman 1978).

This chapter will review the evidence for cognitive impairment in epilepsy and will examine those factors which may contribute to this problem. Useful reviews of many aspects of this subject include those of Folsom (1953), Lennox & Lennox (1960), Pond (1961), Rodin (1968) and Reitan (1974).

METHODOLOGICAL CONSIDERATIONS

Appraisal of the evidence for cognitive deterioration has been hindered by anecdotal and uncontrolled studies, usually of institutionalised or brain-damaged subjects. The accepted view at any time has been moulded as much by the methods available for investigation as by changes in social attitudes or prejudice. Thus the interactions between epilepsy and (a) cognitive function, or (b) personality, became separate areas of study only when relevant psychological tests were developed. The history of epileptic dementia in this century has followed that of psychometrics, and any discussion of the subject must include consideration of the appropriateness of the investigative tools.

Galton (1883) developed the notion that human abilities could be discretely quantified and these measures used to compare individuals. His tests of various skills were not applied to patients with epilepsy, until the original study of Smith (1905), as the search at that time was for an explanation of the process of genius (Galton 1914). However, in 1905 Binet and Simon produced the first test of abilities designed to separate out those in need of special education (Terman & Merill 1960). In the earliest studies of epilepsy most authors were in no doubt about what they were measuring: Dawson & Conn (1929) entitled their paper 'The intelligence of epileptic children' while Patterson & Fonner (1928) at about the same time more cautiously referred to 'Some observations on the intelligence quotient in epileptics'. The following decades saw a great deal of activity in further construction and widespread application of tests intended to measure intelligence, which were generally standardised against the original Binet test and contained similar items. Psychology was coming of age as a respectable, quantitive science. The energy devoted to test construction was not mirrored by efforts to produce a coherent explanation of the psychological concept of intelligence. The group of abilities measured by Binet's tests were quite different to those evaluated in other contemporary psychological laboratories as tests of intelligence. Galton had been concerned with fine sensory abilities such as visual or auditory acuity, as well as motor skills. The more finely developed the perceptive faculties, the greater the intelligence, he argued. At about the same time J. M. Cattell (1890) had produced an intelligence test which included a measure, for example, of grip strength. The widespread acceptance of Binet's test as a measure of intelligence meant for many psychologists that intelligence and intelligence quotient were identical, though this view has had its challengers (e.g. Ryan 1972). Nevertheless, until the late 1950s the usual objective assessment of intellect in epilepsy was the IQ test, whether that of Binet, or Terman & Merill's revision of it, or later the Wechsler scale and its derived forms. Early attempts were made to demonstrate intellectual deterioration in epileptic patients but it was soon found that scores fluctuated widely, some deteriorating and some improving. Efforts were then directed towards identifying factors which distinguished deteriorating from improving epileptics, such as the aetiology, age of onset or duration of epilepsy, the frequency of seizures, psychosocial factors, and abnormal interictal EEG activity.

More recently, the measures used have evolved with the changing focus of investigation. Global assessments of intelligence quotient have given way to tests of more discrete neuropsychological functions e.g. memory, parietal function, etc. The current preoccupation with focal neuropsychological measures of cognitive function would probably appeal to Francis Galton who saw intelligence in terms of the degree of fine development of the senses, and whose tests of discrete motor and perceptual skills a century or more ago find echoes in modern test batteries.

STUDIES OF GENERALISED INTELLECTUAL HANDICAP OR DETERIORATION IN EPILEPSY

During the early years of this century, reports of the intellectual abilities of epileptic patients were based largely on observations of chronically in-stitutionalised patients.

Smith (1905) developed a test battery in the tradition of Galton and J. M. Cattell, measuring grip strength, tremor, visual discrimination, memory and card sorting. He compared six normal subjects, five of whom were attendants at Claybury Asylum, Essex, with 10 epileptic patients from the same institution. The latter were divided into two groups of five, one described as 'comparatively normal', the other showing 'marked dementia'. Tests of sensory discrimination and speed of voluntary movements failed to differentiate these groups, but he did find differences in the recognition test, the immediate memory tests and the card sorting task, all epileptic subjects showing some impairment with the greatest disability in the 'demented' group.

Turner (1907) in his study at the Chalfont Colony, attempted to relate mental deterioration, assessed clinically, to various factors such as the age of onset of epilepsy, the duration of the illness, the classification and frequency of seizures. 29 per cent of his subjects were in the most severely handicapped category, comprising memory defect, poor work capacity and a pronounced degree of dementia. Only 14 per cent showed no mental impairment at all. Thus, varying degrees of dementia were common but not inevitable in this institutionalised population. He also observed that the majority of these patients who had had fits for more than ten years showed a noticeable impairment of memory and a decrease in initiative. He describes them as slow to comprehend and 'lazy, eccentric and passionate'. There were very few cases in which the disease had lasted for 30 or more years without any obvious mental impairment. Turner, too, was influenced by Morel's (1857) concept of degeneracy and reported increasing 'stigmata of degeneration' among his epileptic subjects in proportion to the degree of intellectual handicap.

Following Turner's influential study, the Binet-Simon test was adapted for use with English children by Cyril Burt (1922) and this seems to have been used first by Tylor Fox (1924) as part of a larger battery of tests measuring educational attainment in epileptic children at the Lingfield Colony. The author points out that children were only accepted at Lingfield if they were considered capable of some education and occupation, and that, therefore, mentally defective subjects were not admitted. Consequently he assumed that the average intelligence of these schoolchildren was higher than that of adult epileptic patients in colonies generally. In his total sample of 130, he found that the boys had a median IQ of 71 and the girls 63. The greatest impairment was in tests involving immediate memory, written language, or handling abstract questions which called for concentration and reasoning. He acknowledged the possible influence on the test results of a recent fit, but he seemed committed to the view that epileptic patients show a characteristic mental deterioration with time and 'a progressive narrowing of the mental horizon'. It is noteworthy that even in this early paper the concept of discrete intellectual handicaps in epilepsy is already being entertained.

Patterson & Fonner (1928) repeated the Binet-Simon test in 98 institutionalized epileptic children after an interval varying from 1 year to 3 years 10 months. A notable feature of this study was the marked fluctuation in retest scores. Among their 51 male subjects 20 showed a decline in IQ on retesting, with a maximum fall of 17 points. 13 were unchanged and 18 showed a gain in IQ of up to a maximum of 18 points. Among 47 female subjects, 13 showed a decline, with a maximum loss of 9 points, 18 were unchanged, and 16 improved up to a maximum of 16 points. The authors concluded that the changes in IQ were not related to seizure frequency, nor the use of phenobarbitone.

Dawson and Conn (1929) used the Binet test on 49 non-institutionalised epileptic children aged between 4 and 12 years and compared them with 991 non-epileptic children. The mean IQ for all the children was 90.5, for non-epileptic children 91.7, and for epileptic children 80.6. Among 21 of their 49 epileptic children who were retested between 8 months and 4 years 8 months later, the mean IQ fell from 82.09 to 66.52. This evidence of apparent deterioration may have stimulated the study by Fetterman & Barnes (1934) in 105 epileptic out-patients of all ages. The mean IQ on the Stanford-Binet test was 74. Of the 46 who were retested between one year and two years later 23 showed a decline in IQ but 19 showed an increase. 25 patients were tested three or more times and only two showed a progressive deterioration. The authors contrasted their findings to the more frequent deterioration apparently observed by Dawson & Conn and emphasised the wide fluctuations in retest results which had been previously noted by Patterson & Fonner (1928). This fluctuation was confirmed by Sullivan & Gahagan (1935) who retested 44 epileptic children between 1 month and 4 years 11 months after their first test, and found a total decline in median IQ of only 3.4 points.

The influence of seizure control on IQ was emphasised by Kugelmass et al (1938) who compared 129 institutionalised epileptic children with 91 epileptic children seen in private practice, hospitals or special schools. The median IQ in the latter group was significantly higher (at least 40 points) than in the institutionalised group but in both groups there was a slight rise in IQ in those patients whose seizure control had improved compared to those in whom seizure frequency was unchanged after retest intervals of 3 months to 3 years.

Yacorzynski & Arieff (1942) and Arieff & Yacorzynski (1942) compared adult out-patients with 'organic' and 'non-organic' epilepsy and found significantly higher IQs amongst the latter. Retesting after one to three years revealed no significant change in IQ in the non-organic group, but a significant overall decline in the organic group. In the latter group, deterioration occurred in 37 per cent, while only 11 per cent improved. There was no difference in the degree of deterioration related to various organic factors, which included trauma, tumour, and alcoholism. In their 'non-organic' group they made the now familiar observation that retest scores fluctuate widely. In contras· to Kugelmass et al (1938) however they did not find that better seizure control was associated with an improvement in IQ.

Lennox (1942) (see also Lennox & Lennox 1960) reviewed the mental status, assessed clinically, of 1905 epileptic patients, based on information supplied to him by members of the American Neurological Association and of the Association for Research in Nervous and Mental Diseases. The distribution of the various ratings of mental level are shown in Table 12.1.

Table 12.1 Mental status in 1905 epileptic patients (from Lennox & Lennox 1960)

Above normal	2%
Normal	62%
Slightly reduced	22%
Definitely reduced	12%
Grossly deteriorated	2%

Thus, two-thirds were regarded as mentally normal and one seventh as clearly subnormal. In the combined 'definitely' and 'grossly' deteriorated groups symptomatic epilepsy was three times commoner than idiopathic epilepsy. This difference rose to eightfold in the grossly deteriorated group alone, in which males were twice as common as females.

Apart from the clear influence of organic disease of the nervous system other factors which appeared to be related to lowering of mental status were: the duration of epilepsy (at least in the first fifteen years), the total number of grand mal seizures (seizure frequency was not assessed), and the type of seizure disorder. The proportion of patients with impaired mentation was least with petit mal alone (11 per cent) increasing with grand mal alone, combined grand mal and petit mal, and reaching the highest with psychomotor alone or combined with other seizures (37.6 per cent). As discussed below and in Chapter 19 Lennox also considered that chronic anticonvulsant medication contributed to mental deterioration.

Lennox was well aware of the imperfections of such a crude clinical assessment, perhaps biased by his sources of referral, but nevertheless the overall picture was reasonably well substantiated in his later psychometric study of 400 adults in association with Collins (1951) (see Lennox & Lennox 1960). Utilising the Wechsler-Bellevue Scale they found that mean IQ was significantly higher in epileptic patients seen in private practice, compared to general or veterans' hospital practice. This was in part due to a high proportion of patients with organic epilepsy amongst the latter, but the striking influence of organic lesions was clearly seen even amongst private practice patients (Table 12.2).

Table 12.2 IQ of private practice epileptic patients (from Lennox & Lennox 1960)

	Idiopathic	Organic
Verbal IQ	110.9	99.3
Performance IQ	109.3	97.1
Full Scale IQ	111.2	98.9

The other factors which Lennox's earlier study had implicated were again in evidence, with the exception that patients with psychomotor seizures alone seemed to function relatively better, and with the additional finding that early age of onset of epilepsy carried a worse prognosis for mental function.

A similar psychometric study by Zimmerman et al (1951) in 100 children and 200 adults was in general agreement with that of Collins (1951). The former authors found that the performance IQ was usually lower than the Full Scale IQ in all groups except those with petit mal. Collins (1951) found consistently poor performance on digit span and arithmetic subtests. Excluding these from the verbal scale she found a relatively superior command of language comprehension and integrative abilities, but relatively deficient handling of situations that call for dexterity and concentration.

In a study of institutionalised epileptic patients Reed (1951) used the Terman & Merill version of the standard Binet and the Wechsler-Bellevue scale, and related mental to chronological age to look for evidence of a deterioration in mean IQ with age. He found no decline in the median mental age between the chronological ages of 20 and 45 years and suggested that the widespread belief in deterioration in epilepsy was an artefact of low mentality present from birth. He emphasised that he was using a hospitalised sample in which both epilepsy and mental handicap were closely associated.

Case note data from 296 children, both inpatients and outpatients seen at the Mayo Clinic, were studied by Keith et al (1955). Some patients had had psychometric testing, mainly with either the Wechsler or the Stanford Binet scales, but in a large number of cases intellectual level was assessed clinically. Combining both types of assessment 37.5 per cent were in the 'retarded' range, compared to the expected 9 per cent for the general population. 73 per cent of patients with 'symptomatic' epilepsy were considered 'retarded' as against 22 per cent of those with idiopathic epilepsy. Retardation seemed more common among younger children and among those with a relatively greater seizure frequency. Walker & Jablon (1959) compared, on the Wechsler-Bellevue Scale, brain-injured soldiers who were still having seizures with those whose post-traumatic seizures had ceased. In the former group they found a shift in the IQ distribution curve to the left, i.e. there were more with an IQ of less than 89, and less with an IQ greater than 120. Although this might be taken to imply that the continuing occurrence of seizures is associated with a deterioration in intellectual function, the possibility has to be considered that the persisting seizures reflect a greater degree of brain damage which in turn could be associated with greater intellectual impairment.

In 56 adolescent or adult outpatients Rodin (1968) found a slight but significant fall in performance and verbal IQ on retesting with the Wechsler Adult Intelligence Scale (WAIS) after intervals ranging from 5 to 9 years. Patients with initially high IQs more commonly showed a fall. The performance IQ was more affected than the verbal IQ and seemed to be influenced by seizure frequency. It tended to rise if the patient achieved a remission of at least two years. Other factors which appeared to be related to a falling IQ included: the number of different seizure types in the same patient, 'organic' features on psychological tests, adverse social environmental influences, and EEG background amplitude. He noted a clear influence of age of onset of epilepsy on initial full scale IQ. With onset before the age of 3 mean IQ was 84.8, between 4 and 12 years of age 90.4, and between 13 and 27 years it was 101.3.

Another approach to the problem of intellectual deterioration and epilepsy is the question of the prevalence of seizures in mentally retarded populations. This is reviewed by Corbett in Chapter 11. Epilepsy occurs in 3–6 per cent of children with an IQ between 50 and 70. His own and other studies have shown that with IQs below 50 the incidence of seizures rises steeply in relation to the degree of intellectual impairment (and presumably the amount of brain damage) reaching as high as 50 per cent in those with an IQ of 20 or less (see Table 11.1, Chapter 11). This association is also age-related, the younger the child with brain damage, the higher the incidence of epilepsy (Table 11.2, Chapter 11).

Summarising the literature we have reviewed on general cognitive impairment associated with epilepsy we would draw the following tentative conclusions:

There is a dearth of careful long-term studies especially of a prospective kind in representative (unbiased) populations.

Approximately two-thirds of epileptic patients have normal mental states.

Patients with an organic basis for their epilepy have a significant lowering of their mean IQ, due to the underlying cerebral pathology. In mentally retarded populations there is an increasing prevalence of epilepsy in relation to the degree of intellectual impairment, perhaps reflecting the severity of brain damage. The intelligence of patients with idiopathic epilepsy falls within the normal range but there is evidence in some studies of a slight lowering of mean IQ compared with normal controls.

Several but not all studies suggest that the earlier the onset of epilepsy the poorer is the prognosis for mental function, as noted by Gowers a century ago.

Repeat psychometric testing in epileptic patients shows a remarkable degree of fluctuation in intelligence measures both in an upward as well as a downward direction, in comparison to normal populations. Some studies suggest an overall slight deterioration in mean intelligence with duration of seizure disorder, with perhaps slightly greater emphasis on performance IQ. However no clear picture emerges of the proportion of patients who actually deteriorate whether, to borrow Gowers' terminology, to a conspicuous or slight degree. There is some evidence that it is more likely to occur in patients with organic rather than idiopathic epilepsy.

FOCAL COGNITIVE DEFICITS IN EPILEPSY

Quadfasel & Pruyser (1955) compared on the Wechsler-Bellevue IQ and Wechsler Memory scales, 19 patients with idiopathic tonic-clonic seizures, and 19 with psychomotor seizures associated with anterior temporal spike EEG foci (five left-sided, one right, and the remainder bilateral). Gross brain damage was excluded in all subjects. Whereas the idiopathic group had no specific deficits, the psychomotor group were significantly impaired on tests of 'verbal intelligence', memory, and verbal memory. The authors suggested that the memory impairment was related to a general impairment of verbal functioning.

In the above study there was no clear relationship of the deficits to the laterality of the EEG focus, which is not surprising as most subjects had bilateral foci. However, separate functions for the two temporal lobes were suggested by the findings of Meyer & Yates (1955) who abstracted psychometric data from the case notes of 18 patients who had had temporal lobectomies for psychomotor epilepsy. A learning difficulty occurred if the operation had been performed on the dominant hemisphere but otherwise general intelligence was relatively unimpaired. Dennerll (1964) applied multiple regressional analysis to the results of WAIS tests on 31 patients with right, and 29 with left temporal lobe epilepsy, matched for age, education, full-scale IQ and 'personality'. He calculated regression-weighted scores which could be used to predict which of the patients had a right and which a left-sided lesion. He found verbal abilities were impaired with left-sided lesions and spatial abilities with right-sided lesions. Blakemore et al (1966) examined 32 patients who had had a temporal lobectomy and whose seizures had ceased or greatly improved post-operatively. The variables considered included the pre-operative Wechsler IQ, the handedness of the subjects, and the pathology of the lesion obtained at operation. They found that patients with left temporal lesions in general showed significant impairment on certain sub-tests of the Wechsler scale, i.e. similarities, vocabulary and digit symbol, and there was also a non-significant tendency for left-sided lesions to show impairment in other verbal items. There was, however, also some evidence that impairment on verbal items was more dependent on the frequency of seizures than on the nature of the neuropathological findings. Parsons & Kemp (1960) utilising the WAIS, are the only authors to have found a relative impairment of performance to verbal IQ in *left* temporal epilepsy, in contrast to the more usual observation of a greater impairment of verbal IQ.

Matthews and Kløve (1967) applied the WAIS and items of the Halstead battery to 134 epileptic patients classified as 'major', 'psychomotor' and 'mixed' and each further subdivided into known and unknown aetiology. All subgroups, except psychomotor epilepsy of unknown aetiology, were significantly impaired in comparison to 51 non-neurological controls. In contrast Schwartz & Dennerll (1969) found a short-term visual memory deficit in patients with combined tonic clonic and psychomotor epilepsy, and they considered that the psychomotor component was the most crucial in determining this deficit.

Fedio & Mirsky (1969) examined an out-patient population of 15 children with left temporal lobe epilepsy, 15 with right temporal epilepsy, 15 with centrencephalic epilepsy, and 15 controls. Their battery included the full Wechsler Intelligence Scale for Children (WISC), various memory and learning tasks, and a sustained attention and continuous performance task. All subjects had a minimum full-scale IQ of 80. They found that on the WISC, full-scale, verbal and performance IQs were not significantly different between the groups but by subtracting the performance score from the verbal score for each subject the verbal-performance discrepancy gave a number, the magnitude and direction of which accorded with their predictions about the influence of laterality, i.e. there was evidence of greater verbal IQ impairment in 10 out of the 15 children with left-sided foci and evidence of greater performance IQ impairment in 10 out of the 15 children with right temporal epilepsy. Children with left-sided lesions also had the poorest recall on verbal tasks and those with right-sided lesions had the poorest recall on non-verbal tasks. In contrast the group with centrencephalic epilepsy showed relatively greater impairment on a test of sustained attention.

Glowinski (1973) gave the Wechsler memory scale and an abbreviated version of the WAIS to 30 patients with temporal lobe epilepsy with unilateral foci, 30 with centrencephalic epilepsy and 23 normal controls. Subjects with chronic unilateral temporal lobe epilepsy had more marked short-term memory deficits than the centrencephalic group, especially integrating and memorising meaningful verbal material. These differences were independent of IQ, laterality of the lesion, age of onset of epilepsy or medication. He considered that the memory impairment occurred early in the memory course during registration and consolidation. He speculated on possible effects of 'sub-ictal' discharges on the registration of new information.

Language related memory deficits were also investigated recently by Milberg et al (1980) in 78 patients, 40 of whom had temporal lobe epilepsy (16 left-sided, 10 right-sided, and 14 bitemporal) and 38 generalised epilepsy. The temporal lobe group was matched with the generalised group for age, full-scale IQ and duration of seizure disorder. Utilising the WAIS the authors paid particular attention to certain sub-tests, i.e. information, vocabulary and similarities, from which they constructed a special index. This index differentiated temporal lobe patients from other groups and the results supported the view that in temporal lobe epilepsy there is a language-related memory deficit. However, this did not seem to depend on the laterality of the lesion, although the authors wondered how many of their patients with right-sided foci had undetected left-sided lesions. On the other hand Delaney et al (1980) did find an influence of laterality in their study of 15 subjects with left temporal lobe epilepsy, 15 with right temporal lobe epilepsy, 15 with unilateral frontal lobe lesions and 15 normal controls. All subjects were right-handed. Applying an abbreviated version of the WAIS, the Wechsler memory scale and a word learning task, they found the temporal lobe group as a whole showed more memory impairment than the frontal lobe patients and the latter were not significantly different to the controls. Overall memory impairment was similar in patients with right and left temporal lobe lesions. However, in learning word lists, patients with left-sided lesions were more impaired than those with right-sided lesions, the latter being no different to frontal lobe subjects or to controls. On a test of non-verbal memory the right-sided temporal lobe group were more impaired than the left-sided group, who did as well as frontal lobe subjects and controls.

In summary, interest in the search for discrete cognitive deficits in temporal lobe epilepy has provided information not only about cognitive performance in epilepsy, but also about the normal functioning of the temporal lobes. The general finding of a defect in memory function has been extended to show that this is often language-related. Some but not all studies (Table 12.3) have lateralised language related memory impairment to the left temporal lobe, and non-language related impairment to the right temporal lobe. In most cases studied the subjects were right-handed and the dominant hemisphere may be presumed to be the left. These observations however have not been related to the evidence for more global intellectual deterioration already dicussed.

Factors associated with cognitive impairment

The biological and psychosocial factors that may contribute to a wide range of psychological disorders associated with epilepsy are discussed in Chapters 19 and 20, but some aspects require amplification here in relation to the specific problems of cognitive impairment.

As in the case of psychiatric and personality disorders there is general agreement that heredity, brain pathology, seizures, chronic drug therapy and psychosocial factors may contribute to impairment of cognitive function, but little agreement as to the relative importance of each (Lennox 1942, Lennox & Lennox 1960, Pond 1961, Guerrant et al 1962, Lishman 1978). Table 12.4, from Pond's (1961) review of psychiatric aspects of epileptic and brain-damaged children, summarises the changing view of Lennox between 1942 and 1960, together with Pond's own slightly greater emphasis on psychosocial factors.

One of the difficulties in evaluating the figures in Table 12.4, and indeed in most of the literature we have reviewed on this subject, is that usually no clear distinction is made between the impairment of cognitive function with which the epileptic patient is endowed, either from birth or from the time of any cerebral

Table 12.3 Summary of studies of focal lateralised cognitive deficits in temporal lobe epilepsy (TLE = temporal lobe epilepsy)

Authors	Groups (n)	Tests	Laterality (+) non-laterality (−)	Comments
Quadfasel & Pruyser 1955	Psychomotor (19) Generalised (19)	Wechsler IQ Wechsler memory	−	17/19 psychomotor patients had generalised seizures too
Parsons & Kemp 1960	Psychomotor (15) Generalised (16) Normals (15)	WAIS	+	'performance' tests relatively impaired with left-sided foci i.e. reverse of other studies. 14/16 'generalised' epileptic patients had temporal lobe foci
Dennerll 1964	R TLE (31) L TLE (29)	WAIS	+	R TLE spatial impairment L TLE verbal impairment
Blakemore et al 1966	Post-op lobectomy (32)	Wechsler IQ pre-op	+	L TLE verbal impairment retrospective study (see text)
Fedio & Mirsky 1969	R TLE (15) L TLE (15) Generalised (15) Controls (15)	WISC & other tests	+	R TLE 'performance' impairment L TLE verbal impairment subjects children aged 6–14 years
Glowinski 1973	R TLE L TLE } (30) Generalised (30) Controls (23)	WAIS Wechsler memory	−	variation due to laterality not statistically significant
Milberg et al 1980	R TLE (10) L TLE (16) Bitemporal TLE (14) Generalised (38)	WAIS	−	language-related memory deficit in TLE not dependent on laterality of lesion
Delaney et al 1980	R TLE (15) L TLE (15) Frontal lobe (15) epilepsy Normals (15)	WAIS Wechsler memory	+	R TLE non-verbal memory impairment L TLE verbal memory impairment

Table 12.4 Factors affecting intelligence in epilepsy (from Pond 1961)

| | W. G. Lennox | | D. A. Pond |
	1942	1960	1961
1. Heredity	20%	40%	1
2. Brain lesion a cause	15%	25%	2
3. Brain lesion a result	30%	20%	4
4. Socio-psychologic factors	20%	10%	3
5. Sedative drugs	15%	5%	5

insult which may have led to the seizure disorder, and any *deterioration* in cognitive function which may have followed the onset of the seizure disorder, for whatever reason. Indeed we have found only one *comprehensive* attempt to evaluate factors responsible for impaired mental function in a group of patients who had clearly deteriorated after the onset of epilepsy. Chaudhry & Pond (1961) compared 28 brain-damaged epileptic children who had deteriorated, with a control group of 28 brain-damaged epileptic children from the same institution and outpatient department, but who had not deteriorated. The main significant differences between the two groups were that in the presence of deterioration there was a higher initial seizure frequency and poorer response to anticonvulsant therapy, a more disturbed family environment and an excess of focal combined with generalised EEG abnormalities. There were no significant differences in the age of onset of epilepsy or brain damage, the degree of existing brain damage, family histories of epilepsy or mental illness, or in the amount of anticonvulsant therapy assessed on a simple rating score (before the availability of anticonvulsant drug monitoring).

Seizures

The role of seizure activity in cognitive impairment has never been clearly resolved. As already reviewed, a number of authors have attached varying degrees of importance to seizure frequency, and some, like Chaudhry & Pond (1961) above, have noted a tendency to improved cognitive functioning with improved seizure control (see for example Gowers 1881, Lennox & Lennox 1960, Rodin 1968, Dikmen & Matthews 1977). It is certainly plausible to suspect that the fluctuations in mental performance on re-testing epileptic patients that has been noted by many authors is related to fluctuations in seizure activity. Putative deleterious neuropsychological effects of seizures might also be consistent with the apparent association between mental deterioration and duration of epilepsy, as noted by a few authors (e.g. Lennox & Lennox 1960, Rodin 1968, Dikmen & Matthews 1977). On the other hand, as already discussed, other authors have failed to find any definite relationship between seizure frequency or duration of epilepsy and impaired cognitive function (e.g. Patterson & Fonner 1928, Arieff & Yacorzynski 1942, Reed 1951, Rodin 1968). Some (e.g. Lennox & Lennox 1960) have commented, at least in the case of petit mal (but not petit mal variant) how even very frequent attacks may have little or no impact on cognitive function between attacks (see Chapters 18 and 19 for discussion of psychometric performance *during* spike/wave attacks). It is certain that deterioration may occur in some patients despite good seizure control. It is also possible that the statistical association between impaired mental performance and high seizure frequency simply reflects a greater degree of cerebral damage which is responsible for both. Furthermore, with the recent increasing evidence of subtle effects of anticonvulsants on mental performance (see Chapter 19) this drug factor clearly need to be controlled for before drawing conclusions about seizure frequency or duration of epilepsy, especially as higher seizure frequency or longer duration of epilepsy is likely to be associated with more drug consumption. Finally, the twin studies of Lennox & Lennox (1960), discussed below, also cast doubt on the importance of seizure activity per se on intellectual functioning.

Some of these considerations are discussed, but not excluded, in the recent study by Dikmen & Matthews (1977), who gave the WAIS and Halstead batteries to three groups of adult epileptic subjects with 'major motor epilepsy' classified according to low, moderate and high seizure frequency, but controlled for age of onset of epilepsy and duration of disorder. Several psychological measures showed significant between-group differences with poorest, intermediate and best test results associated with high, moderate and low seizure frequency respectively, suggesting to the authors that increased seizure frequency is associated with increasing levels of adaptive impairment. They also found that the association of early onset and longer duration of epilepsy with high seizure frequency caused a high risk of impaired neuropsychological performance.

The adverse influence of early age of onset of seizures on subsequent mental function has already been emphasised in this review (see also Rodin 1968) and has most recently beeen confirmed by Dikmen et al (1977). Whether this effect is mediated by early brain damage, more prolonged seizure disorder or associated drug therapy and psychosocial influences, or other mechanisms, has not been clarified.

There is some evidence to suggest that the patients with more than one seizure type, especially combined generalised and partial attacks, have more neuropsychological impairment (Lennox & Lennox 1960, Rodin 1968, Rodin et al 1976), but this too could reflect greater brain damage or more anticonvulsant therapy, amongst other mechanisms.

We have not reviewed the literature relating EEG findings to cognitive impairment as, apart from the immediate correlates of spike/wave activity (see Chapters 18 and 19) this has generally proved unrewarding (see Rodin 1968, Wilkus & Dodrill 1976, Dodrill & Wilkus 1976). The neuropsychological deterioration associated with hypsarrhythmia is discussed by Corbett in Chapter 11.

Heredity
The increasing importance that Lennox attached between 1942 and 1960 to genetic factors in relation to mental performance (Table 12.4) is based on his study of twins with epilepsy (Lennox & Lennox 1960). Table 12.5 summarises his data on 74 monozygotic twins and 85 dizygotic twins, of which at least one of each pair had epilepsy. He separated brain-damaged twins from those without brain damage. He was impressed that in monozygotic twins without brain damage there was remarkably little spread between IQs either when both had epilepsy, or, most

Table 12.5 Mean IQ of groups of twins and points spread between co-twins (Lennox & Lennox 1960)

	Twin pairs	Mean IQ		Points spread	
		Most seizures	Least seizures	Net*	Gross†
Monozygotic					
Uninjured					
Both chronic	32	90.9	89.5	−1.4	6.2
Only one chronic	13	100.7	103.2	+2.5	4.2
Total	45	93.7	93.5	−0.2	5.6
Injured	29	76.6	97.9	+21.3	23.5
Total MZ	74	87.0	95.2	+8.2	12.6
Dizygotic					
Uninjured					
Both affected	8	79.2	83.2	+4.0	8.2
Only one affected	39	94.3	103.0	+8.7	13.4
Total	47	91.7	99.6	+7.9	12.5
Injured	38	77.7	101.7	+24.0	27.6
Total DZ	85	85.1	100.5	+15.4	19.3
All uninjured	92	92.6	96.6	+4.0	9.2
All injured	67	77.1	100.0	+22.9	25.8
Grand total	159	86.2	98.2	+12.0	16.2

* Average spread above or below the most severely affected
† Average total spread without reference to whether above or below score of co-twin

importantly, in the 13 pairs in whom only one had epilepsy. Understandably there was a greater spread among dizygotic twins without brain injury, but the spread was greatest in brain-damaged twins, whether monozygotic or dizygotic. The authors inferred from this study that in non-brain-damaged epileptic patients heredity plays a major role in determining intellectual level, and the findings from the monozygotic twins are 'perhaps the first clear demonstration that seizures in and of themselves do not weaken the intelligence'. On the other hand the data from the brain-injured twins emphasises the very striking influence of this factor in determining cognitive function associated with epilepsy.

Brain damage
The very important role of this factor has already been emphasised in the literature review in this chapter, in Chapter 19 on biological factors and the twin studies referred to above.

Anticonvulsant drugs
The evidence that chronic anticonvulsant therapy, at least with certain drugs such as barbiturates and hydantoins, may have an adverse influence on cognitive performance is discussed in detail in Chapter 19. Since the negative conclusion of Chaudhry & Pond (1961) more recent studies, incorporating blood level monitoring of the drugs, have shown that chronic epileptic patients with intellectual deterioration have generally higher levels of phenobarbitone, primidone or phenytoin than in those patients without such deterioration. The suggestion of a causal relationship in at least some patients is reinforced by recent controlled psychometric studies in normal volunteers and epileptic subjects, and by the effects of reducing or withdrawing drug therapy in epileptic patients.

Psychosocial factors
Billod (1843), quoted by Temkin (1971) drew attention to the effects of social attitudes on the performance of epileptic patients: 'Il lit sur tous les visages sa condemnation à l'isolement. ... Il est frappé de mort morale'. ('On all faces he reads his sentence to isolation ... This is death to the spirit'). Fetterman & Barnes (1934) speak of the 'deterioration in spirit' and comment 'the maladjustment of epileptic patients and the behaviour difficulties which they present may arise from frustration, defeat and failure rather than from an inherent cerebral change responsible for a gradually decreasing intelligence quotient'. Despite statements like this which reflected a general recognition of the difficulties in adjustment experienced by patients with seizure disorders, and the resulting effects on psychological performance, there have been very few attempts at objective evaluation in this area. Dodrill et al (1980) produced the Washington Psychosocial Seizure Inventory (WPSI), a self-report questionnaire including scales for family background, emotional, interpersonal and vocational adjustment, financial status, adjustment to seizures and medical management. The authors believe it to be useful in rapidly obtaining a picture of psychosocial adjustment. Batzel et al (1980) applied the WPSI to an adult population divided into employed, underemployed and unemployed, and found that it differentiated more effectively between the three groups than the WAIS or the Minnesota Multiphasic Personality Inventory

(MMPI). Dikmen & Morgan (1980) also investigated 108 adult epileptic outpatients, classified by occupational status. They found that the unemployed group did worse on most items of a neuropsychological test battery especially on measures to test 'flexibility in thinking', 'motor function', and concentration and memory. Unemployment also seemed related to age of onset and duration of seizure disorder, level of educational attainment, and previous experience of socially less desirable jobs, all of which identified a group they describe as being at risk of 'vocational failure'. The authors did not include any non-epileptic control group with 'vocational failure'.

Rutter et al (1970) found that many epileptic children underachieve at school in relation to their apparent intellectual level, as is also discussed by Stores in Chapter 4. Long & Moore (1979) investigated 19 families who had both an epileptic child and one normal sib. Attitudes were assessed by questionnaire and repertory grid techniques from the parents, the epileptic children, their normal sibs and the patient's class teachers. They found that parents expected their epileptic child to attain lower academic levels, to be less able to concentrate, to have fewer employment choices and to be more prone to emotional problems. The parents were also generally more controlling of their epileptic children.

CONCLUSIONS

The conclusions that we can draw from this review of the literature of the last 80 years are disappointingly few. The nineteenth century concept of frequent and inevitable intellectual deterioration has rightly been laid to rest, but it is not possible at this point in time to replace it with a well-founded twentieth-century concept. It is still not clear what proportion of epileptic patients actually deteriorate, or for what reasons. Conspicuous deterioration is probably relatively uncommon, but subtle degrees of cognitive impairment may be more frequent. The importance of underlying cerebral pathology, at least in the endowed or non-progressive neuropsychological deficits associated with epilepsy, seems well established, but the relative contribution of brain damage, seizures, heredity, chronic anticonvulsant therapy or psychosocial factors to subsequent deterioration remain uncertain.

It seems to us more fruitful to consider some of the reasons for the continuing uncertainty in this field in the hope that they may be remedied in future investigations. There has been a persisting tendency to study unrepresentative groups of epileptic patients who have gravitated to institutions or specialised hospital clinics. Even among the latter the investigations have almost invariably been retrospective and uncontrolled, rendering it difficult to distinguish between endowed or static cognitive deficits and any subsequent deterioration following the onset of epilepsy. There is a clear need to study unbiased groups of patients, prospectively on a long-term basis.

We also have the impression that another difficulty is the inadequacy of many of the psychometric tools that have been utilised to study cognitive deterioration. Clinical experience reinforces our view that standard batteries, which have been so widely used, fail to come to grips with so many of the more subtle cognitive difficulties of which many patients complain. There is therefore a need to develop more appropriate neuropsychological techniques.

Finally, in searching for the causes of deterioration almost all studies have failed to control for some, usually many, important variables. Future studies must take into account at the very least: age, sex, age of onset of epilepsy; type, frequency and duration of seizures; presence of brain damage; type, amount and duration of medication; psycho-social and hereditary factors. Failure to do so in the past (sometimes due to lack of suitable techniques, which are now available) accounts for persisting variation in opinion as to the relative importance of these factors. Of course such variables may be difficult to separate. Patients with the most severe brain damage may have the most frequent seizures, of more than one type, and are exposed to more medication and adverse environmental influences. In the end it may be the summation or interaction of such factors that proves the most important, as implied by Gowers a century ago.

References

Arieff A J, Yacorzynski G K 1942 Deterioration of patients with organic epilepsy. J Nerv Ment Dis 96:49–55

Batzel L W, Dodrill C B, Fraser R T 1980 Further validation of the WPSI vocational scale: comparisons with other correlates of employment in epilepsy. Epilepsia 21:235–242

Billod 1843 Recherches et considerations relatives à la symptomatologie de l'epilepsie. Annales Médico-Psychologiques 2:381–423

Blakemore C B, Ettlinger G, Falconer M A 1966 Cognitive abilities in relation to the frequency of seizures and neuropathology of the temporal lobes in man. J Neurol Neurosurg Psychiat 29:268–272

Burt, C 1922 Mental and scholastic tests. King, London

Cattell J McK 1890 Mental tests and measurements. Mind 15:373–380

Chaudhry M R, Pond D A 1961 Mental deterioration in epileptic children. J Neurol Neurosurg Psychiat 24:213–219

Collins A L 1951 Epileptic intelligence. J Consult Psychol 15:392–399

Dawson S, Conn J C M 1929 The intelligence of epileptic children. Arch Dis Child 4:142–151

Delaney R C, Rosen A J, Mattson R H, Novelly R A 1980 Memory function in focal epilepsy: a comparison of non-surgical unilateral temporal lobe and frontal lobe samples. Cortex 16:103–117·

Dennerll R D 1964 Cognitive deficits and lateral brain dysfunction in temporal lobe epilepsy. Epilepsia 5:177–191

Dikmen S, Matthews C G 1977. Effect of major motor seizure frequency upon cognitive-intellectual functions in adults. Epilepsia 18:21–29

Dikmen S, Matthews C G, Harley J P 1977 Effect of early versus late onset of major motor epilepsy on cognitive-intellectual performance: further considerations. Epilepsia 18:31–36

Dikmen S, Morgan S F 1980 Neuropsychological factors related to employability and occupational status in persons with epilepsy. J Nerv Ment Dis 168:236–240

Dodrill C B, Batzel L W, Queisser H R, Temkin N R 1980. An objective method for the assessment of psychological and social problems among epileptics. Epilepsia 21:123–135

Dodrill C B, Wilkus R J 1976 Neuropsychological correlates of the electroencephalogram in epileptics. II The waking posterior rhythm and its interaction with epileptiform activity. Epilepsia 7:101–109

Fedio P, Mirsky A F 1969 Selective intellectual deficits in children with temporal lobe or centrencephalic epilepsy. Neuropsychologia 7:287–300

Fetterman J, Barnes R R 1934 Serial studies of the intelligence of patients with epilepsy. Arch Neurol Psychiat 32:797–801

Folsom A 1953 Psychological testing in epilepsy. I Cognitive function. Epilepsia 2:15–22

Fox J T 1924 The response of epileptic children to mental and educational tests. Br J Med Psychol 4:235–248

Galton F 1883 Inquiries into human faculty and its development. Macmillan, London

Galton F 1914 Hereditary genius. Macmillan, New York

Glowinski H 1973 Cognitive deficits in temporal lobe epilepsy. J Nerv Ment Dis 157:129–137

Guerrant J, Anderson W W, Fischer A, Weinstein M R, Jaros R M, Deskins A 1962 Personality in epilepsy. Thomas, Springfield, Illinois

Graham P, Rutter M 1968 Organic brain dysfunction and child psychiatric disorder. Br Med J 3:695–700

Gowers W R 1881 Epilepsy and other chronic convulsive diseases. Churchill, London

Keith H M, Ewert J C, Green M W, Gage R P 1955 Mental status of children with convulsive disorders. Neurol (Minneapolis) 5:419–425

Kugelmass I N, Poull L E, Rudnick J 1938 Mental growth of epileptic children. Am J Dis Child 55:295–303

Lennox W G 1942 Brain injury drugs and environment as causes of mental decay in epileptics. Am J Psychiat. 99:174–180

Lennox W G, Lennox M A 1960 Epilepsy and related disorders. Little Brown, Boston

Lishman W A 1978 Organic psychiatry. Blackwell Scientific Publications, Oxford

Long C G, Moore J R 1979 Parental expectations for their epileptic children. J Child Psychol Psychiat 20:299–312

Matthews C G, Kløve H 1967 Differential psychological performances in major motor, psychomotor, and mixed seizure classification of known and unknown etiology. Epilepsia 8:117–128

Meyer V, Yates A J 1955 Intellectual changes following temporal lobectomy for psychomotor epilepsy: preliminary communication. J Neurol Neurosurg Psychiat 18:44–52

Milberg W, Greiffenstein M, Lewis R Q, Rourke D 1980 Differentiation of temporal lobe and generalised seizure patients with the WAIS. J Consult Clin Psychol 48:39–42

Morel B A 1857 Traité de dégénerescences physiques, intellectuelles et morales de l'espèce humaine et des causes qui produisent ses variétés maladaptives. Ballière, Paris, vol 1

Parsons O A, Kemp D E 1960 Intellectual functioning in temporal lobe epilepsy. J Consult Psychol 24:408–414

Patterson H A, Fonner D 1928 Some observations on the intelligence quotient in epileptics. Psychiat Quart 31:542–548

Pond D A 1961 Psychiatric aspects of epileptic and brain damaged children. Brit Med J 2:1454–1459

Pond D A, Bidwell B H 1960 A survey of epilepsy in fourteen general practices. II Social & psychological aspects. Epilepsia 1:285–299

Quadfasel A F, Pruyser P W 1955 Cognitive deficit in patients with psychomotor epilepsy. Epilepsia 4:80–90

Reed H B 1951 The intelligence of epileptics. J Genet Psychol 78:145–152

Reitan R M 1974 Psychological testing of epileptic patients. In: Vinken P J, Bruyn G W (eds) Handbook of clinical neurology. Elsevier, Amsterdam, vol 15, p 559–575

Rodin E A 1968 The prognosis of patients with epilepsy. C Thomas, Springfield, Illinois

Rodin E A, Katz M, Lennox K 1976 Differences between patients with temporal lobe seizures and those with other forms of epileptic attacks. Epilepsia 17:313–320

Ryan J 1972 IQ — the illusion of objectivity. In: Richards M, Richardson K, Spears D (eds) Race, culture and intelligence. Penguin Books, London, ch 2

Rutter M, Graham P, Yule W 1970 A neuropsychiatric study in childhood. Clinics in Developmental Medicine. Nos 35/36 SIMP with Heinemann Medical, London

Schwartz M L, Dennerll R D 1969. Immediate visual memory as a function of epileptic seizure type. Cortex 5:69–74

Smith W G 1905 A comparison of some mental and physical tests in their application to epileptic and to normal subjects. Br J Psychol 1:240–260

Sullivan E B, Gahagan L 1935 On intelligence of epileptic children. Genet Psychol Monographs vol 17, 5:309–375

Temkin O 1971 The falling sickness, 2nd ed. Johns Hopkins Press

Terman L M, Merrill M A 1960 Stanford-Binet intelligence scale. Houghton Mifflin

Turner W A 1907 Epilepsy; a study of the idiopathic disease. Macmillan, London

Walker A E, Jablon S 1959 A follow-up of head-injured men of World War II. J Neurosurg 26:600–610

Wilkus R J, Dodrill C B 1976 Neuropsychological correlates of the electroencephalogram in epileptics. I Topographic distribution and average rate of epileptiform activity. Epilepsia 17:89–100

Yacorzynski G K, Arieff A J 1942 Absence of deterioration in patients with non-organic epilepsy with especial reference to bromide therapy. J Nerv Ment Dis 95:687–697

Zimmerman F T, Burgemeister B B, Putnam T J 1951 Intellectual and emotional make-up of the epileptic. Arch Neurol Psychiat 65:545–556

Medico-legal aspects of epilepsy

This paper will be concerned with two medico-legal aspects of epilepsy, (a) the law itself and (b) the epileptic law breaker.

LAWS RELATING TO EPILEPSY

It is of itself of great interest that the law has so much to say about epilepsy. The falling sickness has always been treated with reverence, respect, or fear, and specific laws regarding the marriage of epileptic people, the validity of their court testimony, and the rights of owners of epileptic slaves, may be found as far back as 2000 BC in the Babylonian code of Hammurabi. (Temkin 1945) A clause in the law of Hammurabi said that slaves could only be sold if the purchaser was given a money-back guarantee should bennu appear within the month after purchase. Bennu probably meant fits.

As recently as 1939 a law was enacted in North Carolina to control the marriage of people with epilepsy. The first modern anti-marriage laws for those with epilepsy were probably those devised in Sweden beginning in 1757, but many US states still have such laws on their statute books even although today they are not operated. The laws varied in type, some making marriages void or voidable, others, e.g. those in Washington State, imposing penal sanctions of fines or even imprisonment of up to three years should an epileptic person get married. Twenty-eight of the United States have also had, at some stage, some form of sterilisation law allowing those with epilepsy to be sterilised either by consent, or in some States by court order. However these matters are largely of historical interest as, to the best of my knowledge, no western country now actually uses any statute of this kind. Nevertheless epilepsy is still a bar to immigration to some countries, e.g. Australia.

On the whole, in Western society the law has become progressively less restrictive towards people with epilepsy. As laws, in democratic countries, are largely a reflection of public opinion this surely means that attitudes towards the epileptic are also improving. Tables 13.1 & 13.2 given below indicate that this may be the case. The data shown is a composite of answers obtained by Gallup Poll Ltd to two standard questions used in surveys commissioned both in the USA and the UK at the times indicated. (Caveness et al, Office of Health Economics 1965, Channon 1980).

Table 13.1   Do you think people with epilepsy should be employed like other people?

| | UK | | USA | |
	Should	Should not	Should	Should not
1964			82%	9%
1969	57%	23%	76%	12%
1979	78%	12%		

Table 13.2   Would you object to having your children associate with people who have fits?

| | UK | | USA | |
	Yes	No	Yes	No
1964			15%	77%
1969	15%	68%	9%	81%
1979	5%	88%		

Driving regulations in the UK

One important current restriction to the activities of the person with epilepsy is the limited conditions under which they are allowed to drive. Even here, however, there has been considerable liberalisation in recent years. The Road Traffic Act (1930) prohibited any person 'suffering from epilepsy' from holding a driving licence. Part of the problem for this Act was the difficulty in defining 'epilepsy'. Pond & Bidwell (1960) estimated that at the time of their survey about 15 per cent of adult patients with epilepsy drove, and Phemister (1961) estimated some 20 per cent. Maxwell & Leyshon (1971) reported that of 248 men with a definite history of epilepsy examined in a department of electrophysiology, 42 per cent held driving licences. Putting these figures together Pond & Espir (1976) estimated that there must be at least 15 000–20 000 epileptic drivers in Great Britain.

The Vehicle & Driving Licences Act (1969) altered the law very considerably to the advantage of the epileptic patient. It allowed that a driving licence may be granted to people with a history of epilepsy who, on the basis of medical evidence, have been free from attacks (or have had them only while asleep) for at least three years with or without treatment. However it should be noted that anyone who has had an epileptic attack since the age of three is prevented by law from obtaining a licence to drive a heavy goods vehicle or a public service vehicle, and it is probably better for the epileptic patient to avoid commercial driving altogether.

Epilepsy and the criminal law

Modern development in the law relating to epilepsy as far as criminal responsibility is concerned has been more complex. In English law, unless charged with an act of absolute liability, for example breaking the speed limit, it is necessary to show or assume that the individual charged not only carried out the illegal act but intended to do so. Intent can be interfered with by abnormal mental states, and traditionally there have been two types of mental interference with intent which lead to acquittal. The commoner route, although very uncommon in England now, is for a plea of mental illness to be substantiated so that the accused is found not guilty by reason of insanity. Such a verdict is called the 'Special Verdict', and carries with it compulsory commitment to a mental hospital for an indefinite period at the discretion of the Home Secretary. An even rarer verdict is 'not guilty by reason of non-insane automatism'. This verdict carries no restrictions and is a straight acquittal. The doctrine of non-insane automatism usually applies to sleep walking, confusional states caused by hypoglycaemia, dissociation, and, until 1963, epileptic confusional states on some occasions.

In 1961 a Mr Bratty was charged with killing a girl whom he had taken for a ride in his car. He alleged that at the time of the killing a blackness came over him, and that he just didn't know what he was doing. It was suggested that he might be subject to attacks of psychomotor epilepsy. At his trial the defence asked the jury either to acquit the accused on a plea of automatism, to find him guilty of manslaughter, or to find him not guilty by reason of insanity. The judge instructed the jury to discount the plea for automatism on the ground that there was no evidence to support it. In the event Bratty was convicted of murder, and on appeal the judge's direction on the matter of automatism was upheld and the case went to the House of Lords in 1963 where again the appeal was rejected. In the House of Lords, Lord Denning made an important statement about the distinction between insanity defined as a disease of the mind and non-insane automatism. He said 'It seems to me that any mental disorder which has manifested itself in violence and is prone to recur, is a disease of the mind. At any rate it is the sort of disease for which a person should be detained in hospital rather than be given an unqualified acquittal'.

I think however it is worth noting that Lord Denning was referring to *violent* offences. It may well be that the non-violent offender, e.g. the thief, the indecent exposer, is in exactly the same position as before, and that epileptic or other automatism would be a valid reason for complete acquittal, if proven to the jury's satisfaction. Even when an offence of absolute liability is being considered (i.e. a case, such as driving in excess of the speed limit, in which intention is irrelevant, only the action is considered), altered consciousness to the point of virtual unconsciousness is an acceptable defence. I am personally aware of a recent case in a magistrates' court when a man was charged with dangerous driving after he crashed his car inexplicably, and was later found to be suffering from epileptic seizures. He was acquitted from the charge of dangerous driving on the grounds that he was unconscious at the time of the crash and therefore was not driving.

There has been some further interpretation of this Denning judgment by a later verdict in the Court of Appeal. In the case of Quick & Paddison in 1973, the defendants were nurses at a mental hospital charged with assaulting a patient. Quick was a diabetic, and said that he couldn't remember the assault. On the morning in question he had taken his insulin but had not eaten sufficiently and he claimed, therefore, hypoglycaemic automatism. Following Lord Denning's judgment the trial judge ruled that such a defence was not admissable because the act was violent and might occur again. On appeal however it was ruled that contrary to what Lord Denning had said, disease of the mind did not include transitory malfunction caused by the application to the body of some external factor, such as insulin. So this judgment leaves open the question of whether an epileptic fit can ever be considered as provoked by an external stimulus, e.g.

would a flickering light be considered an external factor? A recent case in Leeds (R v. Owen), drawn to my attention by Drs Kay and Milne, who have kindly supplied me with detailed information, indicates that drug-induced epileptic seizures are elligible for acquittal as non-insane automatism. A man with a history of depression and social inadequacy was prescribed maprotiline HCl 75 mg t.i.d. One evening he had a strange staring attack whilst watching the TV. His mother, with whom he was living and who doted on him, ran next door and asked the neighbours to assist her and to call the police. The subject was found sitting on a settee staring at a disconnected TV screen — he did not answer his name. When he was stared at however he grabbed the other man's hand and said 'I'm going to get thee'. The neighbour left the room, and the subject and his mother together. There was a noise, the mother fell against the door, having been assaulted, and she died. When the police came, the subject was calm and rational, but amnesic for the fatal events. An EEG showed a right-sided temporal lobe abnormality. He had no history of epileptic fits. However the court accepted the submission from the two psychiatrists that the subject attacked his mother during a temporal lobe seizure induced by an antidepressant drug, and acquitted him by reason of non-insane automatism. He was admitted to hospital informally, treated with carbamazepine, and was allowed home after 3 months having had no further attacks. All of which means that drug induced seizures are going to be of increasing medico-legal significance in the future.

THE EPILEPTIC LAW-BREAKER

In discussing the epileptic offender we have to grapple with the strongly held belief that there is a clear connection between epilepsy and crime. Strange to relate there is no data which can definitely prove or refute this claim one way or the other. The few surveys on this subject that have been carried out are conflicting, and of course most of them are conducted in institutions which do not provide a random sample of the epileptic population. Clinic studies, such as that carried out by Juul-Jensen in Denmark (1964), show that neurological clinic attenders are no more or less likely to be criminal than the rest of the population. One really comprehensive survey of epilepsy, because it was a total survey of the well-defined population of Iceland, was carried out by Gudmundsson (1966). He found that of 1169 epileptics, 271 aged 16 years and over had a police record, 33 patients having been convicted of criminal offences. These 33 represented 8.3 per cent of the epileptic population, a rate three times that expected in a general community. However, as far as I am aware, there has been no survey to determine the proportion of people with epilepsy appearing in court.

My own survey of prisoners in England and Wales conducted in 1966 (Gunn 1977) suggested that the prevalence of epilepsy in prison is at least 7.2/1000 when the general population rate is approximately 5/1000. This excess prevalence was not found to be due to the youthful age structure of the prison population, as can be seen by comparing the prison survey with the College of General Practitioners (1960) survey (Table 13.3).

A further survey, carried out in my own unit (Channon, 1980), with a questionnaire sent to prison doctors, confirms the 1966 figure with a prevalence of

Table 13.3   Prison survey compared with the college of general practitioners' survey

Age	Eps	Prisoners Total sentenced	rate/1000	Eps	GP patients Pts	rate/1000		χ^2
15–24	23	2014	11.42	104	17 738	5.86	7.89	P < 0.01
25–34	11	1597	6.89	107	19 521	5.48	0.30	NS
35–46	6	817	7.34	94	20 091	4.68	0.68	NS
45–64	6	627	9.57	119	34 781	3.42	4.99	P < 0.05
65 +	0	41	—	54	13 311	4.06	—	

7.6 undoubted people with epilepsy per 1000 prison population.

A recent American survey of Illinois prisons (King & Young 1978) showed that 1.9 per cent of the prison population are receiving maintenance anticonvulsant therapy. The authors conclude that this is equivalent to a 1.9 per cent prevalence of seizure disorder, although of course this is highly unlikely as anticonvulsants are sometimes prescribed for other conditions, and some people with a seizure disorder will not be taking anticonvulsants.

I had good evidence in the 1966 survey that the 7/1000 figure was an underestimate of the number of epileptic people actually in prison because I also came across undiagnosed epileptics in my search for normal controls. My guess therefore, is that the true figure lies somewhere between 0.7 and 1.9 per cent, a figure probably above that of the general population, although we must be very cautious about drawing too firm a conclusion as the prison figures are only $\frac{1}{2}$-$1\frac{1}{2}$ times those of the general population figures, and there is likely to be a good deal of inaccuracy in any epidemiological survey of this sort.

Even if we take it that there are more epileptic people in prisons than would be expected by chance, this does not prove that those with the disorder are more likely to commit crime. Given that half of all criminal activity, as discerned by British courts, is related to the motor vehicle, such a statement would inevitably be absurd. Even Gudmunsson's excess criminality among his epileptic population does not tell us much about the behaviour of those people. The prison survey figures simply suggest that those with epilepsy are slightly more likely to get to prison than are other members of the population. Furthermore the prison survey (Gunn 1977) did not suggest that there was any association between type of crime and epilepsy, and in particular there was no association between violent crime and epilepsy.

Relationships between epilepsy and antisocial behaviour among imprisoned epileptics

If there really is a tendency for people with epilepsy to be imprisoned more often than others, I would hazard a guess that this is probably more often due to society's inherent bias towards institutional care for the epileptic than to any other factor. There is a long history of social pressure pushing the epileptic towards institutions. Very few disorders have caused specialised institutions to be built for the exclusive use of sufferers from those disorders; mental hospitals are an example, mental handicap hospitals another, leprosy colonies a third, and epileptic colonies a fourth.

Nevertheless epileptic people in prison give a good opportunity to study the possible relationships between epilepsy and antisocial behaviour, and following the census I was able to carry out an interview survey of 158 prisoners with epilepsy who constituted a spot sample of those confined throughout England and Wales in 1967. Six different relationships seemed to be apparent (1) fits causing antisocial acts directly, (2) brain malfunction causing both epilepsy and behaviour disorders, (3) antisocial behaviour in response to the low self-esteem and social rejection suffered by some epileptic patients (4) mental illness, as a result of epileptic disorder, creating antisocial problems, (5) poor environments causing both epilepsy and antisocial behaviour, (6) behaviour disorders leading to accidents producing brain injuries.

1. Fits causing antisocial acts

There is an age-old belief that during lapses of consciousness epileptic patients are liable to do nasty antisocial things. In fact it was very hard indeed to find cases from the survey where the question of automatism could be seriously considered. Knox (1968) showed that an association between automatic behaviour in an epileptic state and violence is very unusual. Of the 158 cases studied in my 1966 survey, only 10 reported having a fit within 12 hours of the offence they were charged with. Examining these 10 in some detail very little direct or automatic relationship between the crimes committed and the epilepsy could be discerned. One man hit out at a policeman after he had been drinking and had had a fit; it was just possible he was in a state of postictal confusion. Another stole goods from a car after he had had a fit. Two cases of serious violence seemed to be rage reactions to frustration. Another man set fire to a building, allegedly in response to instructions from a hallucinatory voice, but as he was a chronic alcoholic as well as having epilepsy it was difficult to attribute the hallucinations to the epilepsy alone. Professor George Fenton did a parallel study of Broadmoor hospital at that time (Gunn & Fenton 1971) and found two cases of men who probably did commit dangerous offences in a state of altered consciousness. The first struck out, during an epileptic fit, at some friends he was visiting and an elderly man died as a result. The other patient developed a fit after an evening of shooting pigeons, and the following morning, in a state of confusion, he rose early, took his shotgun and brandished it in a village street firing shots occasionally, although nobody was hurt. The best example I have personally come across was a man who fell into my 1966 survey but who was missed from the 10 cases I mentioned above as it was not clear, even at the time I saw him, that his crime was related to a fit. He is now a patient of mine (Gunn 1978) and he was a petty recidivist who killed his wife by beating her to death with a hammer. It was later discovered that he had epilepsy, and the pattern of his fits is that a typical tonic–clonic seizure is followed by a prolonged post-epileptic confusional state in which florid paranoid ideas usually develop. In retrospect it was almost certainly in such a paranoid confusional phase that he attacked his wife.

The overall conclusion must be however that automatic behaviour is an extremely unlikely explanation for criminal behaviour in a person with epilepsy.

2. Brain malfunction causing both epilepsy and behaviour disorder

In the prison survey, just over a third of the epileptic group exhibited central nervous system signs but no correlation could be obtained between this measure and the degree of violence exhibited in their offences. Given the complexity of both brain function and violent behaviour, it would be surprising to find such a crude correlation any way. It is more likely that specific types of brain damage (e.g. frontal lobe damage) are related to specific kinds of violent behaviour (e.g. impulsive, disinhibited violence). A case which illustrates the type of association found was a 39-year-old man with an apparently normal childhood in a well integrated working class home who suffered no psychological or social traumata until the age of 29 years. There was no previous history of head injury but at the age of 29 years he was involved in a motor-cycle accident sustaining a severe fracture of his skull which led to meningitis. By the aid of neurosurgery he gradually recovered but he was left with a right-sided weakness and some disorientation. After leaving hospital he attempted to return to his wife and his old job as a welder but he failed completely, soon degenerating into an unemployed drifter, stealing frequently and sleeping either in the street or in hostels for homeless men: Since his accident there were recorded 15 indictable offences, all for stealing, in 10 years.

3. Antisocial behaviour in response to the low self-esteem and social rejection suffered by some epileptic patients

Graham & Rutter, in a survey of children on the Isle of Wight, concluded 'the widespread community prejudice against epilepsy was probably an adverse factor in the epileptic child's development and it may have been one reason for the high rate of (psychiatric) disorder in the epilepsy group'. They pointed out that supportive evidence for this notion came from the slightly higher rate of psychiatric disorder (50 per cent) of those whose physical activities had been restricted, compared with the rate in the remainder (33 per cent). One of the prisoners was a young borstal lad who had epilepsy since the age of 3 years. His home was a stable well-integrated one. There was no family history of epilepsy or behaviour disorder and the origin of his attacks were unknown. He rarely suffered tonic-clonic seizures, but minor focal attacks with twitching of the left side of his face accompanied by numbness of his left arm were very frequent indeed, and at the time of the interview he was having five or six every hour, in spite of medication. He bitterly resented his epilepsy and felt a failure. Although his IQ was in the bright normal range, he was shy and never had a very rewarding job. He complained that he hadn't the chance of a better job because other people soon noticed that he was 'odd' and found out that he was 'epileptic'. Sometimes he even refused to go and look for a job because he felt humiliated. To add to his difficulties his parents always found his behaviour and his condition an enigma, and a probation officer reported: 'His father is very concerned about his status in the community.....his attitude vacillates between outright rejection and protective over-indulgence'. The prisoner had a healthy elder brother who had made a successful professional career for himself and who provided a very unfavourable comparison for the man's own self-image. Several convictions have been recorded from malicious wounding to shopbreaking.

4. Mental illness, as a result of epileptic disorder, creating antisocial problems

It is well known that epilepsy carries an increased risk of mental disorder. (Graham & Rutter 1968, Lishman 1978) In particular schizophrenia-like psychoses, affective psychoses, and suicidal behaviour have all been reported to occur with increased frequency in epileptic populations (Slater et al 1963, Betts 1974, Prudhomme 1941).

The prisoners with epilepsy in my survey manifested significantly more affective symptoms than did their controls, in spite of a high level of such symptoms among the controls. They also complained much more frequently of suicidal ideas (11 per cent of the epileptic men being troubled in this way compared with 3 per cent of the controls), and significantly more (39 per cent) of the epileptic prisoners had made a suicidal attempt (22 per cent controls). Perhaps it is not surprising that no cases with schizophrenia emerged—such patients would have been likely to have been transferred to mental hospitals.

5. Poor environments causing both epilepsy and antisocial behaviour

A number of previous studies have shown an association between maternal care and quality of childhood environments and the likelihood of developing fits (e.g. Miller et al 1960). This association could be mediated through many channels, but child battering is an extreme example which illustrates the point. Kempe et al (1962), in their classic paper on this problem, reported their findings on 302 children who had been attacked by their parents. Of these, 33 had died and 85 had suffered permanent brain injury. In the prisoner survey one boy, seen in borstal, broke down in the middle of his interview and told of frequent beatings from his mother. He said he was convinced that his seizures were due to this as they only began in his teens after a particularly unpleasant episode when his mother had beaten him around the head with a leather strap until he was dazed. One or two other men talked of severe ear infections in childhood which had probably been neglected and even gone on to meningitis in one case. Modelling, or learning by imitation, seems to be a powerful force in determining our behaviour and attitudes. It doesn't seem unreasonable therefore to speculate that a brutal uncaring home environment during childhood will increase the likelihood of, on the one hand, developing brain damage, and on the other of coping with the adult world in a brutal uncaring fashion.

6. Behaviour disorders leading to accidents producing brain injuries

'Len' came from a disturbed background, his parents continually rowing and separating till the final break when he was 9 years old. At the age of 12 years he sustained his first conviction for stealing a lorry and was sent to an approved school. Following his release he was frequently in trouble but he had no suggestion of head injury or brain damage until the age of 17 years when just after joining the Army he smashed up an army lorry and landed himself in hospital for two weeks with a head injury. Following this incident he developed typical tonic-clonic seizures which required medication with phenobarbitone. Clearly his criminality could not be attributed to his epilepsy or any underlying cerebral damage because it antedated the accident. It is much more reasonable to assume that his behaviour disorder led to reckless driving and the subsequent neurological consequences.

Obviously the types of association suggested here are by no means the only ones possible, and some cases showed more than one of the mechanisms acting simultaneously or even additively.

Kligman & Goldberg, in a theoretical analysis, have suggested that a further category should be that the drugs given to control epilepsy may cause aggression in some patients. I have not included this category as I am not convinced that I have seen any such patients myself.

CONCLUSION

No neat general conclusions can be drawn from this mixture of medico-legal and socio-medical problems. However epilepsy does show very nicely that legal and social issues have a considerable impact upon clinical practice. We have found here, for example, that there are special laws drawn up to deal with the consequences of a particular neuropsychiatric condition. A few patients suffering this particular disorder run into legal conflicts as a direct result of their illness. Sometimes offenders are especially predisposed to develop the disorder, because of their antisocial propensities.

Acknowledgements
I would like to thank Shelley Channon for the work she carried out on the recent prison census, and the attitude survey. Gallup Poll Ltd gave permission to quote the attitude survey. The Home Office provided the funds for the recent prison survey and gave access to the prisons for both the earlier and the recent work. The Epilepsy Research Fund provided monies for the census study. The original prison survey was carried out with a grant from the Medical Research Council. Celia Gunn provided details of one court case, Drs Milne and Kay provided another. Dr Pamela Taylor made cogent criticisms of the manuscript and Maureen Bartholomew provided secretarial services.

References
Betts T A 1974 A follow-up study of a cohort of patients with epilepsy admitted to psychiatric care in an English city. In Harris P, Mawdsley C (eds) Epilepsy: proceedings of the Hans Berger centenary symposium. Churchill Livingsone, Edinburgh
Caveness W F, Merritt H H, Gallup G H, Ruby E H 1965 A survey of public attitudes towards epilepsy in 1964. Epilepsia 6:75–86
Channon S 1980 Personal communication
College of General Practioners 1960 A survey of the epileptics in general practice. British Medical Journal 2:416–22
Graham P, Rutter M 1968 Organic brain dysfunction and child psychiatric disorder. British Medical Journal 3:695–700
Gudmundsson G 1966 Epilepsy in Iceland Acta neurologica scandinavica 43:supp.25
Gunn J 1977 Epileptics in prison. Academic Press, London
Gunn J 1978 Epileptic homicide: a case report. British Journal of Psychiatry 132:510–3
Gunn J, Fenton G 1971 Epilepsy, automatism, and crime. Lancet 1:1173–6
Juul-Jensen P 1964 Epilepsy: a clinical and social analysis of 1020 adult patients with epileptic seizures. Acta neurologica scandinavica 40:supp.5
Kay D, Milne H 1980 Personal communication

Kempe C H, Silverman F N, Steele B S, Droegemueller W, Silver H K 1962 The Battered child syndrome. Journal of the American Medical Association 181:17–24

King L N, Young Q D, 1978 Increased prevalence of seizure disorders among prisoners. Journal of the American Medical Association 239:2674–5

Kligman D, Goldberg D A 1975 Temporal lobe epilepsy and aggression. Journal of Nervous and Mental Disease 160:324–41

Knox S J 1968 Epileptic automatism and violence. Medicine, Science and the Law 8:96–104

Lishman W A 1978 Organic psychiatry Blackwell, Oxford

Maxwell R D H, Leyshon G E 1971 Epilepsy and driving. British Medical Journal 3:12–15

Miller F J W, Court S D H, Walton W S, Knox E G 1960 Growing-up in Newcastle-upon-Tyne OUP, London

Office of Health Economics 1971 Epilepsy in society London

Phemister J C 1961 Epilepsy and car driving. Lancet 1:1276–7

Pond D A, Bidwell B H 1960 A survey of epilepsy in fourteen general practices. II Social and psychological aspects. Epilepsia 1:285–99

Pond D A, Espir M 1976 Epilepsy. In Repple A (ed) In: Medical aspects of fitness to drive. MCAP, London

Prudhomme C 1941 Epilepsy and suicide. Journal of Nervous and Mental Disease 94:722–31

Slater E, Beard A W, Glithero E 1963 The schizophrenia-like psychoses of epilepsy. British Journal of Psychiatry 109:95–150

Temkin O 1945 The falling sickness John Hopkins Press, Baltimore

Epilepsy and the mental hospital

INTRODUCTION
In this chapter I want to present evidence to suggest that the study of epilepsy occurring in patients in mental hospitals in Great Britain has been neglected, and that this neglect has lead to certain false assumptions about the type, prevalence and aetiology of mental illness in people with epilepsy.

In the last hundred years since Gower's publication the vast majority of severely mentally ill people in this country, whether or not they have epilepsy, have been treated in mental hospitals. Most of the studies made on the relationship between mental illness and epilepsy, however, have been carried out in specialist, postgraduate or general hospital psychiatric units so that consequent factors of selection have made extrapolation from these studies to the general population of the mentally ill with epilepsy difficult and potentialy biased.

Indeed review of what little literature there is on the subject of epilepsy in the mental hospital over the past hundred years suggests that some of the common syndromes encountered consistently in the epileptic population of mental hospitals, even up to the present day, have been little described elsewhere, and syndromes described in special institutions as especially important seem to occur only rarely in the common ruck of patients in the mental hospital.

In the mental hospital itself the only marked change over the years is that the psychiatrist's original interest and expertise in the *medical* treatment of epilepsy has largely evaporated. This to some extent relates to the trend, already well started in Gower's time, to separate the disciplines of neurology and psychiatry (to the detriment of both and particularly to the person with epilepsy).

It is certainly an interesting historical fact that the development of medical scientific interest in epilepsy began at about the same time as the development of mental hospitals (from 1820 onwards) and that many of the early 'epileptologists' were psychiatrists (Temkin 1971). In the early and mid-nineteenth century people with uncontrolled epilepsy (whether or not they were mentally ill) could be given asylum in mental hospitals, particularly because at that time it was believed that epilepsy and mental illness had a common cause. This view later became extremely unpopular, almost heretical, but it is interesting that in a modified sense, in our ideas on the aetiology of the schizophrenias of epilepsy, and the biochemistry of epilepsy and mental illness, we are returning to it. I doubt that Gowers ever held this idea, but it was certainly current in the asylums of his time.

People with uncontrolled epilepsy who could not support themselves, or who had no family to support them, were readily admitted to mental hospitals in Gower's time, particularly because few other places would have them. To *some* extent this trend has lasted until the present day, particularly if they are also disturbed. In Gower's time the number of people with epilepsy who were also severely mentally ill was almost certainly greater than it is now. This probably related to the mental effects of uncontrolled epilepsy, extreme social rejection, and the deleterious effects of the only effective anticonvulsants at the time, the bromides.

Exactly what these patients with epilepsy were like in the asylums of Gower's time is difficult to determine. Nomenclature was very different from today's: what clinicians regarded as important to describe was also different (today, for instance, a patient's masturbatory habits would be of little import: to the Victorian psychiatrist they would have great significance and would be reported in great detail as would the patient's skull structure and whether he was bald or hairy; the fact that he heard voices talking about him in the third person or was disorientated in time and place might not be commented on).

Symptomatic epilepsy was also more common in Victorian times; many of the patients admitted with epilepsy to the asylums of the late Victorian era had general paralysis of the insane (although most published accounts of people with epilepsy in the asylums of that period are careful to distinguish between patients with and without general paralysis). During this time, too, many patients who were severely subnormal in intelligence were also admitted to mental hospitals, as separate asylums for the mentally handicapped were only just starting [although in 1968–69 in Birmingham I found that 19 per cent of mentally ill people with epilepsy admitted to psychiatric care were still mentally subnormal (Betts 1974)].

In addition most early published accounts fail to distinguish clearly between statistics relating to the mental illnesses occurring in patients freshly admitted to hospital and those who remained in hospital for a long time — a point of importance as we shall see later — and the distinction between acute self-limiting disturbance and chronic mental illness is not always made. Likewise the distinction between mental illness with a clear time relationship to the fit, mental illness accompanied by evidence of an acute brain syndrome and mental illness with no apparent time relationship to the fit was not often clearly made.

By the turn of the century, however, separate epilepsy colonies were in existence (although mental illness could occur in them as well — see Turner 1904) so that the social or medical epileptic admission to the mental hospital was less common (a change supported by psychiatrists): in addition the modern classification of mental disorder was developing, and the clinical descriptions used are easier for us to understand. By 1900 as well, most mental hospitals or asylums had been built. It is therefore appropriate to begin a review of the literature relating to epilepsy and the mental hospital in 1900.

1900–1950

Between 1900 and the outbreak of World War I it is clear that many asylum doctors had a particular interest in the medical and psychiatric aspects of epilepsy, which from the published accounts must have been an important and troublesome problem. Discussion in particular centred on the best medical treatment for epilepsy (social rehabilitative treatment was well recognised and described) and the deleterious effects of bromide is described in several papers. Interestingly enough, the mental state of the patients is almost taken for granted: those few authors who do describe patients' behaviour in some detail are almost apologetic about describing phenomena with which they feel their readers will be only too familiar—what, I wonder, do we take for granted in our present-day clinical descriptions? By and large they were describing severe mental disturbance needing compulsory admission to hospital, but the clinical descriptions have a familiar ring today.

Thus, Raffle (1908) noted that in the Exeter asylum status epilepticus was the commonest cause of death amongst his patients with epilepsy. Barham (1907), describing the epileptic population of Claybury asylum mentioned Ward K, an epileptic ward which I think was probably a common phenomenon in mental hospitals at that time. He painted a vivid picture of the agitation and turbulence of such a ward in which status epilepticus, fights and irritability were common. Interestingly enough he stated that he felt that the commonest mental disorder to be found in epilepsy was melancholia. Like many other writers he noted the problems of using bromides, as did Baugh (1908) who described his experience of the patients with epilepsy admitted to Gartloch Mental Hospital, Glasgow from its opening a few years before.

The figure he gave for the proportion of patients in the hospital with epilepsy is confusing, but suggests that about 11 per cent of those resident had epilepsy. It would appear that of the patients with epilepsy coming into the hospital, a quarter left before a year 'relieved', a quarter died (mainly of pneumonia or status) and half remained as chronic patients (some of these, of course, were mentally subnormal and unlikely ever to get out).

Baugh (1908) reported that 12.6 per cent of his patients recovered from their mental illness (and their epilepsy also improved) after bromides were stopped. He also felt that melancholia was the commonest mental illness to be found in his patients, although Barham's and Baugh's accounts are tantalising in that they give little description of the mental phenomena that their patients displayed. Both authors were concerned with the acute episodic disturbances, often of homicidal violence, that seemed to be common to both their hospitals and which were clearly difficult to manage. Barham in particular noted that both the epilepsy and the mental disorder had to be treated together if satisfactory results were to be obtained: 'only second to the treatment of the paroxysms is the observation and management of the psychic manifestations of this disease and the episodic symptoms occurring in conjunction with the attack or its equivalent . . . in order to arrive at the point where, with a satisfactory diminution of the paroxysms, there is the least disturbance of the mental equilibrium'.

White (1900), describing the City of London asylum, painted a picture of epileptic patients with severe frequent fits, (incidentally he noted that minor seizures led to dementia more often than major seizures), with aggression being common after fits and sometimes before, and religious delusions, hallucinations and violent behaviour frequently occurring together. He made the observation that fits occurring spontaneously in the course of mania or melancholia might lead to recovery from these conditions, an interesting pre-ECT idea. He noted reflex epilepsy (startle and water immersion) to be common in his patients.

His description of the typical patient is worth quoting in full because it gives the best picture of the mental hospital experience of epilepsy at the time and for perhaps the next fifty years.

'Fits having recurred with ever increasing frequency; irritability, loss of self restraint, fits of passion and failing memory have followed — then a maniacal outburst with extreme violence necessitates certification... the patient is mildly demented and often has widely dilated pupils, the speech is drawling, ideation being sluggish... there is marked moral decadence yet often religious fervour... they are most quarrelsome, impulsive and dangerous and often come to blows... frequently they have delusions of a religious nature and of persecution, with hallucinations of one or more of the special senses of the familiar types. These delusions and want of self control often cause homicidal acts'.

White also recognised that bromides could make fits worse and dull the senses: 'the fits may be controlled but the advent of dementia is hastened'. One of the discussants of his paper afterwards said that he gave bromides sparingly as he was sure that 'the constant use of these drugs drove many into the asylums'.

Savage (1912) confirmed White's observations of a chronic epileptic psychosis of a paranoid type — 'a certain number of insane epileptics develop definite delusions and ideas of persecution. Hallucinations are common occurring as aural in some cases'. This concept of an epileptic paranoid state was enthusiastically rediscovered many years later, but was clearly well known to asylum doctors at the turn of the century.

Jones (1912), describing Claybury once again, gave some figures. Ten per cent of all the insane persons in the asylum suffered from epilepsy, and 6 per cent of the fresh admissions had it, suggesting that, as indeed was still so half a century later (Betts 1974), people with epilepsy admitted to mental hospitals have difficulty getting out again. He also gave figures to suggest, but fails to quote his source, that one third of the people with epilepsy in the country at that time were also insane. Jones also made the interesting observation, which had been made by the other authors, that 'when epilepsy is asociated with insanity the tone of the mental condition is that of depression or melancholia rather than that of mania'. Like the others he also describes the suspiciousness, aggressiveness and irritability in people with epilepsy confined to an epileptic ward.

This observation, probably true then, was no longer true when I surveyed groups of chronic epileptic patients in mental hospitals in 1967 but the reputation remained in the minds of their nurses, and was responsible largely for the fear and dislike the nurses had of them.

It is interesting that, after the papers quoted above, no formal examination of the epileptic population of English mental hospitals was carried out again until the 1950s. Much, of course, had happened in the interval. New anticonvulsant treatment had come in, two world wars had profoundly influenced the development of psychiatric ideas, new physical treatments had been introduced. Of particular interest to epilepsy was electroconvulsive therapy, which had been introduced because of the widely held theory in the 1920s that there was a biological antagonism between epilepsy and schizophrenia so that if one gave a schizophrenic patient epilepsy he might improve. It is interesting to speculate that, if careful research had been made in the mental hospitals at that time, the theory might never have developed and, therefore, a useful treatment for depression might not have been introduced.

Indeed in the 1930s it became fashionable to publish papers describing the apparent association between epilepsy and schizophrenia to disprove the biological antagonism theory, in the same way perhaps nowadays that anyone discovering several patients in succession who happened to have schizophrenia and a right-sided temporal lobe epilepsy might be tempted to publish them.

Glaus (1931) and Notkin (1929) both described cases of schizophrenia and epilepsy existing side-by-side, and both noted in almost half their cases that the epilepsy followed the onset of the schizophrenia by some years. Some authors, such as Krapf (1928), could declare that the occurrence of epilepsy with schizophrenia was rare whereas others, such as Esser (1938), could describe the association as quite common. The reason for this difference is that Esser was looking at a population of people with schizophrenia contained in hospital for some time, whilst Krapf was looking at acute cases that had been psychotic for only a short while. Many of Esser's cases developed epilepsy some years after the onset of the psychosis, an important group of patients which seems to have been almost entirely missed by surveys in non-mental hospitals, which have concentrated on patients who have epilepsy and then develop schizophrenia.

One author commenting on the relationship between epilepsy and schizophrenia made an original point for which he has never been given credit, although it anticipates by over 30 years the now fashionable explanation of the relationship between epilepsy and schizophrenia. Falsey (1935), in describing two of his patients who in the course of a schizophrenic illness had typical epileptic seizures, said 'it would appear that the epileptic seizures . . . were the result of the same aetiological factors involved in the exacerbation of the psychosis'.

1950 TO THE PRESENT TIME

Interest in the relationship between epilepsy and psychiatric illness, particularly schizophrenia, seems to have revived in the late 1950s and has been reviewed by Trimble (1981), and Toone in Chapter 10. As some kind of herald to this interest Liddell's (1953) survey of the epileptic population of Runwell Hospital is of interest. This was the first survey of an epileptic population of a mental hospital in Great Britain since Jones' survey at Claybury published in 1912.

Liddell, in fact, was looking for examples of epileptic automatism and his survey was incidental to that purpose. He reviewed all patients in Runwell 'who in an arbitrary period of a month suffered from epilepsy'. All cases had been in hospital for some months at least but he would, of course, have excluded from his study those patients admitted to the hospital years before with epilepsy who had subsequently stopped having seizures. He found that 4.3 per cent of the chronic hospital population of Runwell had epilepsy. This is, of course, much higher than one would expect by chance but, even allowing for patients with general paralysis of the insane, much lower than Jones' (1912) figures.

Liddell divided his patients up into three groups — 18 patients who were mentally subnormal and in hospital for care and protection, a group of 11 who were severely demented and in whom the epilepsy seemed related to the dementia, and a group of 18 he called the automatism group. These were mainly patients admitted because of violent postictal furor, although there were a few in whom admission was precipitated by increasing fits leading to an acute organic paranoid psychosis, which usually settled once the patient was admitted to hospital.

Liddell described very similar behaviour to that described 50 years before, in the automatism group: patients were overactive and restless, had episodes of hallucinations (with an increase in attacks before such episodes). They often showed an ecstatic euphoria and during hallucinatory episodes were disorientated, misidentified their surroundings and had amnesia for events occurring during these acute episodes (except for their hallucinations).

Between the acute behaviour disturbances, aggressiveness, hostility and obsessional features were seen in most, if not all, of the automatism group. Many were solitary and moody. All took offence easily and many were subject to short-lived unprovoked outbursts of violent rage (most had a right temporal focus on electroencephalography). Liddell found, as had the asylum doctors 50 years before, that work helped more than drugs in keeping calm patients who, if not stimulated, became withdrawn, asocial and manneristic with slurred speech and mumbling like chronic schizophrenics and 'when leave is granted to a supposedly stabilised patient a rapid deterioration generally occurs'. 12 out of the 18 had a right temporal focus on EEG, four had a left temporal focus and two had bilateral temporal discharges.

Although Liddell's method of ascertaining his patients had selected out some patients in the hospital who probably should have been included in his survey, it showed clearly the patterns of behaviour of epileptic patients admitted to Runwell had not changed much in 50 years. Factors tending to keep patients in hospital were continuing episodes of violence and a difficult personality.

A slightly different study of the chronic epileptic population of two mental hospitals in the Birmingham region was carried out by myself in 1967: these patients were resurveyed 12 years later (Betts 1980, Betts & Skarrott 1981).

In October 1965, 718 of 13 184 mental hospital beds in the Birmingham region were occupied by patients who were also described as epileptic (5.4 per cent). 306 of the 16 104 patients admitted to these beds in 1965 were similarly described (1.9 per cent).

To investigate these figures further a cross-sectional study of the *chronic* epileptic in-patients of two Birmingham Regional Hospitals was carried out in 1967. Patients were included in the survey if they were reported to have had epilepsy at any time during or before their hospital stay, and had been in hospital for at least one year. All wards of both hospitals were visited, all the notes were looked through, senior nurses were questioned and hospital lists of epileptic patients consulted. Ascertainment was therefore as complete as possible. In one hospital there was still an epileptic ward for disturbed male patients.

About 20 per cent of the patients who were labelled as having epilepsy clearly did not have it at all, but either had something else that had been misdiagnosed or had had one or two fits symptomatic of some other brain disturbance. Although in a research study one can discount such patients, they still appear in, and distort, hospital statistics. In 1967 there had been 105 patients in the two mental hospitals (4.7 per cent of their population) who were labelled as having epilepsy. Of these

105, 78 did in fact have epilepsy or had had it in the past. As far as could be determined, the diagnosis on admission to hospital is shown in Table 14.1.

Table 14.1 Chronic mental hospital epileptic population (1967–1979)

Diagnosis on admission	
Paranoid psychosis	28
'Furor'	20
Paranoid schizophrenia	15
Confusion/dementia	8
Hebephrenic schizophrenia	4
Other	3
	—
	78

It will be seen that roughly half the patients had been admitted originally with some kind of paranoid illness. Most had had a paranoid psychosis: in other words they had delusional ideas of reference and auditory hallucinations, but had had no recognisable first rank symptoms of schizophrenia. Just under half of the paranoid psychoses developed suddenly, often in association with a marked increase in attack frequency, as Liddell had noticed, and, again as Liddell had noticed, in these patients the paranoid symptoms often resolved quite quickly when the patient came into hospital. Some patients, after this recovery, continued to show evidence of organic brain impairment as had been described at the turn of the century.

A few patients did satisfy the diagnostic criteria for paranoid schizophrenia, in that in addition to the symptoms mentioned above they had, or had displayed in the past, clear evidence of one or more of the first rank symptoms of schizophrenia (Mellor 1970). In this group of 15 patients the onset of schizophrenia had occurred first in over half, thus confirming some of the observations made in the 1930s and suggesting that studies of schizophrenic patients with epilepsy in institutions other than mental hospitals, may be biased in the direction of 'epilepsy first'. Most of these patients had temporal lobe epilepsy, and right-sided lesions seemed more common than left.

Another group had been admitted because of episodes of severe aggression, as in the other series, usually appearing as a kind of furor after a fit although occasionally occurring without any obvious relationship to the ictus. Some remained violent after admission to hospital, some remitted. The other main reason for these patients' original admission to hospital was a confusional state or an apparent dementia, confusion often being associated with an acute increase in attack frequency.

Many patients still had a considerable fit frequency, most were taking high doses of three different anticonvulsants: few had been investigated, although it was felt in the survey that about half of the patients would have benefited from further investigation and assessment of their epilepsy.

Twelve years later 34 of the 78 patients were known to be dead, 17 had left hospital, 24 were still in hospital and three had been lost to follow-up. Most of the patients who had successfully left had totally left the hospital's care, and were no longer being followed up. Most patients had died of pneumonia or strokes: status epilepticus no longer seemed to be a problem.

Almost all the patients who had survived, whether they were in hospital or not, were mentally well on follow-up. Paranoid illnesses had disappeared (often after psychotropic drug treatment) and the patients with furor had lost their aggression (some by the passage of time, some by treatment with such drugs as chlordiazepoxide). A number of patients who were carrying the diagnosis of 'epileptic dementia' in 1967 had recovered completely and were certainly not demented 12 years later. What had probably originally been a thought disorder, and which had resolved, had been mistaken for a dementing syndrome and one wonders how many of the patients labelled as demented in earlier studies might also have been examples of this condition.

Even 12 years later, however, many of the patients still continued to have frequent epileptic attacks. All but five of the patients were taking exactly the same anti-convulsant medication in 1979 as they had been taking in 1967. No attempts had been made to monitor blood levels except in one patient, and there were one or two patients in 1967 who had appeared to be intoxicated who were still apparently intoxicated in 1979. It is clear that the interest shown by the old asylum doctors in the treatment of epilepsy had not been maintained.

These latter surveys however, suggest that very much the same syndromes reported in the studies at the turn of the century were still being seen in mental hospitals as late as the early 1960s. This certainly applies to chronic in-patients: what about acute admissions?

An acute epileptic admission survey was carried out in the city mental hospitals and psychiatric units of Birmingham, between 1st November 1968 and 31st October 1969 (Betts 1974). Patients came into ascertainment in this study if they were admitted as in-patients to the adult mental hospitals and psychiatric units of the city and were known to be suffering from epilepsy on admission or had had a history of epilepsy in the past.

93 patients came into ascertainment, internal evidence suggesting that probably most of the patients with epilepsy admitted to psychiatric care in the city of Birmingham during that year were included in the survey. As in the chronic survey some patients (21) were thought not to have epilepsy in the customarily accepted meaning, so that 72 patients were included in the full survey.

As will be seen from Table 14.2 the commonest reason for admission, as in most of the other studies reported in this chapter, was an acute behaviour disturbance. Various types of confusional state were also common reasons for admitting patients.

When one looks at the principle psychiatric diagnosis made on these patients by the survey team it is clear that they were a very different population from the chronic population, depression being the commonest diagnosis, followed by the various organic syndromes. Paranoid psychosis was rare. Increase in fit frequency before admission was significantly associated with both an acute behaviour disturbance and a diagnosis of an organic syndrome (as Liddell found). A

Table 14.2 Epilepsy admission study
1968–1969

Main reason for admission (n = 72)	
Acute brain syndrome (delirium, confusion, intoxication etc.)	16
Acute behaviour disturbance	15
Attempted/threatened suicide	14
Assessment	12
Depression	11
Social reasons	4

Table 14.3 Epilepsy admission study

Main psychiatric diagnosis (n = 72)	
Depressive illness (12 endogenous)	22
Brain syndrome (dementia, intoxication, twilight state etc.)	22
Personality disorder/psychopathy	
Social distress	4
Paranoid psychosis	3
Phobic anxiety	3
Psychiatrically normal	2
Not known*	1

* Absconded before assessment

significant reduction in attack frequency was associated with endogenous type depression.

The patients were resurveyed at the end of a year from their admission — 9 per cent were still in hospital (and had therefore become chronic) and a further 15 per cent had had at least one readmission to hospital in that year. Four patients had died during the survey year. Less than half the patients were rated as improved on follow-up and some were actually worse. Many had already lost contact with the hospital where they had been admitted. The prognosis for the epilepsy was somewhat better.

Although acute behaviour disturbance was a common reason for admission, furor was not really seen. The survey suggests that the population of patients going into a mental hospital with epilepsy is very different from the population of patients who remain in the hospital once admitted (the depressed and confused, versus the furious and paranoid). The clinical features of mental disturbance in people with epilepsy in mental hospitals, which seem to have changed little in 60 years, are very different from those features emphasised in studies looking at non-mental hospital populations. If we are to obtain a clear picture of the mental disorders of epilepsy, both must be considered. What is clear is that a surprisingly high proportion of both the chronic and the acute mentally ill epileptic population have a direct relationship between the epilepsy and the mental illness: in the acute survey it was an increase in attack frequency which lead to behaviour disturbance or confusion, or a decrease in seizures leading to depression: in the chronic population increase in attacks leading to confusion or a paranoid psychosis. Review of the other literature suggests that such epilepsy-related mental illnesses have alway been common.

Has the picture changed since the last study was done? The follow-up of the chronic patients (Betts 1980, Betts & Skarrott 1981) suggests that it may have done. Furor may be dying out, paranoid illness may be more treatable, status epilepticus is not the problem it was. Mentally ill people with epilepsy need better medical care than they are currently getting. What is happening in the mental hospitals now?

References

Barham G F 1907 Notes on the management and treatment of the epileptic insane with special reference to the NaCl-free (or hypochlorination) diet J Ment Sci 53:361–367

Baugh L D 1908 Observations on insane epileptics treated under hospital principles. J Ment Sci 54:518–528

Betts T A 1974 A follow-up study of a cohort of patients with epilepsy admitted to psychiatric care in an English city. In: Harris P, Mawdsley C (eds) Epilepsy: proceedings of the Hans Berger centenary symposium. Churchill Livingstone, Edinburgh, p. 326–336

Betts T A 1980 The mental hospital and epilepsy. Research and Clinical Forums vol 2. 2:129–134

Betts T A, Skarrott P H 1981 A follow-up study of the chronic epileptic population of two mental hospitals (to be published)

Esser P H 1938 Epileptiform seizures of schizophrenics and difficulties of differential diagnosis in borderline region between epilepsy and schizophrenia. Z Ges Neurol Psychiat 162:1–24

Falsey E F 1935 Typical epileptic seizures in course of schizophrenia; two cases. New England J Med 212:153–155

Glaus A 1931 Combinations of schizophrenia and epilepsy. Z Ges Neurol Psychiatry 135:450–500

Jones R 1912 The relation of epilepsy to insanity and its treatment. Practitioner 89:772–792

Krapf E 1928 Rare occurrence of symptomatic epilepsy with schizophrenia. Arch Psychiat 83:547–586

Liddell D W 1953 Observations on epileptic automatisms in a mental hospital population. J Ment Sci 99:732–748

Mellor C S 1970 The first rank symptoms of schizophrenia. Br J Psychiat 117:15–24

Notkin J 1929 Epileptic manifestations in a group of schizophrenic and manic depressive psychoses. J Nerv Ment Dis 69:494–521

Raffle A B 1908 Some notes on status epilepticus and its treatment. J Ment Sci 54:94–105

Savage G H 1912 Some relationhips between fits and mental disorder. Practitioner 89:1–10

Tempkin O 1971 The falling sickness Johns Hopkins Press, Baltimore

Trimble M R 1981 Psychosis in epilepsy. In: Laidlaw J, Richens A (eds) A textbook of epilepsy, 2nd edn. Churchill Livingstone, Edinburgh

Turner W A 1904 The mental condition in epilepsy in relation to prognosis. Lancet 1:982–986

White E W 1900 Epilepsy associated with insanity. J Ment Sci 46:73–79

The long-term outcome of temporal lobe epilepsy in childhood

When parents bring a child with fits to a doctor, they want answers to their many fearful questions. Is it epilepsy? What caused it? Could he die? Must he always take pills? Would an operation cure him? Will he grow out of it? Might he go mad? Can he stay at school? What about work? Will they let him drive? Ought he to marry and dare he have children?

Quite recently we have begun to be able to give truthful answers to these questions. This chapter, which describes some personal enquiries, attempts to show that simple prospective studies, if patiently carried through can cast some light on these matters. (Lindsay et al 1979 a,b,c, 1980)

SEIZURES ARE PAROXYSMAL BEHAVIOURS

'Man' wrote William Lennox 'is built to convulse', and this pithy truth should have put an end to the concept that seizures are signs of an alien presence — epilepsy — which has invaded the patient and from whom that enemy must be expelled by 'anticonvulsant' drugs. Unfortunately Lennox's dictum came at a time when 'antibiotics' had, with spectacular success, begun to cure bacterial diseases. Analogical thinking prevailed. To this day most patients with fits receive blind polypharmacy, often in dangerous combinations, on the basis of false understanding of what is to be treated.

When one lists the behaviours of any animal, one constructs an ethogram. A number of groups readily emerge. Nesting behaviours, threat behaviours, feeding behaviours, agonistic behaviours — all these are easily accepted. Ounsted (1971) has suggested that there is a large additional class. This is the class of paroxysmal behaviours. To this class belong: (1) All forms of seizure (2) Orgasms — both male and female (3) Coughing in all its forms (4) Sneezing (5) Yawning (6) Startle with gasping (7) Hiccupping (8) Laughing (9) Weeping (10) Sobbing (11) Raging (12) Screaming (13) Vomiting (14) Labour.

In all these behaviours, to a greater or lesser extent, we find that the following features are held in common.

Neuronal circuitary genomically specified. The genome specifies the nature and the circumstances in which paroxysmal behaviours proceed. Phylogenetically the genomic message is, for many of these, buried deep. The sneeze of a cat and a baby do not differ greatly, and the fits that can be induced in both are closely similar in behaviour morphology. All human beings show all the behaviours listed, and all human beings can be induced to have grand mal convulsions.

Ontogenetic stability. We will see that certain kinds of seizures characterize certain ages but once a particular form such as grand mal has been established, its nature, given adequate provocation, remains stable over the ontogeny. Similarly every paediatrician will have smiled to notice the old man's yawn in the premature nursery.

Prodrome. Many epileptics have an uncomfortable and restless period before the seizure strikes them. They use this warning in some cases to seek an environment where they will induce the seizure they need by subjecting themselves to intermittent photic stimulation. Prodromes are common in the other paroxysmal behaviours; consider sneezing, weeping, sobbing and vomiting.

Aura. Most of the paroxysmal behaviours including some types of seizures have warnings which are capable of being described. This warning period is a particularly interesting one because it is the time when intervention by self-administered stimuli may inhibit both the epileptic and the other paroxysms. The inhibition of seizures by self-administered stimuli, or by the accidents of state or of the ambient environment are cases in point. In the same way that a whispered word may end a spike/wave paroxysm, so a cry from the nursery can inhibit the act of love.

State. The state of the organism in Prechtl's sense influences the occurrence of all the paroxysmal behaviours including seizures. Thus at a Christmas party, epileptic children rarely convulse and the success or failure of a sermon may be accurately measured, for it is inversely related to the number of coughs and sneezes. Fairweather & Hutt (1970) have quantified the effect of level of arousal on epileptic paroxysms and shown that it is sharp and quantitative.

The absolute system. Once the paroxysmal behaviours have passed the aura phase they all become absolute for a greater or lesser duration of time. That is to say, the sequence of events marches forward regardless of what is done to the organism. Thus there is a 'behaviour' which has now begun and cannot be halted. The similarity between orgasm and seizure here is evident. It is perhaps this inevitability in orgasm, labour and seizure which renders all of them to some persons both repugnant and frightening. It has been suggested that psychodynamically the fear is one of loss of control and the sense of being possessed by forces no longer subject to any form of ego control (Taylor 1969).

Mass reflex of voluntary muscle. In the paroxysmal behaviours voluntary muscles of the limbs and trunk, together with those surrounding the eyes and mouth enter into mass reflex jerking and take the form often of tonic-clonic sequences. The vomiting in mid-Channel is associated with jactitations as violent as those of many fits.

Exocrine secretion. Lacrimation, salivation and sweating are all integral parts of many of the paroxysmal behaviours: any of which attaining major duration are likely to be associated with exocrine activity.

Vascular alterations. Flushing and blanching are a regular feature of the temporal ictus and also occur in many of the other paroxysmal behaviours as do elevation of the blood pressure and the pulse rate.

Contraction of smooth muscle. The contraction of smooth muscle and the relaxation of sphincters can occur in most of the paroxysmal behaviours at their extremes of violence. In the epileptic seizure, voiding of the stomach, the bladder and the bowels are rather less common than is often supposed. When they occur, it is better to regard them as integral parts of that particular person's seizure pattern. They ought not to be related, as some clinicians do, to a mechanical effect of raising intra-abdominal pressure, for many violent bouts of grand mal are accompanied by continence.

Primitive respiratory movements. Primitive respiratory gasping is a feature in nearly all the paroxysmal behaviours including major seizure.

After-glow. After any paroxysmal behaviour including seizures there is often change of mood. Ginsburg's mice were the milder for a fit. The induced seizure may lift a mood from profound depression to euphoria. The after-glow is accompanied by lassitude and by a refractory period.

The list I have given does not cover all of the biological factors which paroxysmal behaviours have in common, but social variables are now briefly considered.

Social recruitment. A characteristic of many of the behaviours listed is that they are infectious in a group. Laughing, yawning and coughing are obvious examples. Virtually all the behaviours associated with happiness, sorrow and anger recruit socially. Apart from the anecdotal feeling that there are 'good' and 'bad' spells in groups of epileptic children, epilepsy is the exception to the rule in this case, as far as I know. I have only seen social recruitment of seizures occur in one pair of monozygotic twins. Social inhibition however, is well attested. On the other hand, hysterical pseudoconvulsions are acutely 'infectious'.

Social unacceptability. In most societies and on most occasions the paroxysmal behaviours at their extreme are contrary to the mores of society. The degree and nature of this rejection is flexible. An 18th-century English gentleman might smile but he would not laugh. Because of their private nature, most paroxysmal behaviours are limited ecologically to private territories where they cannot be observed by conspecifics. The remarkable capacity of the mare, for example, to resist the onset of labour in the presence even of her best-known groom, is well attested. It is here that we come to the possible biological significance of seizures, both in man and other animals. The seizure is disgusting and in this, Chance (1957) suggests, lies its value.

Peromyscus, the deer mouse, is polyethic for seizures. About 5 per cent of the wild population are genetically predisposed to convulsions from which they may die. The timing of this propensity in the ontogeny coincides with the period of habitat exploration and imprinting. It has been proposed that these convulsions, which occur when the mice are predated, train predators to avoid *Peromyscus* and hence reduce predation on the total deer-mouse population. Similarly the seizures of the ep mouse are precisely those that would be adversive to a cat who was tossing the mouse in the air, or holding him in his mouth. When adequately shaken, the ep mouse suddenly stiffens, saliva pours from his mouth, urine and faeces are emitted. He next jactitates in the clonic phase and finally goes limp as though he were dead. He becomes a very unappetizing morsel.

It is a curious fact that man too, at least in childhood, has approximately a 5 per cent propensity to convulse. No homology is intended, but we ought to seek for some biological explanation for the polyethism of man, since these potentially lethal behaviours occur in too great a proportion of the population.

The importance in thinking in this way, is that one demythologizes epilepsy and places it squarely in a biological context.

A PROGRESSIVE STUDY

Rodin (1968) wrote, in his comprehensive review of the prognosis of patients with epilepsy, 'Epilepsy being a condition of such diverse clinical manifestations and markedly varying in intensity, it is apparent that any general rule about what epileptic patients can or cannot do, is bound to be unjust'.

Rodin made a plea for careful prospective studies to tease apart the different factors that bear on final outcome.

We began such a study on 5th July 1948. On this date, the National Health Service began. Everyone since that date, who has been entitled to make use of the service, has received a unique number. This number enables one to trace the biographies of one's patients when they move from one family doctor to another.

We collected a large wholly unselected population of 1000 children with seizures of every kind. The occurrence of some sort of fit was the sole criterion for entry. The global series was ascertained through family doctors, health visitors, and the Paediatric Departments of Oxford, Northampton and Swindon. From this global series a sub-group of children with Temporal Lobe Epilepsy was drawn. This was a continuous unselected sample that satisfied two criteria. These criteria were that the clinical diagnosis had been confirmed by two physicians, and that an EEG had demonstrated a focal discharge in one or both temporal regions. We only allowed ourselves the most parsimonious ascertainment criteria.

In 1964 the data on each child were coded and the findings were published in book form, under the title of *Biological factors in temporal lobe epilepsy*. We refer to these analyses as *The 1964 findings*.

The 1964 analysis

Age at entry into the series. Table 15.1 shows the age at entry into the series. 86 per cent of the children were ascertained before their 11th birthday. No case was

Table 15.1 Age at entry into the series

Age in years	No.
Under 3	17
3–4 years 11 months	11
5–10 years 11 months	58
11–15	14
Total:	100

admitted after the age of 15. All were personal patients and remain so. Many of the patients were ascertained before their first limbic seizure occurred. For example, a child who had febrile status epilepticus in the first three years of life would have been in the follow-up study of children with seizures of all types. If he later developed temporal lobe epilepsy, he would enter the group with which this chapter is concerned.

Coding. 25 factors were coded including the aetiology of the disorder, the intelligence, the age of onset of seizures, grand mal experience, frequency of temporal lobe attacks, the EEG findings, the incidence of hyperkinesis, cataclysmic rages, schooling received and details of the home background and pedigree.

Sex ratio. Males were over-represented in the sample. The sex ratio was 63 males to 37 females.

Three aetiology groups. The series was broken down into three aetiological groups of roughly equal size. 33 per cent of the sample had suffered identifiable brain insults before the onset of the chronic seizure disorder. 32 had suffered from status epilepticus associated with fever, without any other evidence of insult. When the duration of this status was 30 minutes or longer, it was taken as the cause of cerebral damage.

The remaining 33 per cent of the sample had suffered neither insult nor status and were coded as of 'not known' aetiology. These are those patients whom we know, from the classic work of Falconer, Taylor and their colleagues, are later found at operation to have hamartomas, calcified angiomas, oligodendrogliomas, hamartia or no specific lesion when the temporal lobes are examined after temporal lobectomy.

1977 follow-up

In 1977 the sample was re-analysed. No patient had been lost to follow-up. Information was coded on survival and death, institutionalisation, social and economic independence, marriage, parenthood and sexuality, employment, the seizure status of the patient, and his psychiatric problems.

Definition of outcome groups

The patients' circumstances at follow-up varied very widely. Outcome was divided into four broad categories which were defined thus:

A. *Independent* Able to support themselves socially and economically. Seizure-free and not receiving anticonvulsant medication.

B *Independent* Supporting themselves socially and economically but receiving anticonvulsant medication and not necessarily, seizure-free.

C *Dependent* Unable to support themselves, totally dependent on the parents at home, or living in institutions.

D *Dead* The D coding implied death before school leaving age, then 15 years. Patients who were dead at 1977 follow-up and had died after the age of 15 years were coded in the appropriate outcome group that they were in at the time of their death. In all cases the so-called cause of death was found.

When each patient had been coded in 1977, then and only then were the 1964 and 1977 codes for each patient brought together. No retrospective change in the coding was permitted. The reason for this is that, in epileptology, tautological reasoning abounds. Thus one eminent epileptologist maintains that if chronic epilepsy follows a febrile seizure, then the febrile seizure cannot have been a convulsion, since convulsions are known to be benign and a retrospective adjustment of the original diagnosis must be made. Astonishingly, this sort of thinking still abounds. It can play no part in scientific enquiries, and was not employed here.

Outcome distributions and aetiological group

The outcome distributions are shown in Table 15.2 as related to the aetiological composition of each group, as coded in 1964.

Table 15.2 Outcome distribution and aetiological composition of each group

| | | 1977 Groups | | | | |
		A	B	C	D	Table
1964	Insult	5	11	16	3	35
Aetiology	Status	10	8	12	2	32
Codes	Not known	18	13	2	—	33
	Total:	33	32	30	5	100

This table shows that the majority of the A outcome group, came from the not-known aetiology group of children. In the B group where chronic epilepsy still prevailed, although the patients were independent, there was a more even distribution of the three aetiologies. A strong bias towards insult and status epilepticus are seen in the group wholly handicapped and among those who died as children (C and D).

Complete recovery (A). 55 per cent of this group had an unknown aetiology; 30 per cent were from the group who had had febrile status, 15 per cent came from the insulted group. The group consists of 17 men and 16 women, representing 28 per cent of the adult surviving males and 46 per cent of the adult surviving females. The gender difference pervades this, as it does all other aspects of medicine, particularly those which involve the central nervous system. No developmental study is complete unless sex differences are sought.

By definition all patients were seizure-free and receiving no anticonvulsant medication. These persons should be regarded as wholly recovered from their seizure disorder. 75 per cent had remitted their seizures by the age of 14. The men were all in work, having in many cases achieved more success in their careers than their siblings in the same family. The women were all married and either in whole or part-time jobs or at home looking after children. Most of these patients were described in terms such as well, very energetic, 'can turn my hand to anything', and so on. We shall return to this curious phenomenon later in this chapter.

Independent epileptics (B). 41 per cent of this group had been coded in 1964 as of 'not known aetiology'. Brain insult had been coded for 34 per cent and 25 per cent derived their epilepsy from a protracted febrile convulsion in childhood. 24 per cent were men and only 10 per cent were women. All members of this group were capable of employment but there was considerable variability in their employment records. Quite unlike the patients in group A, many were in unskilled jobs and in spite of maintaining their IQ were handicapped by the medical and social stigmata of epilepsy. Two were only maintained in work with the help of very charitable employers. 11 of the group had married and five had produced children.

There were three deaths in this group, which had occurred rather early, between the ages of 18 and 22. This is that large group where temporal lobectomy might have given relief. In fact seven of the 32 had had such operations by 1981 and post-operatively can be regarded as cured.

Grave handicap (C). Gravely handicapped patients most commonly derived from the insulted group (53 per cent); and 40 per cent came from the group with severe febrile convulsions. Only seven came from the not-known aetiology group and, as we shall see, the reasons for these patients' dependence were psychiatric.

In this group there were equal proportions of males and females. The handicaps that had rendered them totally dependent seemed to have over-ruled the operation of gender differences.

Eight of the patients were psychotic. Eight had IQs below 50. 13 patients were handicapped by continuing epilepsy accompanied by behaviour and personality problems together with some degree of sub-normality.

Among the severely handicapped people, 14 were in institutions; 16 were living at home, cared for by their ageing families and often in agonising social predicaments.

Epilepsy as such was never the sole reason for admission to an institution. The death or collapse of the parents had been relatively common. Gross physical handicap, psychiatric disorder and severe sub-normality figured largely and were interconnected. The average period of institutionalisation to follow-up or death was 13 years, by the time of the 1977 coding. These gravely diminished but highly expensive biographies derived their deviations from two main childhood sources: the failure to bring about complete cure in bacterial infections of the brain and failure to arrest protracted febrile convulsions. In a number of cases both meningitis and severe convulsions had occurred simultaneously with the long-understood disastrous effect. It is sad to see in modern texts that the importance of containing paroxysmal behaviours during brain infections is seldom mentioned. It was first described nearly 30 years ago (Ounsted 1951).

Childhood deaths (D). Five children died before reaching the age of 15. One was known to have an astrocytoma, only partially removed, and the other had been diagnosed as Schilder's disease. The remaining three died of status epilepticus.

Adult deaths. Nine of our patients have so far died as adults. One, who was diagnosed at post mortem as suffering from tuberose sclerosis, died in custody when his anticonvulsants were withheld. Table 15.3 shows the age and cause of all 14 deaths. It will be seen that epilepsy figures very largely.

CHILDHOOD BIOLOGICAL FACTORS RELATED TO ADULT OUTCOME

The biological factors coded in 1964 were all of them examined in relation to adult social outcome groups. There were six variables that were found to be of particular relevance. They were: (1) Aetiology (2) Degree of intellectual loss (3) Age of onset of first seizure (4) Severity of grand mal experience (5) Maximum frequency of temporal lobe attacks (6) Side of EEG focus.

Table 15.3 Death: cause and age of death; aetiological and outcome groups

Sex	Age	Aetiological group	Outcome group	Cause of death
Childhood deaths				
M	8 yrs	Chronic insult	D	Astrocytoma
F	8 yrs	Birth injury	D	Epilepsy
M	12 yrs	Chronic insult	D	Schilder's disease
M	11 yrs	Status epilepticus	D	Epilepsy
F	11 yrs	Status epilepticus	D	Epilepsy
Adult deaths				
M	15 yrs	Meningitis	C	Epilepsy
M	20 yrs	Meningitis	C	Accident
F	17 yrs	Status epilepticus	C	Epilepsy
M	21 yrs	Status epilepticus	C	Haemosiderosis — 11 years after hemispherectomy
M	31 yrs	Status epilepticus	C	Coronary thrombosis following seizure
M	19 yrs	Tuberose sclerosis	B	Epilepsy
F	22 yrs	Not-known	B	Suicide
M	22 yrs	Not known	B	Acute myocarditis
M	27 yrs	Not known	A	Road accident (passenger)

In addition there were two behavioural disorders that emerged as of prognostic significance, namely the hyperkinetic syndrome and the occurrence of cataclysmic rage. Two social factors also emerged, namely the necessity for special schooling and the effect of 'disordered home backgrounds'.

Predictive factors in the main group

A number of preliminary analyses suggested that when the proband had first or second degree relatives who were affected with seizures, this had a powerful statistical effect on outcome. We therefore separated the genetic sub-group of survivors, which numbered 23, from the non-genetic group of 72, which we called the main group. The five children who had died before they left school, were excluded from these analyses (Table 15.4).

Intelligence. The intelligence quotient used in the 1964 exercise was the verbal intelligence score on the last test made before a child's data were coded. The median IQ of the whole sample was 90. In terms of adult outcome, an IQ below 90 predicted a poor outcome; 22 of the 35 patients in the C group, twelve of those in the intermediate group, and only one in the A group were below the median. It is just as important to notice that the C group were, as children, intellectually handicapped as to notice that the A group were as children intellectually favoured above the level of the general population.

Age of onset. The coded age of onset, was that biographical moment when the first seizure had occurred, whatever its nature. For the sample as a whole the median age was 2 years 4 months.

There were 32 children in the main group, with an onset below the sample

Table 15.4 Variables coded in 1964 and the 1977 outcome groups main group and genetic subgroup considered separately

		Main non-genetic group n = 72				Genetic group n = 23 adults			
		A	B	C	Total	A	B	C	Total
1964 Codes	*Intelligence*								
	Median 90 & under	1	12	22	35	5	2	4	11
	90 +	21	13	3	37	6	5	1	12
		22	25	25	72	11	7	5	23
	$\chi_2^2 = 32.6$ P < 0.001								
	Age of first seizure								
	Before median 2 yrs 4 mths	3	11	18	32	9	3	3	15
	After median 2 yrs 4 mths	19	14	7	40	2	4	2	8
		22	25	25	72	11	7	5	23
	$\chi_2^2 = 16.1$ P < 0.001								
	Severity of grand mal seizures								
	Severe	2	11	16	29	5	3	4	12
	Mild	20	14	9	43	6	4	1	11
		22	25	25	72	11	7	5	23
	$\chi_2^2 = 14.9$ P < 0.001								
	Frequency of TLE								
	1 per day or more	7	17	16	40	4	3	5	12
	< 1 per day	15	8	9	32	7	4	–	11
		22	25	25	72	11	7	5	23
	$\chi_2^2 = 7.3$ P < 0.02								
	Side of focus omitting bilaterals								
	Left side	3	12	11	26	5	4	2	11
	Right side	13	9	8	30	2	2	1	5
		16	21	19	56	7	6	3	16
	$\chi_2^2 = 6.9$ P < 0.05								

median. 18 of these were totally handicapped in follow-up, 11 were still epileptic but independent and only three had made a complete recovery. This march is reversed for those with an onset after 2 years 4 months, of whom there were 40: 19 were in the A group, 14 in the B group and seven in the C group. As we shall see later, the relationship of age of onset to outcome in no way holds in the genetic sub-group.

Grand mal experience. By criterion all children in this sample had temporal lobe epilepsy, and it is important to note that no less than 88 per cent of the children had, in addition, grand mal attacks. Thus when we speak of studying the outcome of temporal lobe epilepsy we are largely speaking of temporal lobe epilepsy complicated by grand mal, which is clinically much the most common thing to find in unselected series. We coded grand mal experience as severe if five or more grand mals had been coded for by 1964. Less than five was described as 'mild'. Status epilepticus was not used in dichotomising the 1964 codes in this case.

Severity of grand mal experience strongly predicted a poor outcome. 29 children were coded as having severe grand mals in childhood. Of these 16 were in group C, 11 in B and two in A. The march is reversed for those coded as having mild grand mal.

The frequency of temporal lobe attacks. The frequency of temporal lobe attacks in the 1964 coding was taken as the maximum frequency recorded. This varied from median more than 40 a day to less than one a month. The medium in the whole sample was about one a day. As Table 15.4 shows, frequent temporal lobe attacks were a bad prognostic.

Side of focus. There were 25 children in the original sample in whom bilateral foci were recorded. The remaining 75 had a clear right or left focus. Outcome is displayed in Table 15.4. It will be seen that in the main group of 56 who had clear-cut foci, only three out of 26 with a left-sided focus achieved complete recovery. This compared with 13 out of 30 with a right-sided focus.

Hyperkinetic syndrome. This term is now loosely used. We employed it only as defined by us (Ounsted 1955), that is to say, referred to children who had fixed invariant attention spans and activity spans in all situations, a sustained high level of activity when awake and the other features common to this syndrome. Where this syndrome had been coded in 1964, then the outcome was grave indeed. Only two patients attained full recovery. These two children, in fact, probably represented misdiagnoses, but the code must remain inviolate.

Catastrophic rage. In 1964 we coded for 'catastrophic rage', (the term 'cataclysmic' would have been better). 36 children were so coded. Three of these children died before 15 years, all of them gravely handicapped. Rage of this nature was a poor prognostic and was highly linked with low IQ.

Schooling. Table 15.5 shows the social oucome for 63 children who had normal

Table 15.5 Social factors coded in 1964 and 1977 outcome

| | | 1977 Codes | | | |
		A	B	C	Total
1964 Codes	(a) *Schooling*				
	Required special schooling	1	8	23	32
	Normal schooling	32	24	7	63
	Total:	33	32	30	95

$$\chi_2^2 = 39.7 \; P < 0.001$$

schooling, and 32 children who required special schooling. All but one who finally made complete recoveries were educated in normal schools. It will be seen that half those who did receive normal schooling did not attain full recovery in adult life. Closer examination of the reasons for exclusion from normal school showed that this largely depended on behaviour. The objective fact of exclusion is clearly a grave prognostic, for only one of the children so treated fully recovered.

Disordered homes. In the 1964 codes, the sample is dichotomised into those who were found to have come from disordered homes and those who were not. Our criteria were strict. A family was only rated as disordered if one or more of the following five factors was present:

1. Gross poverty in the sense that the family had received National Assistance or had had to place the children in the care of the Children's Officer under the Children's Acts in being at that time
2. Death of the mother at an early age
3. Grossly socially aggressive father
4. Psychosis in one or both parents
5. Gross chronic neurotic illness in one or both parents.

There were 27 children who, by these definitions, were considered to have come from disordered homes. At follow-up two of them were found to have died as children, the remainder were equally divided between the three outcome groups. 27 per cent had fully recovered, and 36 per cent were either in B or C. To our great surprise, therefore, a grossly disordered childhood home, coupled with temporal lobe epilepsy, seems to have no predictive effect on adult outcome.

Adding the adverse factors. These analyses have shown that there are eight factors, in addition to that of aetiology, which prognosed poor outcome and can be ascertained in childhood. The factors are inextricably interrelated. They are:

1. An IQ below the sample median
2. An age of onset below the sample median
3. Frequency of grand mal seizures above the sample median
4. Temporal lobe seizure frequency above the sample median
5. A left-sided EEG focus
6. The hyperkinetic syndrome
7. Cataclysmic rage
8. Special schooling.

Tables 15.6 and 15.7 show that the number of adverse factors suffered by each child relates very significantly to the social outcome in adult life. Among those who had fully recovered by 1977, 30 had three or less adverse factors and 10 had no adverse factor in 1964. In the group wholly dependent (C) the position was reversed: 25 out of 30 had four or more adverse factors. The group which was independent but still epileptic had an intermediate distribution.

It will be seen that 22 patients had more than five adverse factors: none of these achieved full recovery. The prognosis for children with limbic seizures is, in

Table 15.6 Relation between social outcome and numbers of adverse factors suffered by each patient

		1977 Codes			
		A	B	C	Total
1964 Codes	3 or less adverse factors	30	18	5	53
	More than 3 adverse factors	3	14	25	42
	Total:	33	32	30	95

$$\chi_2^2 = 35.12 \; P < 0.001$$

Table 15.7 Number of adverse factors and social outcome

		Social outcome 1977			
		A	B	C	Total
	0	10	4	1	15
	1	7	4	0	11
	2	7	4	2	13
Adverse factors	3	6	6	2	14
(1964)	4	2	5	4	11
per patient	5	1	2	6	9
	6	0	5	9	14
	7	0	1	5	6
	8	0	1	1	2
Total:		33	32	30	95

general, clear before the end of adolescence. A simple count of the number of childhood adverse factors predicts adult outcome at a high level of significance.

CAN HE GET MARRIED? CAN HE HAVE CHILDREN?

The parents of our patients are asking precisely that most fundamental question in evolution: is the fitness of the group reduced? Here we must turn aside for a moment to consider the concept of fitness. David Taylor and I (Ounsted & Taylor 1972) have pointed out that this concept is often used imprecisely, just because it seems so easy to define. Waddington (1957) wrote 'fitness is the capacity to contribute offspring to the next generation'. One may not equate a capacity, which is potential, with an observed frequency which is a matter of fact. Thoday (1953) wrote 'the fitness of a unit of evolution is its probability of leaving descendents after a long lapse of time'. But what are units of evolution? It is reasonable to consider any one of a hierarchy of identifiable entities. One may consider the fitness of a gene, or a group of genes, or a chromosomal aggregate or the modification of a whole organ. Moving further up it would be possible to consider the fitness of a mating dyad, the fitness of a sibship, or a kinship group. One could ask how fit was a particular gene pool, conceived as a whole, or a series of gene pools in an ethnic group. The one element as we ascend that cannot be considered as a unit of fitness, is an individual. Thus Waddington's basic statement: 'We are always concerned to compare the fitness of organisms of one kind with that of individuals of another sort' does not seem to hold. The unit of fitness must be considered a fertile mating pair. Thus we defined a female as she who bears live-born children and a male as he who impregnated her. We shall see in the following analyses that this is not a mere semantic point. We shall show that females, as so often, have the advantage over males when it comes to the basic biological fact of parenthood.

Marriage, marriagability and unmarriagability
The five patients who died as children may be disregarded. The group of 29 who had either died early in adult life or were so handicapped by low intelligence,

frequent seizures and disordered behaviour, that they required total care can be regarded as unmarriageable. None of them have either married or borne a child. We are left with a group of 66 eligible for marriage. 40 of these have in fact married and the remaining 26 single patients are potential spouses: these we refer to as marriageable.

Aetiology. Aetiology as coded in 1964 related strongly to marriage status in 1977. In the combined insult and status group, 62 survived and of these only 17 are married. In contrast among the remainder 23 out of 33 have already married. Table 15.8, ($\chi_2^1 = 15.6\,P < 0.001$).

Table 15.8 Aetiological group and marriage

	Aetiology	1977 Codes Married	Remainder	Total
1964	Insult and status	17	45	62
Codes	Not known	23	10	33
	Total:	40	55	95

$$\chi_1^2 = 15.6\ P < 0.001$$

Sex. In the original series there were 37 girls and 63 boys. In the group rated as unmarriageable this proportion is preserved. Thus though boys are twice as likely as girls to develop temporal lobe epilepsy, males and females with the disease are equally likely to be so handicapped that parenthood is barred to them.

When the residual group of 66 is divided by sex, a highly significant difference is found. Among 41 men 17 were married: of 25 women all but two had already married, Table 15.9 ($\chi_1^2 = 14.6\ P < 0.001$).

Table 15.9 Comparison of married and single in 66 marriageable males and females

		1977 Codes Married	Single	Total
1964	Males	17	24	41
Codes	Females	23	2	25
	Total:	40	26	66

$$\chi_1^2 \text{ (Yates modified)} = 14.6\ P < 0.001$$

It is clear that for girls, provided they survive and are not grossly handicapped, the prognosis for marriage is good. Males, even though not heavily handicapped, more often than not refrain from matrimony.

Early remission of seizures. Remission was said to have occurred in the 1964 codes when a child had had no seizures for at least 6 months. When the age thus coded was 12 years or under, and recovery was found at follow-up to have been maintained, the definition of 'early remission' was applied. Early remission and marriage were strongly linked. Among 29 who had remitted early, 26 were married by 1977 and only three were single: among 37 who did not remit early 14 were married and 23 single. Refer Table 15.10 ($\chi_1^2 = 16.2\ P < 0.001$).

Table 15.10 Early remission and marriage in the marriageable

		1977 Codes		
		Married	Single	Total
1964 Codes	Early remission	26	3	29
	No early remission	14	23	37
	Total:	40	26	66

$$\chi_1^2 \text{ (Yates)} = 16.2 \ P < 0.001$$

More females than males had had an early remission but Table 15.11 shows that the difference is too slight to have statistical significance.

Table 15.11 Sex and early remission in the marriageable

		1977 Codes		
		Male	Female	Total
1964 Codes	Early remission	15	14	29
	No early remission	26	11	37
	Total:	41	25	66

$$\chi_1^2 = 2.4 \ P \text{ n.s.}$$

Married and single women and early remission. Virtually all marriageable females were married. Table 15.12 shows that all 14 women who had remitted early were also married. Thus of the original 37 female-probands there now survive only two who are nubile but not yet married.

Table 15.12 Early remission and marriage in females

		1977 Codes		
		Married	Single	Total
1964 Codes	Early remission	14	0	14
	No early remission	9	2	11
	Total:	23	2	25

P n.s.

Married and single men and early remission. Married and single men were compared. We could not find any difference in median age at follow-up. In the 1964 codes there were no differences between the two groups in median IQ, frequency of temporal lobe seizures or severity of grand mal experience. Although in the group as a whole aetiology affected outcome, within the group of marriageable men it did not. Marriage was not related to the side of the epileptic focus.

We have shown above that eight adverse factors coded in 1964 had an accumulative effect on social status in 1977. Table 15.13 repeats this exercise for marriageable males. No one adverse factor as defined, nor the cumulative count of

Table 15.13 Marriageable males: adverse factors

		1977 Codes		
	No.	Married	Unmarried	Total
	0	2	4	6
	1	5	2	7
	2	3	3	6
1964	3	2	6	8
Codes	4	2	2	4
	5	2	1	3
	6	1	3	4
	7	0	2	2
	8	0	1	1

		1977 Codes		
	No.	Married	Unmarried	Total
1964	3 or less	12 (11.2)	15 (15.8)	27
Codes	4 or more	5 (5.8)	9 (8.2)	14
	Total:	17	24	41

e values in parentheses

factors, differentiates between the married and the unmarried. The two groups differed notably in respect of early remission. Among 24 single men, three remitted early. The group of 17 married men contains 12 who remitted early and five who did not. Table 15.14 shows that these differences are highly significant. ($\chi_1^2 = 14.4$ P < 0.001).

Table 15.14 Early remission and marriage in males

		1977 Codes		
		Married	Single	Total
1964	Early remission	12	3	15
Codes	No early remission	5	21	26
	Total:	17	24	41

$$\chi_1^2 \text{ (Yates)} = 14.4 \text{ P} < 0.001$$

Of the married men who had not remitted by 12 years, three have already suffered marriage break-downs. Four have had psychiatric disorders.

Sexual indifference

Taylor's (1969) classic account of the absence of sexual appetite in adults with temporal lobe epilepsy was paralleled in this study. Batchelorhood and marriage are no proof of sexual attitudes. But at least 14 of our 24 single men clearly had no attraction to sexuality. Their attitude emerged repeatedly in consultations and was evident in the lifestyle of these patients of whom we have an intimate long-term knowledge. They were often in regular employment, but when we talked to them about their sex lives at say, the age of 30, they showed no inclination to leave the parental home and had shown no interest in any girl friends. Where this absence of sexual drive could not decisively be established, it was discounted in the analysis. This sub-group of sexless men was compared with the married group and again early remission was the only discriminant. Only one of the 14 known to be sexless had had an early remission (Table 15.15; $\chi_1^2 = 10.2$ Yates).

Table 15.15 Comparion of early remission in the married and the sexually indifferent males

| | | 1977 Codes | | |
		Married	Sexually indifferent	Total
1964	Early remission	12	1	13
Codes	No early remission	5	13	18
	Total:	17	14	31

$$\chi_1^2 \text{ (Yates)} = 10.2 \text{ P} < 0.001$$

None of these patients were practising homosexuals. Two brief biographies illustrate the difference found.

A boy born 23rd November 1945 had a natural early biography and a healthy pedigree. At the age of 1 year 5 months he developed seizures of a pure temporal lobe type. At no time did he have major seizures. The attacks were stereotyped. The aura was a foul taste in the mouth. He often described how he had an impulse to drink water. His parents described a sudden arrest of behaviour with staring, mouthing and clutching the lips and nose with the left hand. The seizure ended with chuckling and he would often say that he had had 'funny thoughts'. The maximum frequency of such seizures was five daily. They were never convincingly influenced by drugs.

An EEG focus was repeatedly shown in the left anterior temporal region. He was left-handed. His verbal IQ was 110. At the age of 15 his seizures remitted and have never recurred.

When seen in long-term follow-up at his home, he was a strong healthy businessman earning a substantial income. His house was full of sporting trophies, won in many different fields. He was active in neighbourhood affairs. At no time had he had a girlfriend, nor shown any appetitive behaviour towards either sex. To direct questioning on sexual matters, which was both blunt and persistent, he showed neither embarrassment nor interest. His mother and father had been worried when they had detected his sexual indifference. By the time that he was 30 years they had concluded, they said, 'that he would always be married to his cricket bat'.

Another boy in this series again had perfectly normal early development. At the age of 4 years he developed severe otitis media with a high fever. This was complicated by major seizures of generalized nature, lasting about 15 minutes. A year later he developed habitual epilepsy. In each brief attack his face would contort. His eyes would roll upwards. He would stagger and make semi-purposive movements. He would recover in about 10–15 seconds. He was aware that a seizure had occurred but could recall no aura. Treatment with different drugs was probably without influence on the frequency of the attacks. The maximum frequency was 20 a day. He developed an aggressive behaviour disorder and was excluded from school. He was about to be placed in a residential school for epileptic sub-normal children. At this point his father, who was a Yorkshire miner, managed to get the family referred to our hospital. EEG examination showed that there was a frequently firing left anterior temporal lobe focus. Careful in-patient investigation of the family was undertaken. All drugs were withdrawn. No further seizures have occurred. Psychiatric investigation showed that his rages only related to his mother. They were a reaction to her fearful over-protection. They resolved with psychotherapy, both individual and to the family. His verbal IQ was 112. At the age of 9 years he was returned to his home and to his local school and family.

Thereafter as a schoolboy he was notable at sport and played cricket for his county. He married at $19\frac{1}{2}$ years and $5\frac{1}{2}$ years later he and his wife had had two children. His wife described him enthusiastically as 'successful in every kind of sport'. She described their marriage as 'very happy indeed' and said of her husband proudly that 'he could turn his hands to anything'.

Both these patients grew up to be healthy men, entirely free from seizures. Both showed that active extraverted pattern of behaviour so common among those who recover from childhood seizure disorders. The men differed only in that one was wholly sexually indifferent, whilst the other was a happy and contented parent. They differed also in the timing of their remission. The one had occurred after puberty and the other before it.

Parenthood and fitness

Temporal lobe epilepsy impairs an afflicted group's overall contribution to the next generation. Those dead in early life or hopelessly handicapped as adults cannot reproduce. They have been selected out. From those remaining 66 probands, 63 children have so far derived. Since our patients are now in their 30s, this number can be expected to increase as the follow-up continues through its fourth decade. But parenthood differs between the sexes. The 25 marriageable women have had 41 children and the 41 marriageable men have had 22. So the fertility achieved so far from the 37 original female probands averages 1.108 child per proband. If we consider only marriageable women, the figure rises to 1.64, which is approaching the replacement figure of 2. For males the picture is quite different. From the 63 original probands, there are at present only 0.349 young each. Considering the marriageable only, the figure rises to 0.536.

Converting these data into the conventional sex ratio shows:
1. Whole sample: 169.2   males per 100 females
2. Unmarriageable: 183.3   males per 100 females
3. Married: 73.9   males per 100 females
4. Single: 1200.0   males per 100 females

So we see that the biological fitness within a group marked by temporal lobe epilepsy differs sharply between the sexes, and this fact must be born in mind when we come to consider genetic aspects of the study.

The syndrome of sexlessness, as Taylor (1969) described it, was in his words 'a loss of vital synergism' rather than some positive psychiatric syndrome. Careful investigation of this phenomenon may help us to understand the neurological basis of sexual appetite.

In animals with sexual cycles, rhythmic and reciprocal changes in EEG activity in the amygdala and hippocampus have been shown to parallel the rise and fall in sexual drive (Kawakami, et al 1967).

Most of the single men, and virtually all those known to have sexual indifference, had had frequent epileptic disruption of the hippocampal and amygdaloid functions during the developmental period when sexual appetitive behaviour finally develops. Children who had had frequent limbic seizures but who showed early remission before puberty grew up as normally sexually appetitive. Four of the five married men who had not had early remission were found on follow-up to be psychiatrically disturbed and three out of five marriages broke down within a few years. The part played by sexual indifference could not be disentangled from their psychiatric disorders, but we believe it to be contributory.

We have suggested that animal replicas of limbic seizures such as those devised by Mellanby et al (1977) are well suited to test the notion that such seizures differentially disrupt adult sexual appetitiveness, dependent upon the ontogenetic epoch in which they occur.

Many epileptologists have found more afflicted relatives on the distaff than on the spear side of the pedigree of epileptic probands. I suggested (Ounsted 1952) that this might be simply due to the fact that mothers know more about their families than fathers do. A recent prospective study by Annegers et al (1976) shows that this is not the whole truth. In the present study the greater fecundity of females suggests that, in so far as familial traits play an aetiological role in temporal lobe epilepsies, they will have a threefold greater chance of transmission through females than through males.

It seems from these analyses that the likelihood of marriage and parenthood as posed to us by the parents of our children, can be answered by studying a few recognisable biological factors which can be discerned before the end of childhood.

PSYCHIATRIC DISORDERS IN CHILDHOOD AND ADULT LIFE

It will be recalled that our original sample was ascertained on a wholly paediatric basis. Yet we had to report in 1966 that 'only 15 of all the children in this sample are recorded as showing no form of personality difficulty at any time'. This figure cannot be taken to mean that 85 per cent of all children with temporal lobe fits show more or less grave disorders of personality. 'It is likely that many of these children are going through a difficult phase of development and then the epilepsy and its concomitent social and mental disabilities simply added to the difficulty of evolving a mature and stable personality' (Ounsted et al 1966).

Psychiatric disorder in the 1964 codes
The most seriously handicapping conditions in childhood were mental defect, the

hyperkinetic syndrome and catastrophic rage. It must be emphasised that these three commonly coexisted.

a. Mental defect

Nearly a quarter of the sample had verbal IQs of less than 70. Eight of those who had survived into adulthood had childhood IQs under 50 and could not be further psychiatrically assessed. Five were in institutions and the remaining three were wholly dependent and living at home.

A further 13 patients had verbal IQs between 50 and 70. Four of these are in the psychotic group described below. Of the remainder there were only three who achieved independence. Two of those who did not had had hemispherectomies in childhood. Two had died by the age of 22 years.

b. The hyperkinetic syndrome

The term hyperkinetic has now become fashionable. It is often applied to a heterogeneous group of children who seem to adults to be more energetic than is to their taste. The term is used here to mean a very precise syndrome, which was made by Hutt & Hutt (1970) the subject of a sharp and quantitive ethological analysis.

There were 26 children coded as having suffered from the hyperkinetic syndrome. Three factors related to the syndrome:

a. Males were heavily over-represented

b. Cerebral damage from a known insult to the brain or from severe status epilepticus had occurred in 88 per cent

c. The onset of seizures was very early.

Among the hyperkinetics, 81 per cent had started their seizures before the median age. Similarly only two of the hyperkinetics had an IQ above the sample median. The median for the hyperkinetic group was 70 and that for the remainder of the whole sample was 100.5. This gap of two standard deviations means that there was virtually no overlap between the two distributions. We have seen that the hyperkinetic syndrome in early childhood is a strong predictor for poor social outcome as an adult. Four of the five child deaths had suffered from this syndrome.

Only two patients (one male and one female) achieved full adult recovery. We have reviewed these biographies. It seems likely that we would now have coded them differently although this naturally must not let us re-adjust the codes in favour of our theory! One of these patients probably had a drug-induced hyperkinesis and one who came from a heavily disordered home background may well have had her activity driven by anxiety. They had both maintained their IQs at over 100. Of the remaining 14 patients, half had developed some form of psychiatric illness (two were among the psychotic group and five were among the anti-social group in adult life).

The classic hyperkinetic syndrome is now rare. This is probably due to a number of factors. When this series began quite a large number of children were recovering from purulent meningitis and similar insults but were left with heavy brain damage. The main anticonvulsants were phenobarbitone and primidone, both of which can themselves potentiate hyperkinetic behaviour when the appropriate damage and gender are present. Use of these drugs has now been greatly reduced in civilised countries. Certainly any child with epilepsy who develops the hyperkinetic syndrome should be carefully investigated to see whether it relates to his medication which should then be most promptly changed.

c. Rage

Rages were a major problem for 36 of our children. This childhood marker carried a poor adult prognosis in terms of both social and psychiatric outcomes. Boys are more prone to overt physical violence than girls, but there was no significant difference in the incidence between the sexes.

Boys and girls with rage differed, however, in the age at the first seizure: The median for the males was 16 months and for the females 9 months. They also differed in IQ: aggression in the girls was largely confined to the severely retarded group; their median IQ was 58 whilst the boys had a median of 83.5 and they spread out over the whole IQ range.

We have seen that childhood rage was a significant prognosticator for poor social outcome in adult life. In terms of psychiatric troubles, as defined in our three groups below, it was a still more powerful predictor of poor outcome. Of 29 coded as 'rage' in 1964, 16 had entered the psychiatric group by 1977. Table 15.16 ($\chi_1^2 = 13.3$ P < 0.001).

Table 15.16 Childhood rage and adult psychiatric disorder

| | | 1977 Codes | | |
		Psychiatric disorders	No psychiatric disorders	Total
1964 Codes	Rage	16	13	29
	No rage	10	48	58
	Total:	26	61	87

$$\chi_1^2 = 13.3 \text{ P} < 0.001$$

Disordered homes. It was a matter of great surprise to us to find that disordered homes as coded in 1964 bore no significant relationship at all to the likelihood of adult psychiatric problems (Table 15.17).

Table 15.17 Disordered homes in childhood and adult psychiatric disorder

| | | 1977 Codes | | |
		Psychiatric disorder	No psychiatric disorder	Total
1964 Codes	Disordered	9	13	22
	Not disordered	17	48	65
	Total:	26	61	87

$$\chi_1^2 = 1.7 \text{ P n.s.}$$

Adult psychiatric disorders. Three categories of psychiatric disorder were identified. For each category we applied the following operational definitions with rigour so that the rates of psychosis, neurosis and antisocial behaviour are minimal.

Definitions

1. Psychotics: patients both diagnosed by persons other than ourselves and treated in mental hospitals for schizophrenic signs and symptoms.

2. Personality disorders of an antisocial nature: those patients whose antisocial behaviour was unacceptable either to their families or to society. They had either been convicted by the criminal courts or required admission to institutions on account of severe behavioural problems.

3. Neurotic: patients who had received treatment for anxiety and/or depression.

In addition to the five children in our series who died before the school leaving age of 15, we have omitted eight patients, four males and four females with verbal IQs below 50 who were too handicapped to speak of Schneider's first-rank symptoms — see Kolvin (1971). The series therefore numbered 87.

a. Psychosis

The schizophreniform psychosis of temporal lobe epilepsy has so far developed overtly in nine patients. Several additional patients revealed to us first-rank symptoms of Schneider, but since these experiences have not placed them in predicaments requiring psychiatric treatment, we decided that such covert disorders should, for purposes of analysis, be excluded.

In considering the risk of psychosis in the series, some negative and positive points have emerged from the 1964 codings.

Of the 87 patients, nine have so far developed overt psychosis. Eight of the psychotics are male and one female. None of the psychotics had a right-sided focus in the 1964 codes. Seven had a left-sided focus and two had bilateral discharges.

None of the males who had become psychotic had shown early remission. All had continued on anticonvulsants, and all had active seizures. Two later died in status epilepticus. The one female who developed the syndrome had experienced an early remission in the 1964 codes but her epilepsy had relapsed and she was on anticonvulsants when psychotic. All the eight males had been coded in 1964 as having either severe grand mals or frequent temporal lobe attacks.

The following factors of the 1964 codes were not related to the development of psychosis: aetiology, age of onset, rage and the occurrence of the hyperkinetic syndrome.

Taylor (1975) has recently reviewed the evidence linking seizures of the left limbic system with psychosis. Our data strongly support his important conclusions. Since our studies were prospective, ascertainment bias can have played no role. The fact that psychosis was limited to those who as children had had a left-sided EEG focus, yields an internal control system. Taylor points out that as maturation proceeds, social and language functions of the left hemisphere are mediated by a contracting volume of brain. Thus, viewed developmentally, limbic seizures and their associated lesions might be seen as contributing to an increasing noisiness within those territories where perversion of function leads to psychotic behaviour. 30 per cent of males who had left-sided foci, and who continued their fits through puberty, have so far become psychotic.

b. The anti-social group

12 of the 87 patients have exhibited antisocial behaviour as adults. Seven have been convicted by the courts, each of them for more than one offence. In six out of seven cases, aggression in the form of assult or criminal damage figures prominently. The remaining one man had two offences of theft. Five of this group were sufficiently disturbed to have been admitted to mental institutions, either permanently or periodically. There were 10 males and two females. Neither of the females had been convicted.

None in this group had had an early remission of seizure. All were still receiving anticonvulsants at the time of follow-up. Table 15.18 shows that 11 of the 12 with antisocial behaviour had foci contralateral to the preferred hand. When the

Table 15.18 Laterality of focus and anti-social behaviour

	Foci	1977 Codes Anti-social	Normal	Total
1964 Codes	Ipsilateral	1	31	32
	Contralateral	11	11	22
	Total:	12	42	54

$$\chi_1^2 \text{ (Yates)} = 13.9 \text{ P} < 0.001$$

antisocial group are compared with the rest of the sample, who also had a clear-cut unilateral focus, there is a highly significant difference. 10 of the 12 had severe grand mal epilepsy in childhood.

In 1977, eight of the 12 were economically and socially independent. Four were totally dependent socially. Thus in general it seems that a very low rate of antisocial behaviour can be expected in adult life, even given the fact of the gross childhood disturbances and often chaotic intra-familial experiences of this group.

c. Neurotics

Only five patients had been treated for neurotic symptoms as adults. This low rate underlines the concomitant, but unquantifiable, observation that a high proportion of all our surviving patients were energetic, extraverted and successful in sport and in their work achievements.

The surprising and hopeful feature of this new analysis is the fact that so many of our patients are now entirely free from psychiatric handicap as adults. In many cases their plight as children and adolescents was so grave that recovery might have seemed quite hopeless. We found that 85 per cent of our samples had had psychological problems when the childhood data were coded. Yet 70 per cent of the adult survivors had no psychiatric disorder whatever, when severe mental defect was excluded. It would seem that powerful forces exist, which restore homeorhetic patterns of development before adult life is reached in the majority of these children. There was no evidence to support the notion that the bad childhood environments of more than a quarter of our patients potentiated adult psychiatric disorder. Biological factors seen to be paramount.

GENETIC FACTORS, FEBRILE CONVULSIONS AND THE REMISSION OF SEIZURES

In some children, febrile convulsions occur because the affected children carry a genetic predisposition to convulse in fever. In others the convulsion depends only on age and the nature of the infection. In the latter, there is no specific genetic component (Ounsted 1976). Both types of febrile convulsions occurred in the children in this series.

There are four possible outcomes of febrile convulsions: death, full recovery, the subsequent development of epilepy which then in itself remits, and the development of epilepsy which continues in spite of treatment.

We have said that this series of children with temporal lobe epilepsy is drawn from a larger group of children with fits of all sorts. We here refer to that coeval and sympatric group of 438 children who had suffered any kind of febrile convulsion.

Figure 15.1 shows the distribution in our series.

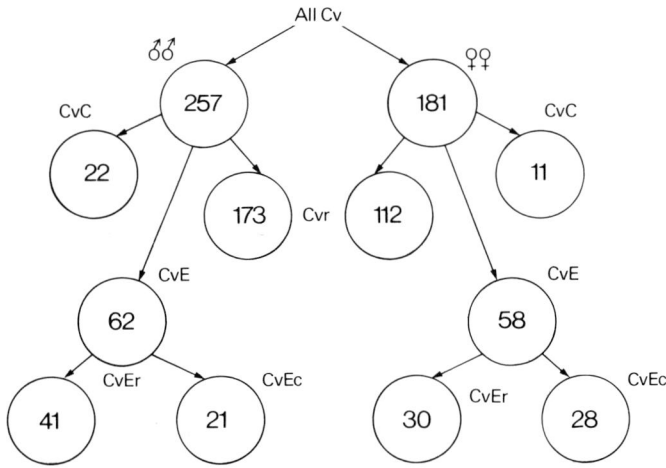

Fig. 15.1 Outcome in 438 children (257 boys, 181 girls) with febrile convulsions, coeval and sympatric with the TLE series:
1. Simple remittent febrile convulsions (Cvr)
2. Febrile convulsions which are followed by chronic epilepsy which remits (CvEr)
3. Febrile convulsions which are followed by epilepsy which continues in spite of treatment (CvEc)
4. Febrile convulsions which continue to death (CvC).

We refer to a family history as positive if one or more relatives have been affected by any form of seizure disorder, including febrile convulsions. We distinguish between first and second degree relatives.

The fact that a family history is positive or negative for affected relatives is no proof either way of the existence or absence of a genetic factor operating in the proband. There must be some misclassifications. In practice we have shown in other analyses of the same data that such a division produces regular and meaningful differences (Taylor & Ounsted 1972). We shall use the distinction here.

We have already shown that a count of the adverse factors when the family history is negative powerfully predicts adult outcome. When the family history is positive this is not the case. Table 15.19 shows that here there is no association between the number of adverse factors and whether in the final outcome the

Table 15.19 Adverse factors 1964, outcome 1977 and family history

+ F.H. (1st degree relatives)	A	B	C	Total
0		2		2
1	4 { 2	4 { 1	0 { –	3
2	2	1		3
3	4	1	1	6
4	7 { 2	1 { –	2 { 1	3
5	1			1
6		2		2
7	0 { –	2 { –	3 { 2	2
8			1	1
Total	11	7	5	23
Mean no. per proband	2.82	2.57	5.80	3.39

Adverse factors	A	B & C	Total
3 or more	7	8	15
Less than 3	4	4	8
Total	11	12	23

Not significant

patient still has epilepsy or not, i.e. is in group A or B. The mean numbers of adverse factors here among those with a positive family history who fully recovered (A) was 2.82, compared with the group which was independent but still epileptic (B), who had 2.57. Why is it that a positive family history seems to yield a benign outcome even when the adverse factors are present?

Febrile convulsions, pedigree, age of onset and remission

The 100 proband biographies were scrutinised, and all those children having a fit in association with fever were extracted. There were 59. No other selection criterion was made. Specifically, infections of the brain associated with seizures were included as were those where the seizures had been complicated and protracted. We did not permit ourselves anything more than the most parsimonious selection criterion. Table 15.20 shows the whole series of 59 arrayed by sex, age at first seizure, whatever its nature, and by final outcome of the

Table 15.20 59 patients from TLE series who had CV with fever. Arranged by age of onset of first seizure and by long-term remission

Nil F.H. n = 32			+F.H. (2nd degree relative) n = 8			+F.H. (1st degree relative) n = 19		
Onset age	Sex	Remitted	Onset age	Sex	Remitted	Onset age	Sex	Remitted
3 mth	F		4 days	F		2 days	M	
5 mth	M					4 mth	F	
7 mth	M					4 mth	M	
9 mth	F					5 mth	M	remitted
9 mth	F					6 mth	F	remitted
9 mth	M					6 mth	F	remitted
9 mth	M					8 mth	F	
9 mth	F					9 mth	M	
10 mth	M					10 mth	F	
10 mth	M					11 mth	M	remitted
10 mth	M					11 mth	M	remitted
11 mth	F							
11 mth	M							
11 mth	M							
1 yr 0 mth	M					1 yr 3 mth	M	
1 yr 3 mth	M					1 yr 4 mth	F	remitted
1 yr 4 mth	M					1 yr 6 mth	M	
1 yr 5 mth	F					1 yr 6 mth	M	remitted
1 yr 7 mth	M					1 yr 8 mth	M	remitted
1 yr 8 mth	F							
1 yr 10 mth	M							
2 yr 0 mth	M		2 yr 0 mth	F		2 yr 0 mth	M	remitted
2 yr 0 mth	M		2 yr 6 mth	F		2 yr 6 mth	F	remitted
			2 yr 10 mth	F		2 yr 9 mth	M	
3 yr 0 mth	F		3 yr 0 mth	F	remitted			
3 yr 3 mth	M							
3 yr 8 mth	M							
4 yr 0 mth	M	remitted	5 yr 2 mth	F	remitted			
5 yr 3 mth	M		6 yr 5 mth	F	remitted			
5 yr 6 mth	M		6 yr 5 mth	M	remitted			
6 yr 7 mth	F	remitted						
6 yr 9 mth	M	remitted						
12 yr 6 mth	M							

temporal lobe epilepsy. The first column lists 32 probands with no affected relatives: only three of these were in remission in adult life. All those who had remitted had an onset after they were 4 years old.

The second column arrays eight probands with second degree affected relatives: four had remitted. All those who had remitted had their first seizure after they were 3 years old.

The third column displays 19 probands with first degree affected relatives: 10 had remitted. The age at first seizure of all 19 showed a sharp cut-off at 2 years 9 months.

In Table 15.21 the series is dichotomised ignoring age of onset and merging the two positive family history groups since remission rate was identical in each. In

Table 15.21 TLE series. Remission of seizures when febrile convulsions are associated with limbic seizures

Probands	+ F.H. (1st & 2nd degree relative)	− F.H.	Total
Remission	14	3	17
Remainder	13	29	42
Total:	27	32	59

$$\chi_1^2 \text{ (Yates modified)} = 10.89 \text{ P} < 0.001$$

the negative group only three out of 32 remitted: in the positive group 14 out of 27 remitted. The difference is highly significant.

So there emerges a clear, if complex, pattern linking genetic endowment, age of onset and a likelihood of remission. In the absence of any indication of the genetic factor, the age of onset covers a wide range and it is only among those of later onset that a few final remissions occur. In the group with first degree affected relatives an onset age cut off at 2 years 9 months and a 50 per cent remission rate are found.

This small intermediate group with affected second degree relatives also achieved a 50 per cent remission rate, but this was confined to those of later onset.

The risk of convulsions among siblings and its nature
Most of the siblings of our probands who convulsed had febrile convulsions of a simple type. Table 15.22 contrasts the risk of simple febrile convulsions as compared with all other types of outcome in 2 groups:

1. In the affected siblings of the temporal lobe epilepsy probands
2. In the unselected global group of 438 coeval and sympatric children with febrile convulsions.

Table 15.22 Proportion of simple benign febrile convulsions in the global febrile convulsion series and in the affected siblings of the probands with TLE

	Siblings of TLE probands		Global febrile convulsion series	Total
Simple febrile convulsions	67%	16	65% 285	301
Convulsions with other outcomes		8	153	161
Total:		24	438	462

$$\text{No significant difference } \chi^2 = 0.025$$

The relative proportions in the two groups are precisely the same. Thus it seems that only one gene is likely to be involved in the promotion of febrile convulsions, whether these are benign or followed by epilepsy. That is to say, genetically the same factor operates in the main febrile convulsions group and in the temporal lobe epilepsy series.

Among the 59 probands with convulsions and limbic seizures, one was adopted. He is here omitted. Of the remaining 58 probands, 17 remitted and 41 did not. These patients had a total of 133 siblings. Table 15.23 shows that when the proband had remitted, then 38 per cent of the siblings have a convulsive disorder.

Table 15.23 Remission of epilepsy in relation to sibs with convulsions in 58 probands with convulsions

		Probands		
		Remitted n = 17	Non-remitted n = 41	Total
Siblings	Unaffected	23	85	108
	Affected	14	11	25
	Total:	37	96	133

$$\chi^2 = 12.2 \; P < 0.001$$

When the proband had not remitted then only 11 per cent of the siblings had a seizure disorder. The difference is highly significant. Here again looking at the same data from another point of view, the genetic risk of convulsions is higher where the prognosis is good. Where the prognosis is bad we are much less likely to have found affected brothers and sisters.

Theoretical considerations

Febrile convulsions vary greatly in provenance, frequency and severity from time to time and from place to place. A study by Thom in 1942 among a working class North American population revealed a mortality of 19 per cent. The Newcastle upon Tyne cohort born in 1947–48 showed a 20 per cent mortality among those who convulsed (Miller et al 1960). Our global series of children with febrile convulsions began in 1948 and the convulsive mortality was just over 8 per cent.

Natural selection in favour of any genetic sub-group capable of inhibiting seizures once they have begun can thus be seen to be operating. The selection pressure towards a benign outcome must be limited to that sub-group in which the propensity to convulse is itself genetically transmitted. Where there is no genetic factor in a febrile convulsion, a phenocopy occurs. Should death, sexlessness or severe handicap follow, then selection will not specifically affect the gene pool in the next generation.

Thus from an evolutionary point of view the superficial paradox of a good outcome with a positive family history makes sense.

The eight adverse factors, which so powerfully predict adult outcome in general, failed to do so when the family history was positive. This suggests that an additional positive factor enters here which can overcome seizures. We suggest that this is simply a genetic instruction enhancing the inhibitory mechanisms within the brain. In this context an obvious but often ignored fact should be noticed. In most persons with epilepsy, the seizures are actively inhibited for nearly all the time. We are suggesting that among those who with a genetic propensity to febrile convulsions, natural selection will serve to promote those genetic instructions which underlie the maturation of inhibitory functions. A further selective factor has been noted. Males having limbic seizures through puberty commonly make no attempt at fatherhood and thus make no contribution to the next generation.

As a scholium we may note that if the proposed genetic instruction to inhibit limbic discharges were parsimoniously coded on a single gene, then half of those with a sequence CvE would receive it and half would not. The observed ratio of CvEr to CvEc among those with a positive family history was 14:13.

These notions are now being put to the test among strains of laboratory rodents having naturally occurring seizures on a simple genetic basis (Glaser, personal communication).

Implications

Like every study, the detailed findings of this one apply only to that group of children ascertained as having temporal lobe epilepsy in the Oxford region in the years following the institution of the National Health Service. This was a period of paediatric transition. For the first time it was proving possible to give active treatment in many illnesses that afflict the brains of young children. Anticonvulsants and the control of status epilepticus were emerging. Are there any more general lessons which should be of wider application? It seems to me that there are. First, it is abundantly clear that there is no answer to the question 'what is the prognosis of temporal lobe epilepsy in childhood'? In this series the answer ranged from complete, and indeed enhanced, recovery in adult life to death and total handicap. Yet when a number of biological factors were closely analysed, prediction emerged as very possible. Something perhaps has been learnt about such unexpected matters as the development of schizophrenia, the development of sexual appetitiveness, the difference in biological fitness between the genders in an afflicted group and the danger of predicting from a bad family background in childhood what the adult will achieve in his life.

Practical considerations

Three major dangers in caring for children with temporal lobe epilepsy are:

1. Continuing drug treatment after that time when lasting remission would otherwise have occurred
2. Operating early on children who are likely to experience natural remission
3. Delaying operation for the relief of seizures so long into adult life that social recovery becomes impossible.

When a child with no affected relatives has temporal lobe epilepsy and febrile convulsions the likelihood that the seizures will persist into adult life is of a high order. This is particularly so in those whose first seizure was in the first three years of life. All such children ought to be considered most carefully before school leaving age to see whether they merit relief by the operation of anterior temporal lobectomy using the method devised by the late Murray Falconer.

Children on heavy medication who continue seizures, particularly if they have had an affected relative, also need most careful investigations. Some of these will be found to have seizures which are dependent on their anticonvulsant medication. Periodic weaning and providing the child with a clean brain for a time is mandatory. Since withdrawal of anticonvulsants can precipitate fatal status epilepticus, it is necessary that such reviews of managment take place in hospital.

Many of the patients in this series, when they have grown up, have asked us about the genetic risk to their children. The data we have presented suggests that the only common risk is for simple febrile convulsions. These can now be controlled and rendered harmless, should they threaten to go into runaway status. Thus these parents can be advised about the true likelihoods. In our experience this often gives great relief and helps to lift that sense of genetic guilt which plays otherwise a major role in the lives of people with epileptic disorders.

ENVOI

Developmental Medicine is the science of biographies. And as Sir Peter Medawar has pointed out, each individual biography is unique. This chapter ought to end with one.

An early biography

In 1970 a boy with temporal lobe epilepsy presented as an emergency. He had attempted to murder his mother and had nearly achieved his goal.

He was born 11th October 1958. He was the only child of his parents, seemed a healthy enough baby and developed well until he was 11 months old. He then went into a severe febrile status epilepticus which lasted 12 hours. He was profoundly cyanosed. Postictally he had transient hemiplegia and postictal blindness. Examination of notes made at the time showed that he had a leucopenia with a relative lymphocytosis. This finding, when associated with febrile convulsions, is strongly suggestive of infection by the virus of Roseola infantum (Exanthem Subitum). As is so often the case, his mother when she witnessed him in the throes of his seizures thought that he was dying. She developed Solnit's syndrome of the 'vulnerable child'. She was already chronically sick with kidney disease. Her terrible anxiety that her son's continued existence could not be guaranteed was reinforced over the next few years by repeated severe fits, major in type. By the age of 5 years, her son had had a total of four more bouts of status epilepticus.

When he was six the patient began to have minor seizures. He had brief epigastric aura and an ictal dysphasia. He was treated with phenobarbitone which seemed to increase the frequency of the fits and was associated with a severe behaviour disorder. The family situation went from bad to worse. The mother became an alcoholic as a reaction to her chronic anxieties. The father was frequently absent from home. The patient was gravely physically neglected. At night he and his mother shared a bed.

He was taken in for some months of very intensive psychotherapy. It became clear that he had a grossly disordered sexual identification. His ambivalent relationships with women exhibited themselves in transvestism and homosexuality. He was anxious, confused, frightened, insecure and aggressive. In hospital he was unpopular with his peers and a social isolate. The mother brought with her a letter written by her son, the morning after he had attempted to murder her. It read thus:

'Dear Mother,

I am very sorry from what I did tonight. I am really. Oh, Mommy please try to forgive me please. Mommy I know that I should have not done it, I know, but Mommy please try to forgive me please. I know I tried to burn myself. I know I jumped out of the window. I know that I am greedy. I know that I am rude. I know that I swear. I know that I hurt you. I know that I kick you. I know that all this hurts you. Mommy, but Mommy please try to forgive Just this once, please Mommy, please, from that boy you really hate, detest.

X.'

In the crisis of this family predicament, psychotherapy proved effective. The mother was told that we were working towards brain surgery. She asked what she could do and was told she must stop drinking. She has not drunk since. The father and she received further marital advice. The boy was given intensive personal psychotherapy and careful educational treatment in hospital. His drug programme was greatly reduced. He was discharged home on trial. Great improvement in the family situation and in the child's behaviour followed, but the frequency of his epilepsy increased so that he was having seizures at home, at school and in traffic.

Investigations had shown a consistent left anterior temporal lobe discharge and on air pictures there was a dilated left temporal horn. The operation of left anterior temporal lobectomy was undertaken when the patient was 13 years and 3 months old. The patholological findings revealed the expected sclerosis of Ammon's horn.

By the time he was 15 it was clear that he had come through a somewhat delayed adolescence satisfactorily. He had had no epilepsy, he had had no medication. He prepared for and passed successfully 8 'O' levels at the age of 16. $8\frac{1}{2}$ years post-operatively the situation was reviewed. The parents were still happily united and the mother had remained free from alcoholism. The patient was leading a normal social life, studying for a diploma in accountancy and described as surrounded by many girlfriends.

Both Oedipus and Hamlet raised their hoary heads early in this young life, but they now seem well sunk below the surface and our patient's future seems likely to conform to a more civilised mode.

References

Annegers J F, Hauses W A, Elveback L R, Anderson V E, Kurland L R 1976 Seizure disorders in offspring of parents with a history of seizures — a maternal-paternal difference. Epilepsia 17:1–9

Chance M R A 1957 The role of convulsions in behaviour. Behaviour Science 2:30–35

Fairweather H, Hutt S J 1969 Inter-relationships of EEG activity and information processing on paced and unpaced tasks in epileptic children. Electroencephalography and Clinical Neurophysiology 27(7):701

Hutt S J, Hutt C 1970 Direct observation and the measurement of behaviour. Thomas, Springfield, Illinois

Kawakami M, Seto K, Therasawa E, Yoshida K 1967 Structure and function of the limbic system. Adey W B, Tolizane T (eds) Elsevier, Amsterdam, p 69–102

Kolvin I 1971 Studies in childhood psychosis. 1 Diagnostic criteria and classification. British Journal of Psychiatry 118:381–384

Lindsay J, Ounsted C, Richards P 1979a Long-term outcome in children with temporal lobe seizures. 1. Social outcome and childhood factors. Developmental Medicine and Child Neurology 21:285–298

Lindsay J, Ounsted C, Richards P 1979b ibid. 2. Marriage, parenthood and sexual indifference. Developmental Medicine and Child Neurology 21:400–433

Lindsay J, Ounsted C, Richards P 1979c ibid. 3. Psychiatric aspects in childhood and adult life. Developmental Medicine and Child Neurology 21:630–636

Lindsay J, Ounsted C, Richards P 1980 Long-term outcome in children with temporal lobe seizures. 4. Genetic factors, febrile convulsions and the remission of seizures. Developmental Medicine and Child Neurology 22:429–440

Mellanby J, George G, Robinson A, Thompson P 1977 Epileptiform syndrome in rats produced by injecting tetanus toxin into the hippocampus. Journal of Neurology, Neurosurgery and Psychiatry 40:404–414

Miller F J W, Court S D M, Walton W S, Knox E J 1960 Growing up in Newcastle upon Tyne. Oxford University Press, London, p 369

Ounsted C 1951 Significance of convulsions in children with purulent meningitis. Lancet 1:1245–1255

Ounsted C 1952 The factor of inheritance in convulsive disorders in childhood. Proceedings of the Royal Society of Medicine 45:865–868

Ounsted C 1955 The hyperkinetic syndrome in epileptic children. Lancet 2:303–321

Ounsted C 1971 Some aspects of seizure disorders. In: Gairdner D, Howle D (eds) Recent advances in paediatrics, 4th edn. J & A Churchill, London, p 363–400

Ounsted C 1976 Genetic messages and convulsive behaviour in pyrexia in brain dysfunction in infantile febrile convulsions. Brazier M A B, Cocceani F (eds) Raven Press, New York, p 279–290

Ounsted C, Taylor D C 1972 The Y chromosome message: a point of view. In: Gender differences: their ontogeny and significance. Churchill Livingstone, Edinburgh, p 241–262

Ounsted C, Lindsay J, Norman R 1966 Biological factors in temporal lobe epilepsy. Clinics in Developmental Medicine 22: Spastics International Medical Publication with William Heinemann Medical Books, London

Rodin E A 1968 The prognosis of patients with epilepsy. Charles C Thomas, Springfield, Illinois, p 348

Taylor D C 1969 Sexual behaviour and temporal lobe epilepsy. Archives of Neurology 21:510–516

Taylor D C 1975 Factors influencing the occurrence of schizophrenia-like psychosis in patients with temporal lobe epilepsy. Psychological Medicine 5:249–254

Taylor D C, Ounsted C 1972 In: Gender differences: their ontogeny and significance. Churchill Livingstone, Edinburgh, p 215–262

Thoday J M 1953 Components of fitness. Symposium, Society for Experimental Biology 7:96–99

Thom D A 1942 Convulsions of early life and their relation to chronic convulsive disorders and mental defect. American Journal of Psychiatry 98:574–580

Waddington C H 1957 The strategy of the genes. George Allen & Unwin, London

The limbic system

INTRODUCTION

Although Willis, in his *Cerebri Anatome*, referred to a section of the brain around the brainstem as the 'cerebri limbus', it was Broca (1878) who defined the comparative anatomy of an area of cortex, which he referred to as 'le grand lobe limbique', which in man included some parts of the hippocampus, and the subcallosal and cingulate gyri. He also noted the close connections of these areas with the olfactory apparatus of the brain, which led to the adoption of the term 'rhinencephalon'. While several contemporary anatomists, including Ferrier and His, objected to this latter name, it remained in use until the middle of this century when the concept of the limbic system was fully elaborated by Papez (1937), Yakovlev (1948), and Maclean (1970).

Papez drew attention to the distinction between the activities of the medial cortex, with hippocampus and cingulate cortex participating in hypothalamic activities, and the lateral cortex mediating general sensory activities via the dorsal thalamus. He outlined the so-called Papez circuit of: hippocampal formation — mamillary bodies — anterior thalamic nuclei — cortex of gyrus cinguli, and suggested it was central to affective experience, forming 'a harmonious mechanism which may elaborate the functions of central emotion, as well as participate in emotional expression'. Yakovlev noted the psychogenetic development of the brain which went pari passu with the development of behaviour. Thus the visceral, expressive and effective motility of an animal had neural correlates as the neuraxis differentiated from a cylindrical hollow with a virtually homogenous structure, to a three-tiered system. The innermost layer was nearest the central canal, and was composed of diffuse short neurones which essentially 'integrates the energy metabolism within the body; it regulates homoeostasis and maintains the steady state of the internal medium.' The intermediate system, which included the limbic system, was more external, more myelinated and more clearly differentiated into nuclear matter, and integrated predominantly axial and essentially postural motility of the outward expression of internal states and emotions. The outmost system, appearing only in mammals, consisted of well-myelinated neurones with cells of origin in the cerebral cortex which connect with long axons to the anterior horn cells of the spinal cord. Yakovlev thus commented: 'The intrinsic synaptic surface of the neuraxis and the behaviour of vertebrates and man evolve thus from within outward as a stereo-dynamic unity.'

Maclean (1970) discussed the 'inherited structure' of three aspects of the human brain — the reptilian, paleomammalian and neomammalian. The paleomammalian brain, representing the limbic system, had similar features in all mammals, had many connections with the hypothalamus and brainstem structures, and played a 'basic role in integrating emotional expression' (see Fig. 16.1).

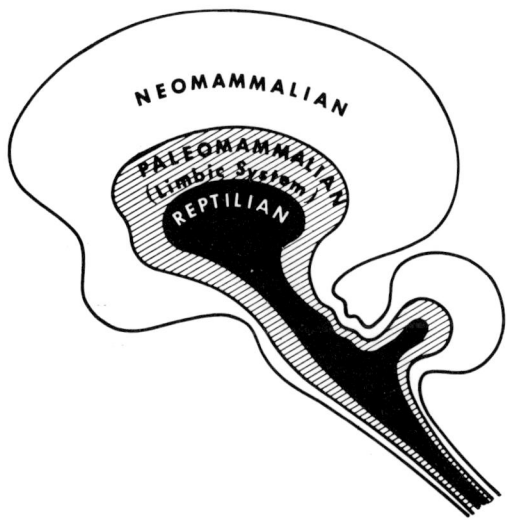

Fig. 16.1   The three basic types of brains which in the evolution of the mammalian forebrain become part of man's inheritance. The paleomammalian brain, corresponding to the so-called limbic system or 'visceral brain', is an inheritance from lower mammals and has been shown to play an important role in emotional behaviour. (From Maclean P D 1970 The triune brain, emotion of scientific bias. Reproduced by permission of Rockefeller University Press.)

With recent development of techniques in both neuroanatomy and neurochemistry, and a change in concepts regarding the way the brain is organised, in particular from anatomy to chemistry and thus away from structure towards function, the limbic system has become of central importance in neuropsychiatry. In particular has been the acceptance of its role in emotional expression and psychiatric illness, the acknowledgement of its close associations with the basal ganglia, especially the striatum, and the discovery that monoaminergic pathways, closely associated with other neurotransmitters, such as peptides are central to its activity.

THE LIMBIC SYSTEM AND ITS DEVELOPMENT

During early embryogenesis, the basolateral part of the hemispheric vesicles develop to form an intraventricular projection which, in the course of its development and with expansion of the brain posteriorly, downwards and then forwards, becomes C-shaped. The more anterior portions develop into such structures as the nucleus accumbens and tuberculum olfactorium, while the caudal portions become the amygdala (see Fig. 16.2). Thus in the adult brain, the striatal system assumes a position adjacent to the lateral ventricles and at least two

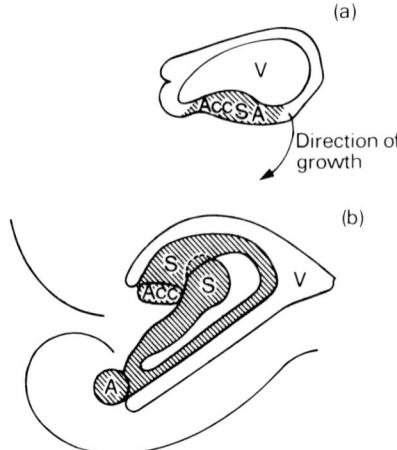

Fig. 16.2 The relationship of the striatum, amygdala and nucleus accumbens, (a) in embryo and (b) in adult. A, amygdala Acc, accumbens S, striatum V, ventricle. (From Nieuwenhuys R 1977 Aspects of the morphology of the striatum. Reproduced by permission of Elsevier-North Holland Biomedical Press.)

of its structures, namely the nucleus accumbens and the amygdala, come into close contact with the limbic system.

The limbic system is generally held to include the phylogenetically older areas of cortex, and related subcortical elements, with the associated tracts and pathways (see Table 16.1). Schematically these are outlined in Figs. 16.2 and 16.3, where some of the important fibre connections are shown. The main nuclei

Table 16.1 Main elements of the limbic system

Gyri	Subcollosal g.	*Nuclei*	Amygdaloid n.
	Cingulate g.		Septal n.
	Parahippocampal g.		Accumbens n.
	Hippocampal formation		Hypothalmic n.
	Dentate g.		Epithalamic n.
	Indusium griseum		Anterior thalamic n.
	Subiculum		Mammillary bodies
	Entorhinal area		Habenula m.
	Prepiriform cortex		Raphe n.
	Olfactory tubercle		Ventral tegmental area
			Dorsal tegmental nucleus
			Superior central nucleus
Pathways	Fornix		
	Mammillothalamic tract		
	Mammillotegmental tract		
	Stria terminalis		
	Stria medullaris		
	Cingulum		
	Anterior commissure		
	Medial forebrain bundle		
	Lateral and medial longitudinal striae		
	Dorsal longitudinal fasciculus		

comprise the hippocampal formation, the amygdala, the hypothalamus and the septal area. The hippocampal formation is composed of archicortex and forms a ring structure in the medial wall of the cerebral hemisphere. It includes the hippocampus, the dentate gyrus, the subiculum and its thin extension the

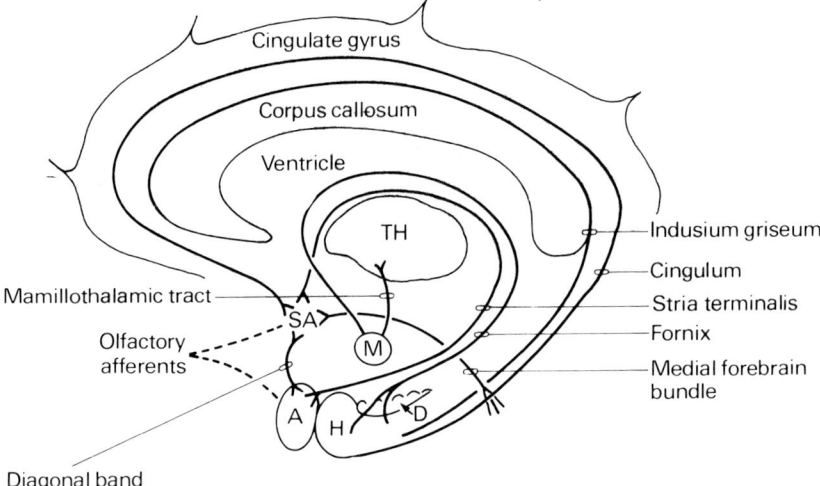

Fig. 16.3   The limbic system and the fibre tracts connecting its parts. A, amygdala D, dentate gyrus H, hippocampus M, mammillary body SA, septal/accumbens region TH, thalamus. (From Trimble M R 1981 Neuropsychiatry. Reproduced by permission of John Wiley & Sons Ltd.)

indusium griseum. The hippocampus itself lies in the floor of the temporal horn of the lateral ventricle, and because of an infolding of its structure, it assumes a complicated shape, the more medially placed dentate gyrus being positioned next to Ammon's horn, which itself is continuous with the subiculum. The indusium griseum passes over the whole extent of the corpus callosum carrying two fibre tracts, the medial and lateral longitudinal striae.

The amygdala resides at the tip of the temporal horn of the lateral ventricle, just rostral to the hippocampus, and has two well-defined nuclear divisions, the corticomedial and basolateral.

The septal area, not to be confused with its thin dorsal extension, the septum pellucidum, is a collection of nuclei situated in the medial wall of the anterior horn of the lateral ventricle, adjacent to the nucleus accumbens. Its ventral group of neurones comprises the bed nucleus of the stria terminalis, and ventromedially the nucleus of the diagonal band of Broca. Another group of neurones forms the lateral septal nucleus (see Fig. 16.4).

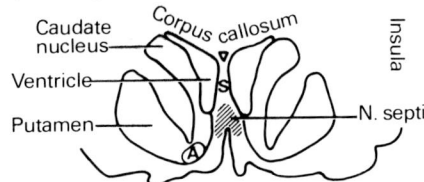

Fig. 16.4   The septal area — coronal section.
A = Accumbens nucleus
S = Septum pellucidum

The hypothalamus is situated in the floor and lateral wall of the third ventricle, posteriorly merging with the rostral midbrain. It has several well-defined nuclear masses, and is connected to the pituitary gland via the infundibular stalk.

The main fibre tracts of the limbic system include the fornix, the stria terminalis, the medial forebrain bundle, and the thalamo-cingulate pathways. The fornix curves round the thalamus and runs forwards under the corpus callosum, carrying information from hippocampus to nucleus accumbens and septal area and vice versa. It divides over the anterior commisure, its pre-commisural fibres ending mainly within the septal nuclei, nucleus accumbens, rostral hypothalamus and diagonal band, while the posterior ones pass to the mamillary bodies of the thalamus, or join the medial forebrain bundle to descend to the brainstem. The precommisural fibres mainly originate from Ammon's horn and terminate in both the accumbens and lateral septal nuclei, while the post-commissural fibres derive mainly from the subiculum, and carry information to the mamillary body, bed nucleus of the stria terminalis, and the anterior thalamic nucleus (Nieuwenhuys et al 1979). The stria medullaris carries information from the rostral limbic structures to the habenula nuclei. The stria terminalis, which passes alongside the caudate nucleus, interconnects the amygdala with the septal area, efferent fibres also ending in the anterior hypothalamus and related nuclear groups.

The cingulate gyrus runs above the corpus callosum, and embedded in it is the cingulum, a fibre bundle that passes backwards to the parahippocampal gyrus and hippocampus. The thalamus is connected to the cingulate gyrus by the thalamocingulate pathways, arising largely from anterior thalamic nuclei which themselves receive projections from the mamillary body via the mamillothalamic tract of Vicq d'Azar.

The medial forebrain bundle forms a large fibre system extending anteriorly from the septal area, amygdala, and olfactory trigone, passing through the hypothalamus to the ventral tegmental area caudally. While not strictly limbic in morphological terms, and probably representing an extension of the reticular activating system, it links the rostral limbic structures to the brainstem, and has been designated 'the mesolimbic system' by Ungerstedt (1971).

It can be seen from these descriptions that the septal area forms a key-point of limbic system activity. It is connected to the hypothalamus, nucleus accumbens, hippocampus and amygdala, and via the medial forebrain bundle to the midbrain tegmentum and brainstem. In addition, efferent septal fibres pass to the habenular nuclei and mamillary bodies. Of all the septal nuclei, the bed nucleus of the stria terminalis has widespread descending projections, through the stria terminalis to the amygdala, and via the medial forebrain bundle to nucleus accumbens, hypothalamus and ventral tegmental area, reticular formation and central grey substance of the midbrain (Swanson 1978). It is therefore a relay station for information from the hippocampus and amygdala to reach the hypothalamus and the limbic midbrain. In addition, since many fibres to the septal nuclei derive from the amygdala, Ammon's horn and the adjacent subiculum, it can be seen that clearly delineated connections exist between the basomedial temporal lobe structures, and the diencephalon and midbrain.

The neurochemistry of the limbic system

Within the brain neurotransmitters are not equally distributed, and the demonstration that some (in particular the monoamines such as dopamine, noradrenaline and serotonin) have a restricted distribution being concentrated mainly within the brainstem and limbic system, has emphasised their central role in the regulation of emotion and behaviour. Of particular importance in neuropsychiatry are dopaminergic neurones, since of all the neurotransmitters, dopamine has been shown to be the most linked with behaviour. One major dopaminergic tract is formed by nigrostriatal pathways, passing from the pars compacta of the substantia nigra to the caudate nucleus and putamen, another being the mesolimbic system which originates in the ventral tegmental area, medial to the substantia nigra. The fibres of this system ascend in the medial forebrain bundle, and are distributed principally to the bed nucleus of the stria terminalis, the olfactory tubercle, the nucleus accumbens, and the lateral septal nucleus (Ungerstedt 1971). Additional projections from the same area project to the anteromedial part of the frontal cortex, anterior cingulate cortex and entorhinal cortex (Bjorklund & Lindvall 1978).

Noradrenergic projections arise from pontine and medullary tegmental areas, in particular the locus coeruleus, and pass, in part within the medial forebrain bundle, to the rostral limbic structures such as hypothalamus, amygdala, hippocampus, and cingulate gyrus. Unlike the dopaminergic system, these noradrenergic neurones have a diffuse projection to the neocortex. Similarly, serotonergic neurones from brainstem areas, in particular the raphe nuclei, ascend to influence wide areas of cerebral cortex, and in addition hypothalamus, substantia nigra, the habenula, and thalamic, limbic and caudate nuclei. Recently it has been shown that several neuropeptides are closely interlinked with some of these monoamine nuclei. In particular the hypothalamus and the amygdala are areas containing high amounts of peptides, and a cholecystokinin-like peptide is found in a sub-population of dopamine neurones from the substantia nigra and ventral tegmental area (Hökfelt et al 1980).

THE LIMBIC SYSTEM AND BEHAVIOUR

Since the earlier discussions of Papez (1937) and Yakovlev (1948), the relationship between the limbic system, and in particular emotional behaviour, has become clear. One of the first demonstrations of this was the dramatic behaviour changes produced in monkeys by bilateral temporal lobe lesions, since referred to as the Klüver Bucy syndrome (Klüver & Bucy 1939). The animals showed hypermetamorphosis, diminished aggressiveness, hypersexuality and visual agnosia, and a similar picture in humans has since been described (Benson & Geschwind 1975).

A number of experiments, in particular using electrical stimulation or surgical destruction of selective neuronal tracts in animals, have emphasised the importance of the limbic system with regard to many different behaviours. These include alteration of food and water intake, particularly following hypothalamic lesions; disturbances of neuroendocrine regulation, mainly through alteration of hypothalamo-hypophysial releasing and inhibitor factors; memory disturbances, especially of the Korsakoff type following hippocampal lesions; and alterations of aggressive, sexual and motivational behaviour. Electrical stimulation of the amygdala leads to a variety of autonomic changes, interruption of on-going behaviour as if the animal had been aroused by some stimulus, and, at high intensity, fear, defence reactions, and aggression. Destruction of the amygdala leads to hypoactivity and a decrease of aggressive activity. Stimulation of the septal area, by contrast, leads to apparently gratifying effects, such that animals with implanted electrodes in this region will continue self-stimulation for considerable periods of time (Olds & Milner 1954), the results of which, in humans, are interpreted as pleasurable (Heath 1977a). Septal lesions often lead to transient episodes of aggression and emotional lability, particularly in rodents, which tends to dissipate with time, and exaggerated responses to painful stimuli, increased water uptake, weight loss, increased locomotor activity, especially in novel environments, and impairment of normal inhibitory responses to punishment thereafter (Grossman 1976). In addition, lesions of the bed nucleus of the stria terminalis in animals have been shown to result in loss of dominance and impairment of competitive fighting in food competition tasks (Miczek et al 1974). In humans it is of interest that of the neurosurgical operations which have been used clinically for treatment of psychiatric illness, leucotomy, particularly lesions which interfere with frontolimbic connections, or those which are placed in the sub-caudate region around the septal area, have been the most successful in influencing the emotional state of patients (Kelly 1976).

It was earlier emphasised that the limbic system had some close striatal connections. The striatum, comprising the caudate nucleus and putamen, is by far the largest nuclear mass in the mammalian brain, and has traditionally been linked primarily with motor activity. As emphasised above, both nucleus accumbens and amygdala are embryologically closely related to the striatum, and thus both striatum and limbic system share some common connections which include the nucleus accumbens itself. In addition, extensive neocortical afferents exist to both limbic system and corpus striatum, either via direct corticostriatal fibres, or via cortico-cortico connections from primary sensory areas, which ultimately converge on temporal cortex and the amygdala/entorhinal area, the major source of afferents for the hippocampus (Nauta & Domesick 1978). Recognition of such connectivity, and experimental behavioural analysis in animals following striatal lesions, has led to a new understanding of the functions of the basal ganglia, in particular their role in sensorimotor coordination (Nauta 1979), and the mediation of emotional expressive behaviour.

In discussing limbic system activity, Maclean (1970) commented how the lower parts of the limbic system 'ring' were primarily concerned with emotional feelings and behaviour that ensure self-preservation, whereas structures such as the septum, in the upper part of the ring, were involved in expressive and feeling states related to procreation and preservation of the species.

Smythies (1967) has emphasised the role of the limbic system in programming of behaviour, particularly in integrating neocortical and thus environmental, with hypothalamic and midbrain, hence visceral, activity. He commented on the widespread convergence of all sensory modalities on the neurones of the hippocampus and the amygdala, emphasising how these structures could correlate environmental with visceral data.

A number of recent experiments have emphasised the close relationship of the monoaminergic limbic and striatal systems to the regulation of behaviour. In particular, the production of stereotypic behaviour in animals by dopamine agonists or amphetamine has been related to nigrostriatal dopamine pathways, while stimulation of the mesolimbic tracts, chemically or electrically, has been shown to increase locomotor activity and motivational arousal (Iversen 1977). Abnormal dopaminergic activity has also now been associated with psychotic behaviour in humans. The evidence for this has been reviewed by Crow et al (1977), whose own work in animal models suggests that neuroleptic drugs exert their therapeutic action in schizophrenia, especially on 'positive' symptoms such as delusions, hallucinations and thought disorder (Johnstone et al 1978), by dopamine receptor blockade at the nucleus accumbens. In addition, the examination of post-synaptic dopamine receptors in post mortem brains by spiroperidol-binding has shown increased activity in the nucleus accumbens, putamen and caudate nucleus of schizophrenic patients (Owen et al 1978). These data implicate mesolimbic dopamine systems in the pathogenesis of human psychosis. It is of interest that earlier work, using implanted cerebral electrodes in psychotic non-epileptic patients, indicated that spike-wave activity could be recorded from the septal region, which spiking seemed to correlate in some patients with exacerbation of the psychotic state (Heath 1977b). In addition, in epileptic patients with implanted electrodes, the pattern of spread of seizure activity has been consistently noted to occur from the hippocampus and amygdala to the septal region (Heath 1976), and thus the same neuroanatomical sites have been implicated with the spread of epileptic activity in patients with epilepsy, with mechanisms of emotional expression, and with psychotic illness in non-epileptic patients.

THE LIMBIC SYSTEM IN EPILEPSY

Evidence from several sources has indicated a high incidence of psychopathology in patients with epilepsy, in particular those with temporal lobe lesions. This has been discussed in earlier chapters of this book (see Chapters 2 and 10), and the evidence has also been presented elsewhere, especially with reference to personality disorders and psychosis (Trimble & Perez 1980; Perez & Trimble 1980). In particular, paranoia, as a reflection of a personality change, and schizophreniform psychosis, especially with Schneiderian first-rank symptoms and often classified as paranoid schizophrenia, has been linked with left-sided temporal lobe dysfunction. Several authors have pointed out that the psychosis usually occurs after the epilepsy has been present for several years (e.g. Beard & Slater 1962), and that the emergence of the psychosis is associated with diminution of seizure frequency (e.g. Flor-Henry, 1969). Recently Kristensen & Sindrup (1978) have shown an association between psychosis and patients who have automatisms, as opposed to 'superficially initiated fits'. The former are said to originate in the uncinate region, which includes the amygdaloid nucleus, and peri-insular regions of the temporal lobe (Jasper 1958). The known connections between the amygdaloid neurones, and the septal nuclei and the mesolimbic dopamine system discussed above would thus form an ideal neurological substrate for the development of psychiatric changes in patients with complex partial seizures.

An electrophysiological mechanism was suggested by Symonds (1962), who referred to 'the epileptogenic disorder of function'. He said:

'Epileptic seizures and epileptiform discharge in the EEG are epiphenomena. They may be regarded as occasional expressions of a fundamental and a continuous disorder of neuronal function. The essence of this disorder is loss of the normal balance between excitation and inhibition at synaptic junctions. The epileptogenic disorder of function may be assumed to be present continuously, but with peaks at which seizures are likely to occur. This background disorder may cause symptoms other than seizures.... The presence and nature of such interictal symptoms as do occur are related to the epileptogenic focus. It is not loss of neurones in the temporal lobe that is responsible for the psychosis, but the disorderly activity of those that remain, and that this disorderly activity is of the kind that is also likely to cause seizures.'

This explanation does not entirely explain the delay in onset of the psychosis, but does emphasise the common origin of both seizures and behaviour disorder. The recent development of kindling as an experimental model of epilepsy may provide a bridge to help us further explain these phenomena. Thus in animal models, repeated sub-threshold stimulation to certain areas of the brain leads to convulsions, which eventually may occur spontaneously. This phenomenon has been observed in a variety of species, and obtained with a variety of experimental agents. Seizures are most easily kindled in the limbic system, the most responsive area being the amygdala, and consequent neuronal changes which develop appear to be persistent (Goddard et al 1976). The higher an animal in the phylogenetic scale, the more difficult kindling becomes, suggesting that in man the process may take many months if it occurs at all (Wada 1976). Of particular importance is that kindling of dopamine systems leads not to convulsions, but to marked behaviour changes. For example, stimulation of the ventral tegmental area in cats has been shown to result in fear reactions, with increased aggressive behaviour and loss of affection (Stevens & Livermore 1978). These changes are inhibited by drugs that are dopamine receptor antagonists and presumably represent neuronal excitation in limbic areas. Since dopamine agonism protects against convulsions and raises the seizure threshold, generalised spread of seizures in response to kindling in these sites may be inhibited, but increased and continuous sub-ictal local activity may occur leading to changes in behaviour and ultimately to chronic alteration of neuronal function in the limbic system. One possibility worthwhile of further exploration therefore, is that certain patients with chronic temporal lobe lesions and persistent subclinical ictal activity in limbic circuits develop behaviour changes over a period of time by a process similar to kindling, which in some results in personality changes or in others leads to the pattern of psychosis which phenomenologically is indistinguishable from process schizophrenia. Testing such a hypothesis depends on further careful documentation of the clinical picture in epileptic patients with psychiatric illness, especially those with psychosis, and on demonstration of altered activity within their mesolimbic dopamine pathways, especially at the septal nucleus/nucleus accumbens axis, which region seems central to the regulation of affective responses in both epileptic and non-epileptic patients.

References

Beard A W, Slater E 1962 The schizophrenia-like psychoses of epilepsy. Proc R Soc Med 55:311–316

Benson D F, Geschwind N 1975 Psychiatric conditions associated with focal lesions of the central nervous system. In: Reiser M F (ed) American handbook of psychiatry, vol IV. Basic Books, New York, p 208–243

Björklund A, Lindvall O 1978 The meso-telencephalic dopamine neurone system. A review of its anatomy. In: Livingston K E, Hornykiewicz O (eds) Limbic mechanisms. Plenum Press, New York, p 307–333

Broca P 1878 Anatomie comparée des circonvolutions cérébrals: le grand lobe limbique et la scissure limbique dans la série des mammifères. Révue Anthropologie. Série 2, 1:385–498

Crow T J, Deakin J F W Longden A 1977 The nucleus accumbens — possible site of antipsychotic action of neuroleptic drugs. Psychol Med 7:213–221

Flor-Henry P 1969 Psychosis and temporal lobe epilepsy. Epilepsia 10:363–395

Grossman S P 1976 Behavioural functions of the septum: a reanalysis. In: De France J et al (eds) The septal nuclei. Plenum Press, New York, p 361–422

Goddard G V, McNaughton B L, Douglas R M, Barnes C A 1976 Synaptic change in the limbic system: evidence from studies using electrical stimulation with and without seizure activity. In: Livingston K E, Hornykiewicz O (eds) Limbic mechanisms. Plenum Press, New York, p 355–368

Heath R G 1976 Brain function in epilepsy: midbrain, medullary and cerebellar interaction with the rostral forebrain. J Neurol Neurosurg & Psychiat 39:1037–1051

Heath R G 1977a Modulation of emotion with a brain pacemaker. J Nerv Ment Dis 165:300–317

Heath R G 1977b Subcortical brain function correlates of psychopathology and epilepsy. In: Shagass C, Gershon S, Friedhoff A J (eds) Psychopathology and brain dysfunction Raven Press, New York, p 51–67

Hökfelt T, Johansson O, Ljungdahl A, Lundberg J M, Schultzberg M 1980 Peptidergic neurones. Nature 284:515–521

Isaacson R L 1974 The limbic system. Plenum Press, New York

Iversen S 1977 Striatal function and stereotyped behaviour. In: Cools A R, Lohman A H M, van den Berken J H L (eds) Psychobiology of the striatum. Elsevier, North-Holland, p 99–118

Jasper H H 1958 Functional subdivisions of the temporal region in relation to seizure patterns and subcortical connections. In: Baldwin M, Bailey P (eds) Temporal lobe epilepsy. Charles C Thomas, Springfield, p 40–57

Johnstone E C, Frith C, Crow T J, Carney M W P, Price J S 1978 Mechanism of the antipsychotic effect in the treatment of acute schizophrenia. Lancet 1:848–851

Kelly D 1976 Neurosurgical treatment of psychiatric disorder. In: Granville-Grossman K (ed) Recent advances in clinical psychiatry, vol 2. Churchill Livingstone, Edinburgh

Kluver H, Bucy P C 1939 Preliminary analysis of functions of the temporal lobes in monkeys. Arch Neurol Psychiat 42:979–1000

Kristensen O, Sindrup E H 1978 Psychomotor epilepsy and psychosis. Acta neurologica scandinavica 57:361–369

Maclean P D (1970) The triune brain, emotion of scientific bias. In: The neurosciences, second study program. Rockefeller University Press, New York, p 336–349

Miczek K A, Brykczynski T, Grossman S P 1974 Differential effects of lesions in the amygdala, periamygdaloid cortex or stria terminalis on aggressive behaviour in rats. J Comp Physiol Psychol 87:760–771

Nauta H J W 1979 A proposed conceptual reorganisation of the basal ganglia and telencephalon. Neuroscience 4:1875–1881

Nauta J H, Domesick V B 1978 Crossroads of limbic and striatal circuitry: hypothalamo-nigral connections. In: Livingston K E, Hornykiewicz O (eds) Limbic mechanisms. Plenum Press, New York, p 75–93

Nieuwenhuys R 1977 Aspects of the morphology of the striatum. In: Cools A R, Lohman A H M, van den Bercken J H L (eds) The psychobiology of the striatum. Elsevier-North Holland

Nieuwenhuys R, Voogd J, van Huijzen Chr 1979 The human central nervous system. Springer-Verlag, Berlin

Olds J, Milner P 1954 Positive reinforcement produced by electrical stimulation of septal area and other regions of rat brain. J Comp Physiol Psychol 47:419–427

Owen F, Crow T J, Poulter M, Cross A J, Longden A, Riley G J 1978 Increased dopamine-receptor sensitivity in schizophrenia. Lancet 1:223–226

Papez J W 1937 A proposed mechanism of emotion. Arch Neurol Psychiat 38:725–743

Perez M M, Trimble M R 1980 Epileptic psychosis — diagnostic comparison with process schizophrenia. British Journal of Psychiatry 137:245–250

Smythies J R 1967 Brain mechanisms and behaviour. Brain 90:697–706

Stevens J R, Livermore A 1978 Kindling of the mesolimbic dopamine system. Animal model of psychosis. Neurology 28:36–46

Swanson L W 1978 The anatomical organisation of septo-hippocampal projections. In: Functions of the septo-hippocampal system: Ciba Foundation Symposium. Elsevier-North Holland

Symonds C 1962 Discussion: the schizophrenia-like psychosis of epilepsy. Proc R Soc Med 55:311–316

Trimble M R 1981 Neuropsychiatry. Wiley & Sons, Chichester (in press)

Trimble M R, Perez M M 1980 Quantification of psychopathology in adult patients with epilepsy. In: Kulig B M et al (eds) Epilepsy and behaviour 1979. Swets & Zeitlinger, Liese

Ungerstedt U 1971 Stereotaxic mapping of the monoamine pathways in the rat brain. Acta physiol scand supp 367:1–48

Wada J A 1976 The clinical relevance of kindling: species, brain sites and seizure susceptibility. In: Livingston K E, Hornykiewicz O (eds) Limbic mechanisms. Plenum Press, New York, p 369–388

Yakovlev P 1948 Motility, behaviour and the brain. J Nerv Ment Dis 107:313–335

Brain lesions, surgery, seizures and mental symptoms

INTRODUCTION

'I trust I have not wasted breath:
I think we are not wholly brain,
magnetic mockeries:...'
Tennyson, *In Memoriam*, CXX

Some years ago, Professor Corsellis drew my attention to the derivation of the word hamartoma which had been used to describe certain small tumour-like abnormalities found in the resected temporal lobes of some people with temporal lobe epilepsy. The derivation is through *hamartia* meaning the tragic flaw. (Random House English Dictionary). The essence of Greek tragedy was that some imperfection in man's make-up waits to reveal itself in his ineluctable destiny (Taylor & Marsh 1977). Considering the awful lives of many of the people whose hamartomas we were studying, the term seemed particularly apposite though few people today would conceed too close a correspondence between the flaw and the outcome. Yet Gowers' contemporary, Hughlings Jackson, who met his famous patient Dr Z in 1877, waited until 1894 for post mortem examination to reveal the indolent lesion of the left uncus which had ruined Z's life and abetted his tragic death (Taylor & Marsh 1980). Modern epilepsy surgery would have saved Dr Z's life and Dr Jackson's time.

Temporal lobectomy as a treatment for chronic temporal lobe epilepsy provides, as a by-product, a unique perspective on such relationships as may exist between certain brain lesions and mental symptoms. The unique perspective derives from the facts that can be ascertained by careful neuropathological examination of the resected specimen, from detailed analysis of the preoperative mental state and history of the patient (who, if deserving of surgery, is highly likely to have been disturbed), and from opportunities to study changes over time following surgical treatment. The chance to make such analyses is rare in psychiatry. The purpose of this chapter is to show that, even so, the relationship between lesions and symptoms is complex and that superficial analyses, especially those without benefit of a developmental viewpoint, are likely to be glib and wrong.

In seeking the relationships between cerebral lesions and mental symptoms we are heirs to a series of unfortunate and unprofitable traditions. According to Bleuler (1951), 19th-century alienists were looking for specific disease entities in brain which were supposed to be manifest in specific psychopathologies. As a result of this way of thinking even epilepsy itself came to be regarded as a *functional* psychosis because of its lack of correspondence with any one particular underlying brain disorder. Most of the cerebral locationists were seen to be following the discredited Dr Gall even though the localisation of lesions responsible for neurological symptoms was respectable. As a result of these failures to find specific brain diseases underlying psychiatric syndromes, or to provide specific psychiatric syndromes to match localised brain disease the search has been, largely, abandoned. There is now a general preference for chemical rather than structural or organisational models of severe mental disturbance. There is little interest in neuropathological studies in psychiatry. It is true that they proved unrewarding but there is almost no criticism of the failure of neuropathological method as being the basis of this failure. Another reaction to this failure has been to assume that cerebral abnormality plays little part in the genesis of mental symptoms. The alternative, presumably, is that the mental symptoms derive as normal reactions to situational and experiential distress. These views are continually being reinforced by finding gross cerebral abnormality in people who appear to be functioning quite adequately, and finding no apparent abnormality in the brains of grossly abnormal people. But as Bleuler (1951) reminds us, what we *regard* as psychiatric or psychological symptoms, as opposed to neurological symptoms, represent only the minor adumbrations of cerebral disorder or a minor component of a cerebral catastrophe which is overwhelmingly neurological. Consider for example the gross case of extensive right hemisphere damage leading to hemiplegia.

There may also be denial by the patient of the left side of his body, although he can see it perfectly well. The self concept is, apparently, in conflict with what seems to be available to the patient by way of external validation. The left hemiplegic is deprived, by the right brain lesion, not only of the use of the left limbs but also of all capacity to register that fact in the describing part of the brain. The self therefore retains the impression of an intact body even though it is severely dysfunctional. The patient, therefore, is not only in error, he is incorrigible. The situation provides a nice model of a morbid conviction. The persistance of a phantom limb creates a converse case. The image of the limb persists after its amputation. Thus we can argue that the 'self concept' is not easily modified by information coming in acutely through the special senses. Nor, if we think about it, should it be. But it does allow for the persistence of inner convictions which are not corrected by external falsification.

For cerebral lesions to produce disorders which would be of interest to psychiatrists as psychopathological syndromes they would have, at once, both to distort the self concept and not produce symptoms that render the picture overwhelmingly neurological. Such lesions would therefore be small, subtle, and insidious. They would also be placed in the brain in loci where they are liable to influence psychic events. Lesions of the temporal lobes, such as those discovered in the neurosurgical treatment of epilepsy provide precisely such lesions.

The problem of the level at which psychological symptoms should be codified has been mentioned by Geschwind (1979). The variety of material produced by patients can easily lead to idiosyncratic codifications of fragments of behaviour, reminiscent of the worst excesses of those interested in the 'epileptic personality'. Indeed the 'hyper-religiosity' and 'preoccupations with philosophical matters' perceived by Bear & Fedio (1977) were common epithets in that context. At the other extreme, the constraints produced by traditional psychiatric categories may weaken potentially valuable insights. For example, hypergraphia had no place in traditional psychiatry (Waxman & Geschwind 1975). It has been very difficult therefore to provide reliable evidence on the nature of psychic functioning with which to correlate cerebral lesions when seeking to establish whether or not they have exerted an effect.

Further, two radically different views about the effects of focal cerebral lesions might be entertained by those doctors who deal with developed or deteriorating brains, who conceive in terms of acute losses, as opposed to those who deal with patients in the process of development where damage is made evident over time through failures to achieve expected performances. The same applies as between those who deal with acute as opposed to insidious processes.

Certain things follow from a recognition that the organisation of cerebral function is a developmental task to be achieved rather than something given at a particular moment. First, development must be regarded as having a goal or a high point. Second, this has to be achieved over a given period of time. Third, that some processes will be dependent on, and modified by, the prior existence of other processes, what embryologists and Erikson called epigenesis. Fourthly, the whole will be susceptible to various constraints, limitations, and even enhancements, due to intercurrent events which will vary in effect dependant upon the degree of development achieved before the time of their operation. Moreover, it is likely in survivors that reparative, homeorrhetic processes will have been deployed to make good deficits wherever possible. In essence the developmental viewpoint is the perspective of time. These considerations place great constraints upon what sorts of things we choose to regard as similar when we come to group together lesions as bases for our correlations with outcome. This chapter will illustrate, through examining some results, the way in which developmental variables interact in a particular group of patients with epilepsy and psychiatric symptoms, whose brain lesions were discovered and verified through surgical treatment.

METHOD

The principal datum in this analysis will be the Verbal Scale score on the Wechsler tests. This represents one reliably measured aspect of psychic function which might be modified or constrained by a cerebral lesion. Verbal IQ will be considered in relation to age at onset of epilepsy, to performance scale scores, and will be related to aura experience. Certain correlations between cerebral lesions and aspects of mental state will then be considered.

The population studied was some of the 300 patients who underwent temporal lobectomy for the relief of temporal lobe epilepsy by the late Mr Murray Falconer over a period of 25 years. A standard approach to the management of these patients was rapidly established which included rigorous history taking, psychiatric and psychological evaluation, and long-term follow-up. The method of lobectomy was also standardised and neuropathological study of the resected lobe was always of the highest order.

The first analysis is made on a population about whom much has already been written. This is 100 consecutive English-speaking patients on whom an holistic evaluation of outcome was published in 1968 and whose mental state was described in 1972 (Taylor & Falconer 1968, Taylor 1972). That study included an extensive correlation analysis which was, in effect, a search for meaning and for association which might guide future analysis. Of the variables then considered, age at onset of epilepsy, and other age-dependent factors showed very large range correlates.

FINDINGS

Bias of time

I like the physical analogy of *bias* for developmental effects—as in a lawn bowl—in which the propensity to vary from the straight path is incorporate and inapparent except while in movement.

Let us consider first the relationship between Verbal IQ and age at onset of epilepsy: then the distribution of different sorts of lesions over time.

Figure 17.1 illustrates the correlation between age at onset of epilepsy and Verbal IQ as measured on the Wechsler tests *before* operation. (In the original analysis when IQ was allocated to a five-point scale the product moment correlations had been F.S. r = 0.45, P.S. r = 0.48 and V.S. r = 0.45.) In a correlation between age of onset of epilepsy and actual Verbal IQ for all the cases illustrated in Figure 17.1 the overall correlation is 0.34.

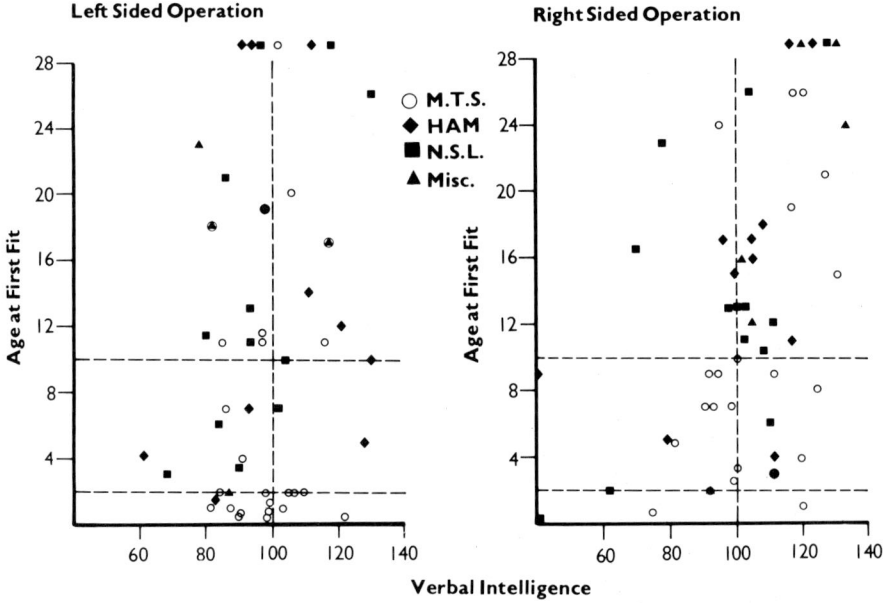

Fig. 17.1   Factors influencing verbal IQ in temporal lobe epilepsy.

In terms of neuropathological findings, the population is divided into four. There are 47 patients who showed mesial temporal sclerosis (MTS) in the resected lobe (including six with other associated lesions); 25 patients showed no clear-cut pathological change in the resected specimen (NSL); there were 22 'small focal tumours' or 'hamartomas' (HAM)[a group of lesions now called Alien Tissue (AT) in our publications]; and 12 cases with miscellaneous changes such as scars, infarcts, etc. (MISC).

The clear tendency for the MTS patients to have early onset epilepsy has proved to be due to the fact that the lesion is actually produced by prolonged local seizures during a limited phase in ontogeny, though it may have other unknown causes. The relevance of this being an important lesion was actually strenuously denied by Gowers (1881). It was probably this view which influenced Penfield to disregard the lesion in the early years of his work.

Bias of side
The correlation diagram is however divided between left- and right-sided operations. Inspection suggests that the overall correlation between age of onset and verbal IQ derives from only the right-sided lesions. Left-sided lesions reduce the mean verbal IQ and they do so irrespective of the age of onset of epilepsy. The coefficient of correlation between age of onset and verbal IQ on the left is 0.14 (NS) and on the right is 0.5 (P < 0.001). Alternatively, divided by the median age of onset (10 years) and by the median IQ (100.0), χ^2 (with Yates correction) yields 5.8 overall; 0.02 for the left operations and 7.1 for the right operations.

It was the distribution of MTS between the two sides as revealed in this diagram that gave rise to the 1969 hypothesis that some maturational change occurred differentially between the hemispheres around the age of two years. Before the age of two most cases occur on the left. After that age they occur on the right (Taylor 1969).

Bias of sex
The different vulnerability to MTS between the hemispheres also proved to be differently expressed by the two sexes. By adding to this material cases of Ounsted's who had suffered status epilepticus in early childhood and also had a lateralised focus in the EEG the distribution was produced which is shown in Figure 17.2. The left brain is more at risk in convulsions occurring before the age of two years. The vulnerability of males persists longer than that of females (Taylor & Ounsted 1971).

The correlation between Verbal IQ and age of onset in Figure 17.1, as expressed on the right side, when reanalysed by sex of patient proves to be contributed only by males.

Female left	r = 0.45 (NS)	Females right	r = 0.03 (NS)
Male left	r = 0.08 (NS)	Male right	r = 0.70 (P < 0.001)

Thus, in so far as there is any correlation between age of onset and Verbal IQ in females it concerns the left brain. The powerful significant correlation is confined to the right brain of males.

Thus, lesions of the left brain are associated with a reduction of Verbal IQ.

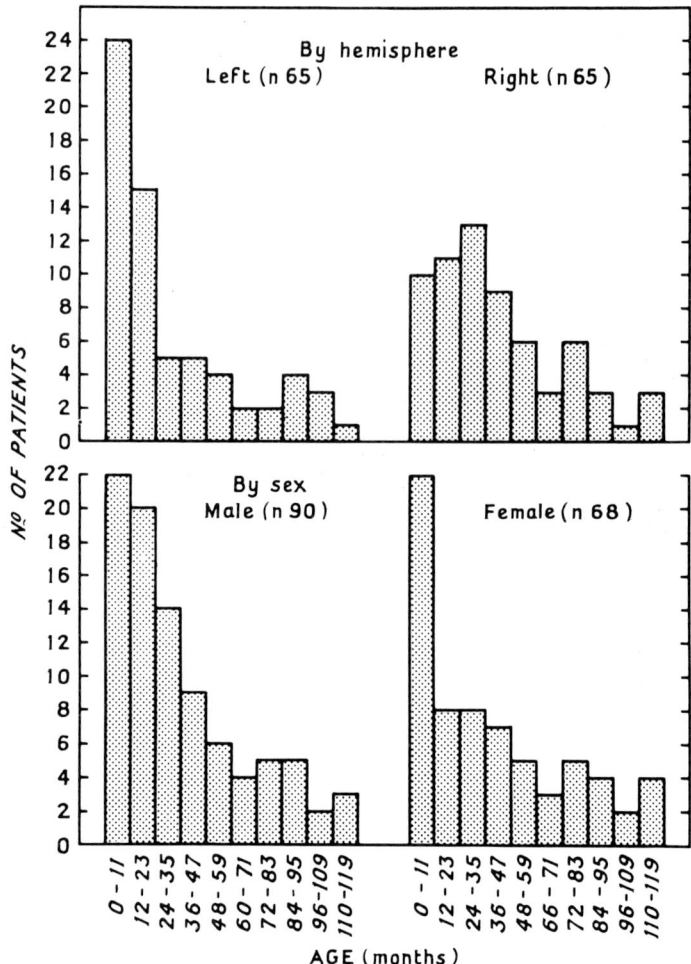

Fig. 17.2   Age at onset of first fit in patients with mesial temporal sclerosis or prolonged convulsion with fever, by sex and by side of lesion or EEG focus.

Epilepsy from right brain lesions in males also reduces Verbal IQ if the epilepsy starts early. But the slope in the right-sided operations' diagram suggests that a lesion of right brain might even be enhancing of Verbal IQ in males provided the epilepsy starts late. The suggestion that this might prove to be the case was made by Ounsted in his Shorvon Lecture of 1969 (unpublished).

Bias of lesion
In more recent studies this MTS group (reduced to 41 cases with MTS alone) has been contrasted with all the available AT lesions drawn from the whole Falconer series up to case 255, 47 cases in all (Taylor 1975).

Table 17.1 reveals that for males a 19 point difference in Verbal IQ exists between AT lesions on the left and right sides favouring the right side [113.8 to 94.8; SE = 8.41 (significant 5 per cent level)]. There is no difference in Verbal IQ between the sides for MTS lesions.

Table 17.1 Verbal intelligence in 87
patients with temporal lobe epilepsy.
Lesion and side, groups in order of verbal
IQ by sex

Males			Females		
AT	R	113.8	MTS	R	108.1
MTS	L	102.4	AT	R	101.4
MTS	R	101.3	AT	L	101.0
AT	L	94.8	MTS	L	87.8

AT = alien tissue   MTS = mesial
temporal sclerosis   R = right   L = left

For females it is in the MTS group that a 20.3 Verbal IQ difference opens up as between the two sides of the brain [108.1 to 87.8; SE = 5.01 (significant 0.1 per cent level)]. There is no difference in Verbal IQ as between the side of the AT lesions.

As would be deduced from the sex by side onset histogram (Fig. 17.2) the few females with left-sided MTS are affected early and severely by their convulsions and this is associated with reduced Verbal IQ.

Bias of side of operation
This same population of 88 patients also illustrates the effect of side of lesion and also any increased bias that might be produced by the lobectomy. In similar correlation matrices (Fig. 17.3) but now between preoperative Verbal IQ and preoperative Performance IQ it can be shown that there are more people for whom Verbal IQ exceeds Performance IQ for right-side lesions; and more with the reverse, Performance IQ greater than Verbal IQ, for left-sided lesions. [These complex biases which have been disputed by psychologists for many years were illustrated by Meyer & Jones (1957) using the first 31 cases operated on by Falconer. They were discussed by Benton (1962). They are explained in detail by Taylor (1976).]

Although these biases exist pre-operatively they are *not* in fact grossly enhanced after operation. Surprisingly most of the effects are in the P + V + and P − V − axes (Fig. 17.4, Table 17.2). Changes in the 'lateralising' axis P − V + are few and all but one of the P + V − cases are confined to the group of operations on AT in the left temporal lobe (the exception is a left-handed male with schizophrenia). These patients are also older at the time of operation.

One interpretation of this is that if the surgical removal of the lobe makes little increased difference where the left temporal lobe had been damaged by MTS, then there must have been a subsequent reorganisation of functions. The effect of the surgical lesion on Verbal IQ is more pronounced in the case where small left-sided alien tissue lesions have been removed in the lobectomy which suggests that they have had a rather more insidious effect within a lobe which was still functional pre-operatively. Removal of the lesion may in itself improve cerebral function and cerebral function may also be improved with relief of epilepsy. Either may account for the post-operative increases in scores. The least likely event is for the Verbal IQ to increase after left-sided alien tissue operations and this also suggests that the tissue lost was functional before the operation. Milner

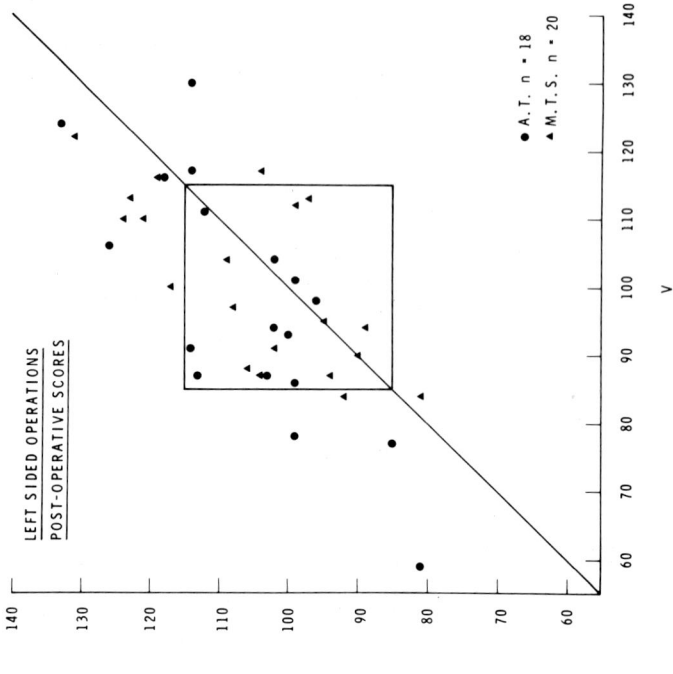

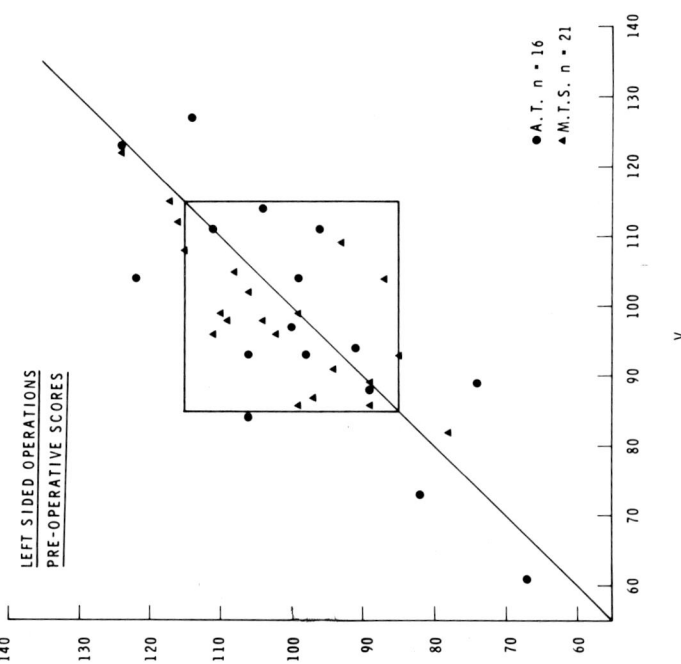

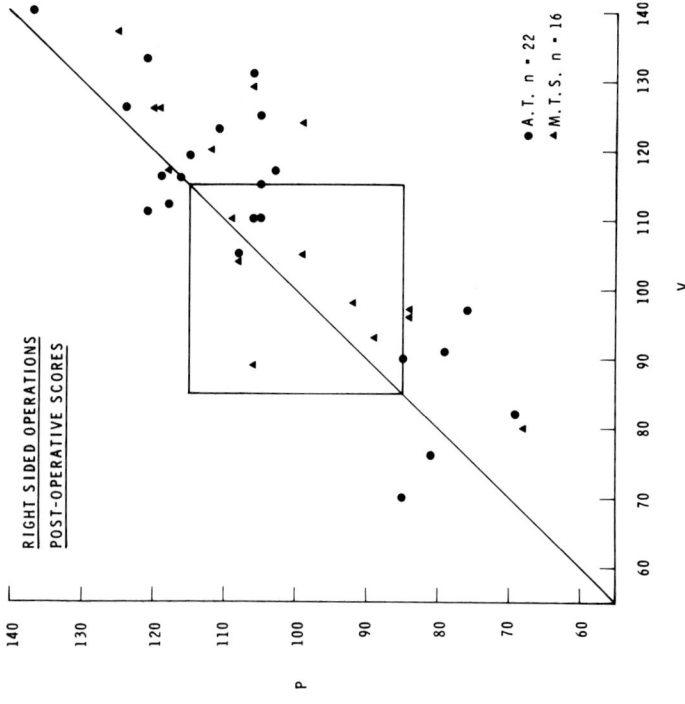

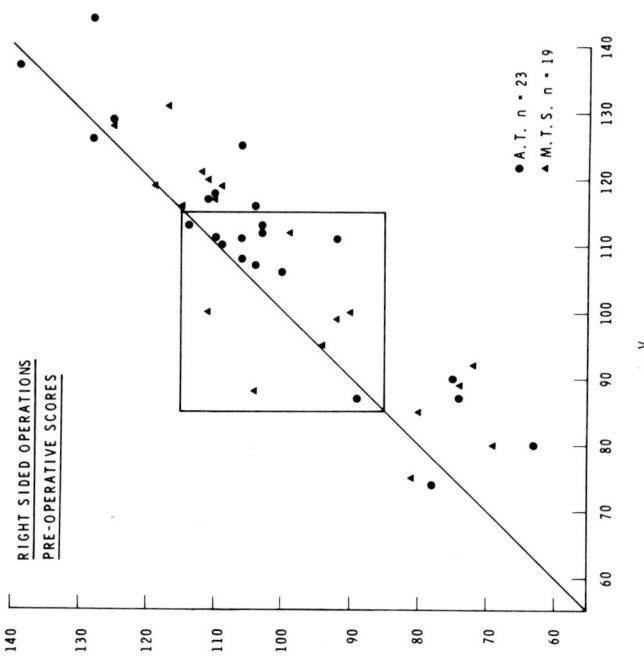

Fig. 17.3   Correlation of verbal and performance IQ before operation in patients with AT or MTS lesions confirmed after temporal lobectomy.

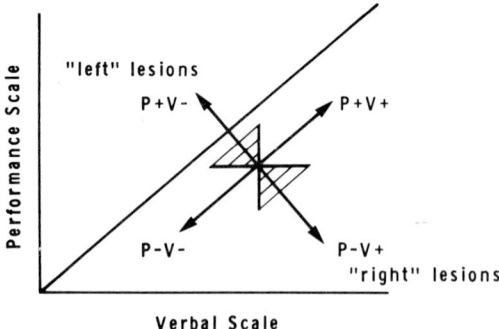

Fig. 17.4 Gains and losses on verbal and performance scale scores produce shifts in the locus of points on the V − P correlation diagram. The diagram illustrates the theoretical possibilities for changes in P and V IQ after surgical removal of the temporal lobe.

Table 17.2 87 patients with temporal lobe epilepsy. The number of patients making gains or losses of verbal (V) and performance (P) IQ scores of 10 or more points on Wechsler tests following temporal lobectomy for epilepsy

Group		P+ V+	P− V−	P+ V−	P− V+	Total
MTS	Left	5	2	0	1	8
	Right	4	1	0	3	8
AT	Left	1	1	7	0	9
	Right	4	4	1	0	9
Total		14	8	8	4	34
Both groups	Left	6	3	7	1	17
	Right	8	5	1	3	17

(1975) attributes this loss of Verbal IQ post-operatively to an effect of age. But no late operated patient with MTS has shown an increase in Performance IQ together with a loss of Verbal IQ to a degree where either change was ten points or more. All eight patients who showed P + V − had AT lesions, seven of them were operated on the left side. This rather supports the argument that the temporal lobe with the AT lesion in it still had verbal functions up to the time of the operation.

Aura and intelligence
Aura is a brief precognisance of some epileptic fits. It is a self report of remembered psychic events which precede the loss of awareness associated with the further spread of the seizure discharge. The range of the experiences described varies from simple vegetative events, feelings in the epigastrium, to the inchoate 'indescribable feelings in the head', to complex relivings of moments in the past. Some incorporate the madness of a dream. If these reports accurately describe the initial events of the seizure then they may vary with the site, timing, and nature of the lesion or give some clue to the organisation of complex cerebral functions. Some people have wondered if the continued recurrence of complex

auras would presage the development of schizophrenia-like psychoses. They offer another possibility of correlating brain lesions with an aspect of psychic functioning.

A detailed study of auras was made in 88 patients with MTS and AT lesions. Only nine of the 88 patients had no aura. The other 79 patients described a total of 215 auras. One patient was untestable for Verbal IQ. The initial classification of the 215 auras was into 21 varieties. For the purposes of this analysis they were reduced to three major categories 'simple primitive auras' (what Gowers called pneumogastric auras) (99), auras in 'special senses' (41) and 'intellectual' auras (75) (Table 17.3).

Table 17.3   Auras described by 88 patients with temporal lobe epilepsy

No aura	9	
Epigastric neutral	23	
Epigastric fear	24	
Nausea	12	Simple primitive (99)
Cephalic	27	
Rectal	1	
Penile/Vaginal	7	
Peripheral sensory	5	
Taste	10	
Smell	10	
Microposia/Macropsia	13	Special senses (41)
Microcusia/Macrocusia	3	
Rotation/Vertigo/Tinnitus	5	
Hallucinations	10	
Doppelganger	3	
Intensification	5	
Depersonalisation/derealisation	9	
Anaesthetic	2	Intellectual (75)
Time anomalies	4	
Jamais vu	4	
Déjà vu/Panoramic memory	16	
Idiosyncratic	22	

Preliminary analyses suggested that aura varied, principally, with intelligence. But again the relationship proves to be complex. If the group is divided by Verbal IQ into those with a Verbal IQ of 99 and less, and those of 100 and above, simple primitive auras are described by 86 per cent of the less intelligent and by only 55 per cent of the more intelligent patients ($\chi^2 = 7.4\,P < 0.01$). Auras in the 'special senses' are equally represented between the two groups. 'Intellectual' auras were reported by 64 per cent of the higher IQ group as opposed to 31 per cent of those with lower IQ ($\chi^2 = 6.9\,P < 0.01$).

Since Verbal IQ depends upon sex, side, and lesion type, the mean number of auras of each of the three types and the mean total number of auras per patient can be examined in eight subgroups (Table 17.4).

For males (Table 17.4a) the mean frequency of report of each type of aura and the mean total number varies precisely with the mean IQ of the subgroup. The total number of auras of all types per patient correlates with Verbal IQ ($r = 0.47\,P < 0.0001$).

Table 17.4 Aura and IQ in 87 patients with temporal lobe epilepsy. Lesion, side groups in IQ order by mean number of auras per person

Group		Simple primitive	Special senses	Intellectual	Total	V. IQ	'N'
a. *Males*							
A.T.	R	1.1	0.5	1.5	3.1	113.8	18
M.T.S.	L	1.2	0.4	0.7	2.3	102.4	16
M.T.S.	R	0.9	0.4	0.5	1.8	101.3	10
A.T.	L	0.6	0.2	0.4	1.2	94.8	10
b. *Females*							
M.T.S.	R	2.0	0.4	0.8	3.2	108.1	9
A.T.	R	1.1	0.9	0.4	2.4	101.4	9
A.T.	L	0.9	0.5	0.9	2.3	101.0	10
M.T.S.	L	1.6	0.4	1.8	3.8	87.8	5

For females (Table 17.4b) there is no such association, many complex auras are reported by the group with the lowest IQ. The correlation between total number of auras of all types and their Verbal IQ is -0.08 (NS).

Considering side of lesion, there is a correlation of 0.32 between total number of auras and Verbal IQ for right-operated patients ($P < 0.05$) and of 0.04 (NS) for those operated on the left side. By nature of lesion, the correlation between Verbal IQ and total number of auras per person for males is 0.6 ($P < 0.01$) for the AT group but 0.2 (NS) for the MTS group. Neither correlation is significant for females.

Thus, the closest relationship between IQ and aura richness would be for males with right-sided AT lesions. These different relationships between aura and intelligence might suggest (or reflect) different cerebral organisation between sexes or else a different attitude towards vouchsafing these intensely personal experiences. In men the reports on the number and the complexity of auras increase with intelligence and they lateralise probably as a reflection of preserved Verbal IQ. Complexity of aura will not relate to the development of schizophrenia-like psychosis in males in this sample of patients as aura is most intense in the group least vulnerable to schizophrenia. It might be different for females.

Mental state and intelligence

Let us return to consider the population of 100 consecutive patients. Certain associations exist between the four mental state categories used in the 1968 and 1972 analyses (normal, psychopathy, neurosis and psychosis) and the variables illustrated in Figure 17.1. 'Normal' at the post-operative follow-up correlated with low intelligence but also with having a Verbal IQ at least seven points superior to Performance IQ.

'Psychopathy' as a pre-operative diagnosis related to younger patients, to males, to operations on the left side, and to lower full scale IQ. This was the group most susceptible to change to normal after operation, largely due to loss of aggression.

'Neurosis' was a diagnosis given to older, more intelligent patients both before and after operation. A tendency for them to have right- rather than left-sided operations just fails to reach significance. Because the number of 'psychotic' patients in this group of 100 was small the association with AT lesions and later onset epilepsy discovered here has been followed up in the larger sample of AT lesions and reported in several publications. In summary, the most susceptible patients proved to have small AT lesions, in the left brain, giving rise to later onset epilepsies, especially in females, and associated with left-handedness (Taylor 1975, 1977).

DISCUSSION

It is worth remembering that these findings are not the results of an experiment but are an aspect of painstaking clinical work extending over a period of 25 years. The surgical treatment of temporal lobe epilepsy in the type of patients considered here was not, originally, primarily directed at the removal of lesions. On the contrary, the Gibbses prevailed upon Percival Bailey in 1948 to undertake lobectomies in patients who had EEG foci but no apparent lesion, with a view to relieving their social and mental distress. It was a parallel exercise to that of Penfield who began by operating on people who had accessible cerebral scars. Falconer's first operation in this series was in February 1951. Each neurosurgeon discovered previously undiagnosable lesions in the resected lobe. Penfield and Falconer became aware of improvement in the well-being of a sufficient proportion of their cases to encourage them to continue. Bailey and Gibbs were discouraged. Only briefly was there a period of unwarranted extension of the treatment in less judicious hands. We are fortunate that the clinical teams at the Guys/Maudsley Neurosurgical Unit supporting the decision to operate were so painstaking. It has greatly reduced the error in the material.

But to what extent may we argue that if a patient's mental and social problems improve after removal of a brain lesion, that the lesion had caused the problem? We should also have to say it was not the cause if the patient did not improve. The having and relieving of epilepsy has been regarded as the most important intervening variable. It may be. The more intervening variables we can find the better defended we are against any sort of cerebral determinism. Unlike the ancient Greeks we, mostly, do not believe ourselves bound by ineluctable fate. Mary Brazier (1973) reminds us that there was similarly a rejection of the original findings that the application of electrical currents to the brain led to movements of limbs without the interposition of man's will. This anxiety is reflected in the next lines of my opening quotation (published almost contemporaneously with Gowers' book on epilepsy):

'Not only cunning casts in clay:
Let Science prove we are, and then
What matters Science unto men,
At least to me? I would not stay.'

Some feminists in the late sixties preferred to deny sex differences in the brain for fear they might limit the realisation of their true potential. Perhaps we too fear to believe that our faculties, personality, character, the nature or chance of mental breakdown should be, to any significant degree, shaped by so banal a circumstance as a small imperfection in brain.

Yet several people who have thought profoundly about the integrative functions of the temporal lobe, Le Gros Clark, Papez, Kubie, Denis Williams among them, have come near to the suggestion that therein lies the neural basis of self. Denis Williams (1968) most explicitly talked of the 'I am' function of the temporal lobe. Kubie (1953) recognised that the correlation of internal and external worlds included setting the appropriate emotional tone. Accepting the idea that the self had a localised neural basis would allow the possibility of its developing, or maldeveloping, becoming limited or warped by a variety of circumstances, including the effects of adjacent dysfunctional tissue without the necessity of global cerebral dysfunction and without obvious loss of other skills.

I have given prominence in this presentation to Verbal intelligence, which can be regarded as a summary statement of certain modes of response, an aspect of psychic function, which can be seen to have been biased in subtle ways by the interaction of several factors. Could not similar variation obtain under similar circumstances, to account for the biases and the warping in what we summarise as psychopathology? Even so, temporal lobe lesions may only represent time markers, or event markers, they may promote disruptions in the organisation of brain. This may merely facilitate psychopathology rather than meaning a direct association between lesion as cause and psychiatric symptoms as effect. I have argued previously, in the case of schizophrenia-like psychoses, that we may have to curtail very considerably what we regard as similar events before correlations with psychopathology become really interesting (Taylor 1977).

Temporal lobe lesions produce biases in the response to Verbal IQ tests which depend upon their precise nature (perhaps related mainly to their time of origin and how they arise), the age of onset of epilepsy, the side on which they occur, and the sex of the patient. Despite all the constraints mentioned in my introduction some associations are being depicted which are being confirmed in other ways in other material. I think they are worth pursuing.

Acknowledgements
This work was undertaken under grants by the locally organised research fund of the Oxford A.H.A.(T). I am grateful to Mrs Susan Marsh and Mrs Eileen Pugh for secretarial help. Dr Alex Barr gave statistical advice and help.

References
Bear D M, Fedio P 1977 Quantitative analysis of interictal behaviour in temporal lobe epilepsy. Archives of Neurology 34:454–467
Benton A L 1962 Clinical symptomatology in right and left hemisphere lesions. In: V Mountcastle (ed) Interhemispheric relations and cerebral dominance. Johns Hopkins Press, p 253–263
Bleuler M 1951 Psychiatry of cerebral diseases. British Medical Journal ii:1233–1238
Brazier M A 1973 The role of electricity in the exploration and elucidation of the epileptic seizure. In: Brazier A (ed) Epilepsy: its phenomena in man. Academic Press, New York, ch 1, p 1–7
Geschwind N 1979 Behavioural changes in temporal lobe epilepsy. Psychological Medicine 9:217–219
Gowers W R 1881 Epilepsy and other chronic convulsive diseases: their causes, symptoms and treatment. American Academy of Neurology Reprint Series, Dover Publications, New York, vol 1, p 166
Kubie L S 1953 Some implications from psychoanalysis of modern concepts of the organisation of the brain. Psycholoanalytical Quarterly 22:21–52

Meyer V, Gwynne Jones H 1957 Patterns of cognitive test performance as functions of the lateral localization of cerebral abnormalities in the temporal lobe. Journal of Mental Science 103:753–772

Milner B 1975 Psychological aspects of focal epilepsy and its neurosurgical management. In: Purpura D P, Kiffin Penry J, Walter R D (eds) Advances in neurology. Raven Press, New York, vol 8, p 299–322

Taylor D C 1969 Differential rates of cerebral maturation between sexes and between hemispheres. Lancet 2:140–142

Taylor D C 1972 Mental state and temporal lobe epilepsy. A correlative account of 100 patients treated surgically. Epilepsia 13:727–765

Taylor D C 1975 Factors influencing the occurrence of schizophrenia-like psychosis in patients with temporal lobe epilepsy. Psychological Medicine 5:249–254

Taylor D C 1976 Developmental stratagems organising intellectual skills: evidence from studies of temporal lobectomy for epilepsy. In: Knights R M, Bakker D J (eds) The neuropsychology of learning disorders: theoretical approaches. University Park Press, Baltimore

Taylor D C 1977 Epileptic experience, schizophrenia and the temporal lobe. McLean Hospital Journal, special volume, June, p 22–39

Taylor D C, Falconer M A 1968 Clinical socioeconomic and psychological changes after temporal lobectomy for epilepsy. British Journal of Psychiatry 114:1247–1261

Taylor D C, Ounsted C 1971 Biological mechanisms influencing the outcome of seizures in response to fever. Epilepsia 12:33–45

Taylor D C, Marsh S M 1977 Neuropathology and social pathology: the effects of small lesions in the temporal lobe. In: Wink C S A (ed) Proceedings on tegretol in epilepsy. Geigy, Basle

Taylor D C, Marsh S M 1980 Hughlings Jackson's Dr Z. The paradigm of temporal lobe epilepsy revealed. Journal of Neurology, Neurosurgery and Psychiatry 43:758–767

Waxman S G, Geschwind N 1975 The interictal behavioural syndrome of temporal lobe epilepsy. Annals of General Psychiatry 32:1580–1586

Williams D 1968 Man's temporal lobe. Proceedings of the Royal Society of Medicine 61:355–356

EEG studies

INTRODUCTION

One of the most significant discoveries that has helped our understanding of epilepsy is the finding that clinical seizures are accompanied by abnormal electrical discharges in the brain. These discharges in the majority of cases can be monitored by measuring the changes in the electrical field on the surface of the scalp. Hans Berger, a German psychiatrist, was the first person to study these fields in detail and in 1929 published the first paper on the electroencephalogram or the EEG. Since that time monitoring of the scalp EEG has become routine. Changes in technology now allow the recording of the electrical rhythms of the brain throughout the 24 hours, during both waking and sleeping. Of more significance, modern telemetry and light weight tape recorders allow the EEG to be recorded during the day away from the hospital at home or at work. This flexibility has opened up an entirely new field as it now allows a much more accurate picture of seizure frequency and type to be defined; but of more significance it has allowed the relationship between cognitive functioning and abnormal brain rhythms to be explored.

Advances in neurosurgery brought about the possibility of recording the electrical activity of the surface of the cortex, the electrocorticogram. Depth electrode recording from leashes of chronically implanted electrodes has revealed the presence of seizure discharges in the deep structures of the brain, in particular the amygdala and hippocampus. Behavioural correlates of these abnormal discharges have led to a better understanding of the functioning of these limbic structures and their possible role in psychomotor epilepsy.

Advances in video-tape recording and split screen viewing so that the EEG and the patient can be viewed side by side has led to a precise correlation between the behavioural changes during a seizure and the abnormal electrical discharges. Finally, the expansion in computing facilities and the application of mathematical methods to signal analysis have allowed features of the EEG to be extracted and quantified. This has led to a better understanding of the cognitive changes which occur during the presence of abnormal cerebral activity. For the future it will be important to study the way that abnormal cerebral activity can be modified at will by biofeedback and other methods.

GENESIS

The electrocorticogram measured on the surface of the cerebral cortex is the spatial average of the underlying dendritic fields of the cells in the superficial layer of the cortex. These dendritic fields are generated by the inhibitory and excitatory post-synaptic potentials (IPSP or EPSP). Micro-electrode recordings from the cell bodies of cortical neurones show that the hyper- and hypo-polarization of the cells which are related to the IPSPs and EPSPs can be detected outside the cells so long as the recording electrode remains within the vicinity of those cells. As soon as the electrode is withdrawn beyond the dendrites then the potential fields of neighbouring cells interfere and the original correlation is lost (Creutzfeldt et al 1966).

Creutzfeldt also showed that the wave form of these potential fields depended on the cells which generated them. Thus at a cellular level there is information about cell type and neural activity coded within the EEG wave form. The spatial average of these dendritic fields all of which have random phase to each other could be expected to sum to zero as predicted by the central limit theorem. However, this does not occur because groups of cells become synchronised, and it is this activity which forms the electro-corticogram (ECoG) (Elul 1972). Calvet et al (1964) showed that in the lightly anaesthetised cat there are at least three generators situated at different layers in the cortex giving rise to cortical spindles; one is probably dentritic in origin and the other two are possibly from the dendrites and the cell bodies. Similar results have also been obtained for man by Peronnet et al (1972).

If spindles of coherent activity are the potentials which go to make up the electrocorticogram, what systems are responsible for this spindling and synchronisation of these cell populations. Several groups of workers (Anderson & Sears 1964, Andersen & Andersson 1974) have shown that spindle activity in the non-specific nuclei of the thalamus is transmitted to the thalamic projection areas of the cortex. Thus the EEG generators can be regarded as thalamo-cortical in structure; although the actual potential fields are created by the cells in the superficial layers of the cortex, the synchronisation of those cells is derived from the thalamus. What then controls thalamic activity?

Thalamic activity is modulated by a tonic bombardment from the reticular activating system of the mid-brain and brain stem. Depression of reticular tone leads to synchronisation of the thalamic rhythms and so to synchronisation and slowing of the cortical rhythms. An increase in reticular tone leads to desynchronisation of the EEG due to a breaking up of thalamic spindle activity. (Andersen & Andersson 1968).

The relationship between the electrocorticogram and the scalp EEG has been studied by several groups of workers including Abraham & Ajmone-Marson (1958), De Lucchi et al (1962) and the most important paper by Cooper et al (1965). In summary they showed that the ECoG shows a difference in electrical activity from point to point on the surface of the cortex even when these points are only 1–2 mm apart. This indicates a lack of spread of activity within the cortex, similar activity of two or more electrodes being due either to an underlying synchronisation of the cortical generators or to a physiological connection between them. The scalp EEG is a spatial average of the activity of these small cortical areas, the larger the cortical area involved in synchronised activity the higher the amplitude of the EEG. An estimate given by Cooper et al is that it requires 6 cm^2 of coherent activity on the surface of the cortex to be 'seen' in the scalp EEG.

Although the above description relates specifically to the ongoing background activity or to the spontaneous EEG, it does also hold true for evoked activity. Evoked potentials are measured by repetitively stimulating the subject in one sensory modality and recording the EEG for a fixed period before and after the stimulus. These recorded segments of EEG are then summed together. In these segments of summed EEG random phase components of the background activity will tend to sum to zero while constant wave forms, the cortical response to the stimulus, will sum out of the background activity. The stimulus enters the central nervous system by the specific sensory pathways, relays in the thalamic nuclei and is then transmitted to the cortex. Wide pools of cortical neurons are synchronised by the stimulus and it is the activity of these pools which is seen as the evoked response.

One further group of potentials should also be mentioned and these are the slow cortical potentials. In a forewarned reaction time task a negative shift in cortical potential develops between the warning stimulus and the second imperative stimulus to which a motor response is mandatory. This shift in potential is enhanced by the method of averaging as described above for the evoked response. These negative shifts in potential are called the Contingent Negative Variation or CNV, and are thought to relate to cortical excitability (Walter et al 1964, Tecce 1972).

Thus the scalp EEG shows, par excellence, patterns of synchronisation of cortical activity and is thus suited for the investigation of epilepsy.

DEVELOPMENT

It is now known that brain activity in man starts in utero as early as 24 weeks after conception although the regular activity does not begin until the 26th to 32nd week. From birth rhythmic activity in the delta and theta bands is seen which progressively increases in frequency until by the age of about eight the final alpha rhythm frequency is usually established, although population studies show 13 to be the final age of development. As the dominant rhythm increases in frequency, so the amount of delta and theta rhythms decreases until the adult pattern is reached at the age of about 25 years (Smith 1937, Lindsley 1939, Smith 1941, Corbin & Bickford 1955).

Genetic factors are known to play a major part in the determination of EEG patterns. Lennox et al (1942) showed that in a group of 41 monozygotic normal twins the EEGs were judged identical in 35 pairs. In another group of 53 normal twins concordance in the EEGs agreed with concordance as judged by physical traits in 87 per cent. A more recent study by Dummermuth (1968) using spectral analysis of the EEG of identical twins, showed that there was very little difference between the spectral profile of identical twins compared to the very different profiles showed by binovular twins. This genetic component determining the

EEG is important as many abnormalities seen in the EEG of patients with epilepsy are also inherited.

INHERITANCE OF EEG ABNORMALITIES IN EPILEPSY

An excellent review of this subject is given by Metrakos & Metrakos (1974). In summary, early studies looking at concordance rates for EEG abnormalities in monozygotic twins found them to vary from 40–90 per cent, while for dizygotic twins the concordance rate ranged from 5–20 per cent. In 1961, Metrakos & Metrakos put forward the hypothesis which still stands, that the encephalogram characterised by 'centrencephalic' EEG abnormalities, i.e. 3 per second spike and wave, is inherited as an irregular autosomal dominant gene of variable penetrance. They found that for the siblings of epileptic probands, 37 per cent showed abnormal EEGs while only 6 per cent of the controls did. They found that the penetrance of the gene varied with age. It was not fully penetrant at birth to $4\frac{1}{2}$ years (first low risk period) but rose rapidly from $4\frac{1}{2}$ to $16\frac{1}{2}$ years, so that about 45 per cent of the siblings showed this trait (high risk period). It then started to wane until it was nearly absent by about age 40 years (second low risk period).

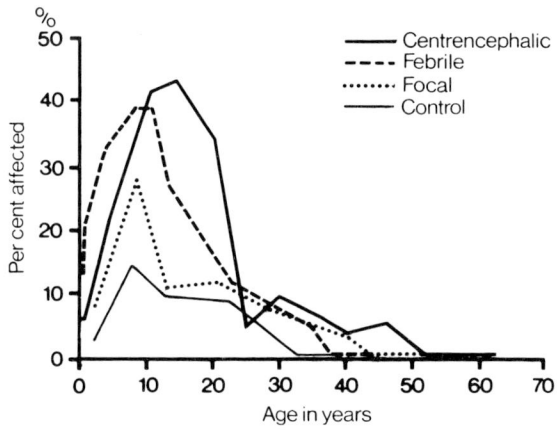

Fig. 18.1   3 c/s spike-and-wave trait. Age distribution of near relatives with the centrencephalic EEG trait for centrencephalic, febrile, focal and control groups. (After Metrakos K, Metrakos J D 1974. Reproduced by permission of North Holland Publishing Co.)

Focal epilepsies can also be inherited. Lennox (1951) found that the prevalence of seizures is 3.6 times higher for the near relatives of the epileptic probands than for the near relatives of the proband controls. Bray & Wise (1965) and Rodin & Gonzales (1966) have reported an increased prevalence of EEG abnormalities among the near relatives of probands with focal epilepsies.

The observation that both centrencephalic and focal epilepsies have a genetic component led Niedermeyer (1966) to suggest that 'there is no clear-cut distinction between the acquired and predispositioned types of convulsive disorder and that the time-honoured distinction between idiopathic and symptomatic epilepsy can be accepted only with some reservation'. This is reinforced by Metrakos & Metrakos (1974) who say that at least in three very divergent forms of epilepsy—centrencephalic, febrile and focal—a common genetically-controlled predisposing factor exists.

This evidence reinforces the practice that the diagnosis of epilepsy is a clinical one and that epilepsy should *never* be diagnosed on the EEG alone. If, in the worst case, 45 per cent of the near relatives of epileptic probands have abnormal EEGs but no seizures, how can one ever be certain that an abnormal paroxysmal EEG can indicate more than a tendency to epilepsy, without a clinical history?

ABNORMAL EPILEPTIC WAVEFORMS

Spike and wave

The traditional view, supported by Penfield (1938) and Penfield & Jasper (1954) and encouraged by Gastaut & Fischer-Williams (1959) as well as many other workers, was that the brain stem reticular formation was responsible for the generation of the spike and wave of the generalised epilepsies. These waveforms were then said to be projected via the thalamic projection system to the cortex. Because of the involvement of subcortical structures and their assumed primary role, these discharges were called subcortical and the epilepsy 'centrencephalic'.

It was suggested that the reticular formation initiated a spike and the thalamus a subsequent inhibitory 'breaking' wave; although in petit mal epilepsy Gastaut & Fischer-Williams (1959) saw the caudate nucleus as being the primary slow wave generator. An excellent review of the subject is given in various papers presented at a symposium on the spike wave discharge (1968). More recent work has thrown these earlier concepts into some doubt. Petsche & Rappelsberger (1973) from their animal work point out that the spikes and waves travel over the cortex at different speeds: spikes faster, at 1–7 m/s, than slow waves, 4–5 m/s. Different points of origin were found for both spikes and slow waves, usually at the junction between frontal and parietal cortex and near the frontal and occipital poles. The speed of spread was related to the density of pyramidal cells in layer V of the cortex and this was not dependent on thalamic pacing.

Evidence from other workers has confirmed the importance of the cortex for the genesis of spike and wave activity. Penicillin and other drugs, placed on the surface of the cortex bilaterally and asymmetrically can induce spike and wave activity and can give rise in monkeys to clinical attacks, resembling petit mal (Marcus & Satson 1968, Mutani et al 1973). Intra-carotid injections of metrazole, which reaches the cortex and not the thalamus, can evoke both clinical and electrical petit mal attacks in man. Intra-vertebral metrazole, which goes to the thalamus, should enhance spike and wave activity, but does not; but it may, in fact, reduce it (Cobb 1975). Intra-cerebral stimulation in man produces both clinical and electrical petit mal attacks when only the frontal lobes and, occasionally, the mesial orbital surface, are stimulated; but this does not occur with stimulation of the deeper structures (Bancaud et al 1974). An excellent review on the use of the term 'centrencephalic' has been compiled by Cobb (1975).

Recent work by Musgrave & Gloor (1980) confirms and extends these previous observations. They propose, arguing from the genesis of spike and wave activity in cats in response to intra-muscular penicillin, that spike and wave activity is generated in the cortex. Spike and wave is an abnormal cortical response to 'normal' thalamic recruiting volleys. Section of the corpus callosum desynchronises the two hemispheres. However, the reticular formation still has a role to play as reticular depression enhances spike and wave activity and reticular stimulation tends to abolish it.

Thus, spike and wave involves the cortex actively rather than passively and the concept that these discharges have an exclusive reticular formation and thalamic genesis must now be abandoned, together with the term centrencephalic. Centrencephalic suggested that the spike and wave activity was arising in the midline structures of the brain; but, as the evidence for this is now rather slim, can we deny what Cobb (1975) said, 'We should be wiser and more honest if we ceased to delude each other with the high-sounding term centrencephalic and admitted that the origin of absence epilepsy remains still cryptogenic', or if not cryptogenic, then more cortical than central.

During a spike and wave discharge, large numbers of cortical neurons are activated and it would be surprising, as mentioned by Gastaut & Fischer-Williams (1959), if 'cognition were not impaired'.

Clinical conditions

During a spike and wave episode, the child may have a classic petit mal attack. Usually the child's eyes may flicker, he may look upwards, but nothing else may be seen. If the child is doing anything when the attack occurs, he will cease his activity for 4–5 seconds or for the duration of the attack and will look blank. Frequently he may have no memory for the episode. Penry and colleagues (1975) have studied children by filming them on video tape when they were having petit mal seizures. They report that ictal automatisms are very common and are found in 90 per cent of attacks. Various workers have looked into the detailed changes in cognition which occur during a spike and wave burst. Some good reviews of the early work are given in a paper by Goode et al (1970) and an overall review by Penry (1973), starting with the work of Schwab (1939). Schwab measured the response and reaction time to auditory and visual stimuli given during spike and wave bursts, by asking the subjects to squeeze a rubber bulb. He found that reaction time was normal with bursts of spike and wave up to 2 seconds, but was then proportionally delayed with longer bursts. Later workers used more sophisticated equipment. It was found that during verbal tasks and mental calculations, the spike and wave activity was more likely to interrupt complex rather than simple tasks. Jus & Jus (1962) found that the mean retrograde amnesia associated with spike and wave attacks varied from 4–15 seconds, but this was absent in attacks lasting less than 1–2 seconds. Tizard & Marjerison (1963), using a complex reaction time test, found that if spike and wave bursts lasted longer than 1–1.5 seconds, then responses were omitted. If the spike and wave lasted for less than this time, then all subjects worked more slowly during the burst and one subject made significantly more errors. They suggested that brain capacity to process information was reduced during spike and wave activity.

Mirsky & Van Buren (1965) showed that on a continuous performance test, when patients with spike and wave had to respond to a letter display, the percentage of correct responses was reduced from 84.8 per cent during normal EEG activity to 24.1 per cent during spike and wave. They noted that these

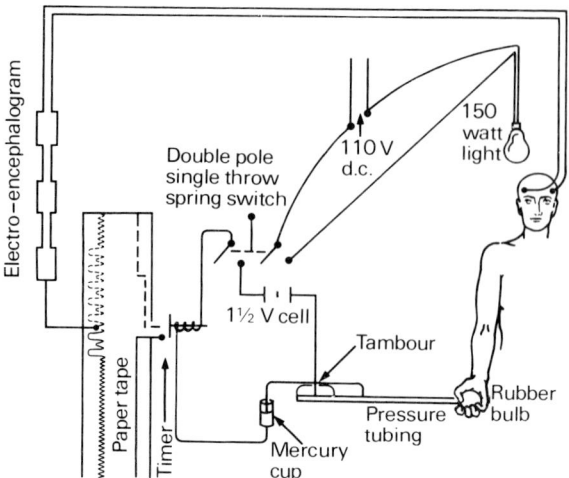

Fig. 18.2   Diagram showing connections of the reaction time apparatus with the electro-encephalographic apparatus. (After Schwab R S 1939 Archives of Neurology & Psychiatry 41:215–217. By permission of the American Medical Association).

behavioural effects preceded the spike wave burst by 1–1.5 seconds. Browne et al (1974) investigated the relationship between the onset of spike and wave and cognition by measuring reaction time. They found that only 20 per cent of reaction times were normal if stimuli were given 0.5 seconds into the spike and wave burst. They also found that the degree of generalisation of the spike wave burst was important. Paroxysms which were generalised from the start produced greater impairment of responsiveness than those which were incompletely generalised. Goode et al (1970) found with a pursuit rotor test that, although

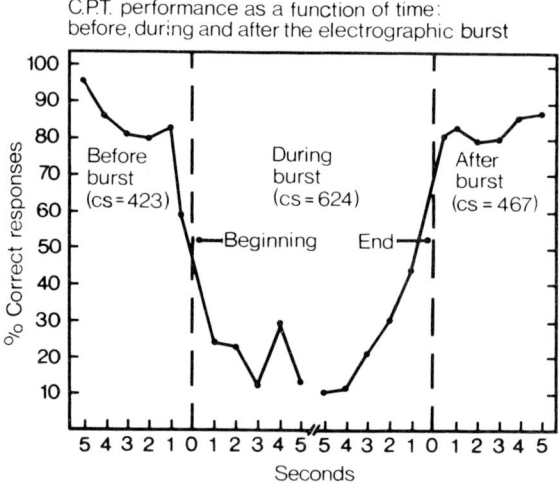

Fig. 18.3   Relation between level of performance on the Continuous Performance Task and onset, development and termination of the electrographic burst. CS refers to the number of correct stimuli. (After Tizzard B, Margerison J H 1963 Journal of Neurology, Neurosurgery & Psychiatry 26:308–313. Reproduced by courtesy of the Editor.)

performance was impaired during a spike wave burst, it was not as impaired as in the other tests already mentioned. They noted a previously-reported finding that attention decreases the incidence of spike and wave activity. This possibly explains the findings of Jus & Jus (1962) that children who were passively listening to an observer showed longer retrograde amnesia after a spike and wave burst than those who were actively engaged in a task. Photoconvulsive responses, produced by photic stimulation, have been shown by Ounstead et al (1963) to produce changes in cognition similar to those caused by generalised spontaneous spike and wave bursts. Thus, spike and wave activity seriously alters cognition and may severely handicap the patient. A recent paper by Stores et al (1978) suggests that the effect of spike and wave activity on the capacity of children to attend in the classroom may not be as serious as laboratory studies suggest for girls, although boys were impaired. An interesting finding is that distracting stimuli *improved* the performance of the boys and girls. Children with spike and wave activity attended better than children with other EEG abnormalities.

We have been discussing spike and wave activity in patients known to have clinical seizures. It would be interesting to know whether or not the *non* epileptic relatives of an epileptic proband who have spike and wave activity in their records show cognitive changes during the presence of the abnormal activity. If they do, then clearly the borderline of epilepsy will need to be extended.

Focal spikes and sharp waves

It has been pointed out by several authors that cortical spike activity is part of the normal functioning of the central nervous system. Examples of normal spikes usually quoted are 14 and 6 positive spikes recorded from the temporal lobes in adolescents, a few children show parietal spikes, which are thought to carry no pathological significance. Some of the normal phenomena of sleep show a spike-like wave form, K complexes and the spikes of stage three and four sleep are good examples. Outside of these contexts, spikes are certainly abnormal.

Stevens (1977), in an interesting article proposing a hypothesis to explain the presence of photosensitivity in the population, also suggests that spike activity is a normal method of communication within the CNS. 'An outstanding quality of the spike mode of transmission is the uncompromising fashion in which the spike coded message preempts access to cerebral circuitry by swamping and displacing ongoing activity.' She suggests further that spikes occur naturally in the neuroendocrine and reward systems and that spikes are contained within these systems by the activity of the cortical monoamine pathways. A disturbance in this system which contains physiological spiking leads to the spread of epileptic activity.

Local sharp waves or spike activity are some of the commoner forms of abnormal epileptic discharges seen in the EEG. Pathological spikes may originate in either the deep or superficial brain structures, frequently arising from the area surrounding an acute or chronic brain lesion. The spike has a short duration up to 70 m/s, but slower, sharp waves may frequently occur with a duration of up to 500 m/s.

Brazier (1955) initially suggested that epileptic spikes and sharp waves may have their origin in the discharges of the apical dendrites of the large pyramidal cells, which project upwards from the depth of the cortex. Petsche & Rappelsburger (1973) extended their observations when they examined the genesis of spikes evoked from penicillin lesions or metrazol activation in rabbits. They found that the spikes originated in the cortex, were conducted vertically, and were maximal in amplitude in the deep pyramidal cell layer. Frequently, while single at the surface, they were multiple deeper in the cortex and showed a high degree of independence at different electrode sites.

The presence of spike activity in the EEG does not always indicate that a structural lesion is present. Even if a lesion is present, spike activity cannot always be relied on to give a precise localisation. Spike activity may be projected remotely from the original cortical lesion, or it may arise in deep structures and be projected to the cortex.

It is also not unusual to have a spike focus develop in a homologous area in the other hemisphere, in response to continual bombardment from the primary focus across the corpus callosum or other major inter-hemisphere pathways. This 'mirror' focus may become independent or it may disappear once the original focus has been removed by surgery (Morrel 1960). Brazier (1973) describes how abnormal activity in the deep temporal lobe structures may pace the cortex and may determine where and how the cortical spike focus is seen. She also points out that the appearance of abnormal waves in the cortical EEG may signal the cessation and not necessarily the start of a psychomotor seizure.

An interesting hypothesis has been put forward and reviewed in detail by Lockard (1980). This hypothesis suggests that the neurones involved in an epileptic focus are deafferented and unable to fire normally. They fire in only a bursting, paroxysmal or epileptic mode. These are called group 1 neurones. Group 2 neurones surround the focus and are partially deafferented so they can fire in both the epileptic and normal modes. Spikes are thought to be generated by the synchronization of large pools of group 1 neurones. When group 1 neurones are able to recruit group 2 neurones, a mass of neurones of critical size firing paroxysmally is created and this can lead to either a focal seizure or, if the normal neurones surrounding the group 2 neurones are recruited, then a secondary generalised seizure can result.

In summary, although the spike focus appears dramatic in the EEG, it requires careful consideration before it can be accepted as indicative of the site of the epileptogenic lesion.

Clinical correlations

In contrast to spike and wave activity, very little work has been done on the cognitive changes which occur during the presence of cortical spiking. It is thus not possible to say with confidence that the presence of a cortical spike does alter cognition. Studies of cortical lesions of the motor area frequently show a spike focus, which does not necessarily result in a disorder of movement. The cortical spikes associated with myoclonic jerks do not appear to change cognition (Halliday 1967). Lairy and co-workers (1967) have described the presence of cortical sharp waves, mainly parietal, in populations of children with psychiatric disorders but without epilepsy. Improvement in the child's mental state resulted in a disappearance of the spikes. More recently Baird et al (1980) have studied a group of epileptic under-achieving children and normal controls. They concluded that almost all the children with epilepsy 'display abnormal sharp waves, as frequent, severe and anatomically widespread in those who do well as in those who do poorly'. The poor school performance is not therefore related to occasional sharp waves; they add that a high incidence of sharp waves was noted in the control children with learning difficulties but who did not have epilepsy. They suggest that the sharp waves may be related to underlying brain dysfunction, a conclusion already arrived at by Lairy (1967), and that spikes are not necessarily related to seizures. However an interesting paper has recently been given by Peterson (1980) showing that children who were given a reaction time test frequently missed the stimulus if the latter was triggered from a parietal spike. Thus cognitive changes with spike activity clearly occurs, although more work is still required on the subject.

Recently, Lockard and colleagues (1980) have been studying the effect of interictal spikes on the cognition of monkeys whose epilepsy has been induced by the application of alumina gel to the cortex. They have found that there is a relationship between the number of interictal spikes and the monkeys' performance in both conditioned avoidance and reward programmes. This work is of interest as it clearly has significance when applied to patients with interictal spike foci and the cognitive changes which may be caused by this activity. Again using the alumina gel monkey preparation they have also shown that there is a relationship between anxiety, generated in a social situation, and the firing of cells which have been made epileptogenic. This observation provides the link between the often reported increase in seizure frequency in social situations which are anxiety-provoking and the epileptic process itself.

Angeleri and co-workers (1980) report a study of 16 patients with partial seizures in which they automatically counted EEG spikes while the patients were sleeping and waking. They report a cyclical variation in the number of spikes throughout the night with frequencies between $\frac{1}{2}$ to 1 cycle per hour. The 10 patients who showed the shortest cycles were responsive to pharmacological control while the remaining six were not. Clearly detailed analysis of the spike and the way it fires will repay further study.

Electroclinical correlations of spike and wave and focal EEG changes
The two preceding sections have studied the cognitive changes found in either spike and wave discharges or focal discharges. This section looks at studies comparing the two. Nuffield (1961) studied 322 children who had passed through the Maudsley Epilepsy Unit. They were aged 1 to 15 years with the majority between 7 and 15. He classified their EEG according to whether they showed spike and wave, focal or mixed EEG activity. The correlation of EEG with seizure type was found to be much as expected. Regular spike and wave activity was correlated with petit mal epilepsy, atypical spike and wave with grand mal epilepsy and psychomotor seizures with temporal lobe foci. He compared the EEG classification with the children's interictal behaviour. This was rated for aggressive manifestations and antisocial conduct. The following table is from his paper.

The main findings were that the temporal lobe group is by far the most

Table 18.1 The relationship of aggression and neuroticism to EEG category in 236 children (from Nuffield 1961)

EEG category	Aggressivity score	Neurotic score	No. of cases
Temporal focus	6.35	2.10	40
PCOF (spikes)	3.8	3.0	30
3/s spike wave	1.6	4.8	28
Irregular spike wave	4.0	4.1	44
Diffuse spikes	4.5	3.3	32
Non–specific abnormality	4.4	3.6	33
Normal	3.7	3.7	29

aggressive, but also the least neurotic; while the true petit mal children are the least aggressive, but the most neurotic. They found, however, that no real correlations with EEG type were seen for the antisocial conduct disorders. Finally, they point out that the EEG is a more effective classifier of psychiatric morbidity than seizure type.

Stores & Hart (1976) looked at the changes in cognition and behaviour between children with focal EEG abnormalities and a matched group of children without epilepsy, but matched for age, sex and general behaviour. The outcome showed that against prediction 'the progress of children with generalized epilepsies is, on the whole, no worse than that of their non-epileptic controls. In contrast, persistent focal discharges appear on average to be associated with impaired reading accuracy'. They also point out that some of their children had long bursts of spike and wave activity in their EEG every time these were recorded in the EEG Department, but the children were well in advance with their reading and comprehension skills. Thus, the predicted cognitive deficit expected to be produced by frequent spike and wave bursts was not seen in their series. 'The inferior performance of the focal group as a whole is largely attributable to those children with left hemisphere focal spikes, and these are predominantly boys.' 'The reading skills of epileptic boys are worse than epileptic girls. This sex difference was not seen in the non-epileptic controls. Phenytoin is associated with lower levels of reading skills.' It is, however, difficult to be certain about the relationship of medication and reading skills, as no serum levels were measured.

Mirsky et al (1960) and Landsell & Mirsky (1964) compared adult patients with focal and 'centrencephalic' epilepsy on tests of memory and on a continuous vigilance task, their Continuous Performance Test. They demonstrated that patients with focal temporal lobe lesions were not impaired on the tasks of attention, but did show definite memory deficits; while those with diffuse EEG abnormalities did not show the same memory deficit, but were impaired on the Continuous Performance Test. They suggested that temporal lobe integrity was necessary for specific intellectual capacities, while intact functioning of those structures involved in 'centrencephalic' epilepsy is required for sustained, attentive behaviour.

It is now clear from numerous studies that dominant temporal lobe pathology, shown by dominant temporal lobe spikes, is associated with verbal memory deficits; while non-dominant temporal lobe pathology and non-dominant temporal lobe spikes are associated with visuospatial memory deficits (Chapter 12).

This was also shown to be true for children. Fedio & Mirsky (1969) studied four groups of 10 children, two groups with temporal lobe spikes — right and left, a group of children whose records showed generalised symmetrical 3/second spike wave and a normal control group. Their results confirmed the previous findings. The left temporal group show memory deficits on verbal tasks, with unaffected non-verbal tasks: the converse being true for children with right temporal spikes. The 'centrencephalic' children showed no significant memory deficit, but lower scores on the test of sustained attention. Taylor (1972), in a review of the cases with temporal lobe epilepsy seen at the Maudsley Hospital for temporal lobectomy, noted an association between anti-social behaviour and left temporal foci. Neurotic symptoms were more commonly seen with right foci. Bear & Fedio (1977) have recently suggested that there is a difference in personality between patients who show right or left temporal lobe epilepsy. Their hypothesis is reviewed in detail in Chapter 8.

Ictal and postictal changes
Petit mal status
This condition presents with clouding of consciousness and confusion. It lasts from a few minutes to several days and it may wax and wane in intensity, sometimes ceasing abruptly for several minutes. There is a rapid onset and the attack is often terminated by a grand mal seizure. The patient is usually uncoordinated, confused, perseverative and slowed. Not infrequently, the patient appears stuperose and out of contact, remaining motionless and withdrawn.

The EEG record is dominated by spike and wave activity, which is very seldom classical. Frequently, it is degraded spike and wave and polyspike activity. The names 'spike and wave status', as suggested by Niedermeyer & Khalifeh (1965), or 'spike and wave stupor' are to be preferred. In its classical form, this is an illness of children or young adults, only occasionally reported in mature adults (Schwartz & Scott 1971). In the older age group, it may mimic a retarded depression or a dementing illness.

A similar clinical state is not infrequently seen after one or more grand mal seizures, when the EEG is dominated by diffuse atypical spike and wave activity, the continuous abnormal epileptic EEG activity indicating status epilepticus.

Automatic states
Automatisms commonly arise during and following the partial phase of temporal lobe seizures, although Falconer & Taylor (1970) have reported that they may also occur with discharging lesions of the inferior frontal region or the cingulate cortex. A good review of automatisms is given by Fenton (1972). The automatism can be divided into three phases, early, middle and late. During the early phase, the subject carries out small stereotyped movements, such as lip smacking or small hand movements. This is accompanied in the EEG by, firstly, a flattening and then by the appearance of low-voltage theta activity at 6–7 Hz, which increases in amplitude and slows in frequency. During the middle phase, the automatisms are more complex, such as handling objects on a table or fumbling with clothes. The EEG during this phase shows the abnormal theta discharge, which slows and generalises to the opposite hemisphere. In the late stage of the automatism, the

patient's behaviour becomes more complex and gradually merges into that of everyday life. The EEG shows a postictal picture, with bilateral delta waves that frequently have a fronto-temporal distribution (Gastaut 1953). However, it is not uncommon for the EEG to show marked differences between patients and not to follow this standard scheme in detail.

Postictal states
Following a grand mal seizure, the patient is confused, disoriented and irritable as he regains consciousness. He may lapse into natural sleep or his initially clouded sensorium may slowly clear until full consciousness is regained. The postictal state commonly lasts for 5 to 10 minutes, with a period of sleep following this. Occasionally, full consciousness may remain impaired for hours and, rarely for days or weeks. Immediately after the fit, the EEG is dominated by generalised high-voltage delta activity, which slowly decreases in amplitude until the normal background rhythms have returned. During prolonged twilight states or abnormal states following a seizure, the EEG frequently shows either focal or generalised delta activity.

The effects of a grand mal seizure in some patients may not be trivial. A patient in the Maudsley Epilepsy Unit with dominant temporal lobe spikes showed changes in verbal fluency for two weeks following an isolated grand mal seizure. He was totally unaware of the change in his verbal fluency and claimed to be back to normal after only two days. Deteriorated cognitive states are frequently seen after grand mal seizures, lasting for several days, in either elderly patients or patients who have significant associated brain damage. Thus, the response to a grand mal seizure will depend on the location of the epileptogenic lesion and on any other associated cerebral pathology.

EEG changes in postictal, twilight or psychotic states
The most comprehensive study is that of Dongier (1959) who edited the data presented at a meeting in Marseille in 1956 by workers from most countries in Europe. He analysed 536 psychotic episodes in 516 epileptics which occurred between clinical seizures. The onset was preceded by a seizure in a quarter and terminated by one in 10 per cent; surprisingly 6 per cent passed from the episode into a psychotic state. Some clouding of consciousness was present in two thirds, changes of affect were seen in 43 per cent, delusions in one third and hallucinations in 23 per cent. Nearly half the episodes lasted for days and a third for weeks, 40 per cent of the episodes were in patients with 'centrencephalic' epilepsy and 44 per cent had psychomotor epilepsy. The presence of confusion was highly correlated with generalised diffuse delta waves or nearly continuous bisynchronous spike and wave discharges. When focal epileptic discharges disappeared the clinical confusion improved. Affective symptoms were seen more frequently with temporal lobe cases (45 per cent) than with 'centrencephalic' (24 per cent). As would be expected from the above, delta dysrhythmia correlated more frequently with a normal affect as did bisynchronous spike and wave. Patients who lost their spike activity during the psychotic episode were usually depressed. There were no EEG changes which correlated with heightened affect. With regard to behaviour, patients with petit mal status were nearly always calm. Both the

patients with temporal lobe lesions and the remaining patients with a 'centrencephalic' discharge were as agitated and aggressive as each other (44 per cent and 34 per cent respectively). Delusions were seen most frequently amongst those with temporal lobe epilepsy, but they were altogether lacking in those patients who had petit mal status. In the patients with temporal lobe epilepsy delusions were found most frequently amongst those whose focal discharge disappeared during the psychotic episode or in those whose EEG did not change and was the same as in the control period prior to the episode. In summary, spike and wave in the EEG produced a confused mental state while temporal lobe spikes were mainly associated with delusions, hallucinations and changes of affect.

Bruens (1974) has suggested that all the above-mentioned abnormal states can be divided into the three clinical types, postictal twilight states, 'absence' status and psychomotor status. These states frequently have definite EEG correlates. The postictal twilight state is characterised by a disorganised record dominated by slow wave activity and very little evidence of epileptic waveforms. 'Absence' status shows 3/second spike wave and is readily responsive to i.v. diazepam. Psychomotor status shows a varied picture with or without temporal lobe spiking but nearly always an EEG with either excess delta or theta activity. It is frequently worthwhile in the author's experience giving i.v. diazepam as this may either normalise the record or limit the spike activity to the affected side. Bruens' classification has yet to be superseded.

Heath (1977) has reported on scalp and depth electrode studies in patients with interictal psychotic episodes. He reports the most interesting finding that the intracerebral electrodes were dominated by abnormal activity, bursts of spikes and slow waves, in the deep temporal nuclei (hippocampus and amygdala) during the psychotic episode. When the septal region was not involved then the patients were not psychotic.

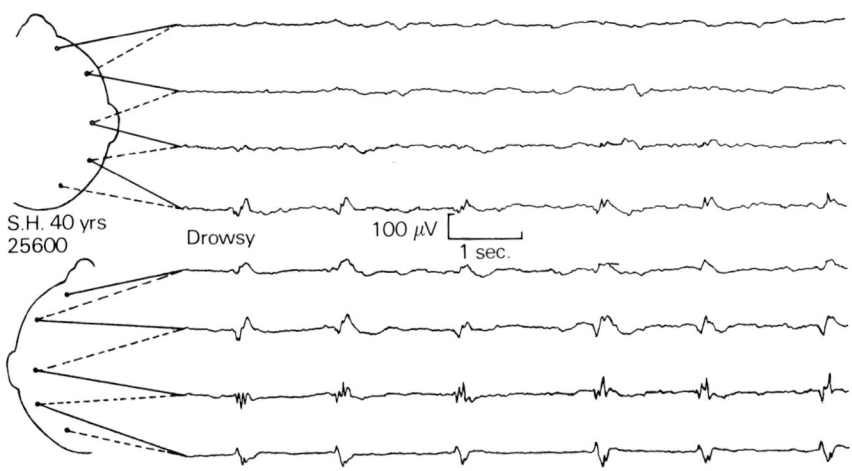

S.H. 40 yrs
25600

Drowsy

100 μV

1 sec.

Fig. 18.4 EEG record of psychomotor status epilepticus in a patient aged 40 who is drowsy, confused and disorientated.

This finding is highly relevant as it indicates that the abnormal activity in the deeper temporal lobe structures is of prime importance in the genesis of the psychosis. Scalp leads may or may not reflect the underlying discharges and so may or may not be of importance in the clinical diagnosis.

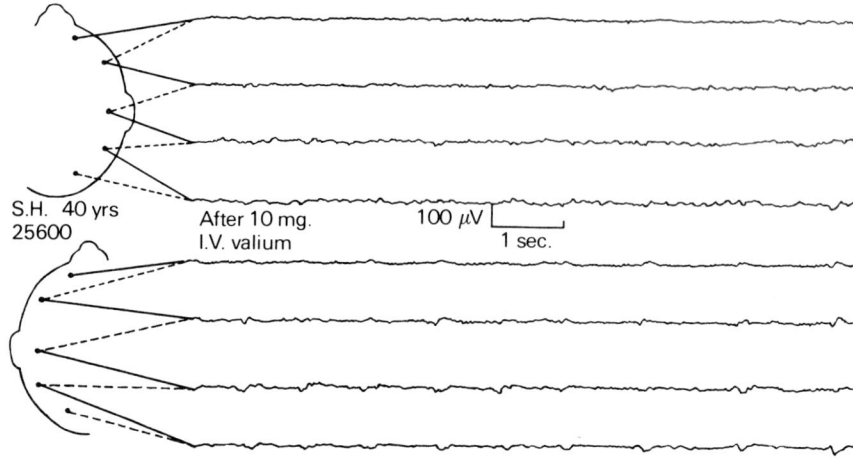

S.H. 40 yrs
25600

After 10 mg.
I.V. valium

100 μV

1 sec.

Fig. 18.5 The same patient as in Fig. 18.4 after the injection of 10 mg of diazepam by intravenous injection. The injection only partially normalised both the EEG record and the patient's mental state. 20 minutes after the injection the EEG and patient's mental state were again abnormal.

Forced normalisation

This was a concept initially introduced by Landolt (1953, 1955, 1956, 1958). He observed that the EEGs of a proportion of patients with epilepsy who developed psychotic episodes become less abnormal during the period of the psychosis. Thus a normal EEG correlated with a psychotic episode while an abnormal EEG with the presence of mental normality. This finding has been confirmed by several other authors [for a review see Bruens (1974) and Glaser (1964)]. However, most of the authors did not carry out their studies with the idea that non-specific factors may be involved. Admission to hospital and better anticonvulsant compliance may be responsible and without measurement of serum anticonvulsant levels this cannot be excluded.

No study attempted to quantify level of anxiety or arousal, both of which could be expected to increase during a psychotic episode and both of which could help to 'normalise' the EEG. Without frequent EEG recordings both before and after the episode it is possible that the effects noted are due to sampling error. Finally, Glaser (1964) studied 37 patients with psychomotor-temporal lobe seizures all having clearly defined clinical episodes of psychosis not considered to be actually part of the seizure complex. He says 'we did not observe any "normalisation" of the electroencephalogram during episodes of psychoses. In four instances psychotic reaction was increased along with improvement of the electro-encephalogram.' He states in summary that 'Electroencephalographic correlates with interictal psychotic episodes are only occasional and then usually consist of more intense focal temporal or bilateral paroxysmal discharge. At times, however, the electroencephalogram improves or becomes normal during a psychotic state.

However, it is possible that these personality and behaviour disturbances may be due at least in part to sub-ictal cerebral excitation'.

Thus the evidence is not compelling that normalisation as an entity really exists. Brazier's (1973) observations relating to the variability of deep structure and cortical activity should be borne in mind. As already described above the normalisation of cortical rhythms can correlate with limbic system discharges, and as Heath (1977) has shown, normal scalp activity can be seen while frequent spiking is occurring in the amygdala and hippocampus. Thus the term 'forced normalisation' is misleading and is probably better dropped.

EEG EPILEPTIFORM ACTIVITY IN PSYCHOTIC ILLNESS AND IN THE PSYCHONEUROSES

Stevens' (1977) quotation that 'All that spikes is not fits' is particularly true in psychiatry. There are many studies which show a correlation between paroxysmal EEG activity, abnormal personality, behaviour disorders, aggressiveness and psychotic episodes in patients without epilepsy.

Personality disorders and psychoneurosis

It had always been hoped that the EEG could contribute to the diagnosis of patients with personality disorders. Unfortunately, the recording of an EEG in any particular patient frequently confuses rather than clarifies the problem. Non-specific abnormalities are common in groups of control subjects said to be normal (from 5 per cent to 10 per cent) and in patients with a psychoneurotic illness (up to 26 per cent) (Williams 1941). The changes seen are usually non-specific increases in theta activity, particularly on the borders of sleep. It is usually very difficult to say exactly what these changes mean in terms of clinical pathology. The psychopathic personality was initially said to have a specific EEG correlate — posterior temporal slow activity. This waveform has now been shown to be normal in adolescents and children, but is abnormal in adults. The EEG studies are reviewed by Hill & Parr (1963). Posterior temporal slow activity can occasionally carry a sharp focal discharge and has frequently been mistaken for a posterior temporal epileptic focus. Posterior temporal slowing was said to be found in conjunction with aggressive psychopaths, homosexuals and those patients who had explosive outbursts. The presence of these focal changes and general paroxysmal abnormalities led Hill (see Hill & Parr 1963) amongst others to use the term 'latent epilepsy'. Some of these patients do show a low seizure threshold (Williams 1944). However, because of the confusion the term latent epilepsy can cause, it is now best avoided. Fenton et al (1974) studied the diagnosis of a group of patients in a special hospital for violent offenders who had been selected by the presence of a posterior temporal slow wave abnormality in their EEG. There was no correlation between the diagnosis of psychopathy and posterior temporal slowing. The authors concluded that this was a non-specific finding in populations who were liable to multiple cerebral insults. Williams (1969) reviewed patients in his practice who were investigated by him before standing trial for violent criminal offences. After having removed all those cases who had associated cerebral pathology, a large proportion of the remainder had abnormalities in their EEGs. 17 per cent of patients who showed habitual aggression had abnormal EEGs compared with only

12 per cent of the non-aggressive normals. He summarises the non-specific nature of the EEG changes seen in personality disorders by quoting the American poet, Adelaide Crapsley (Chapter 5, page 54).

Psychosis

Ever since Kraepelin described schizophrenia there has been an association of 'epileptic' phenomena and psychosis. Early workers noticed that this occurred predominantly in catatonic states (Jasper et al 1939). The paroxysmal EEG activity seen in schizophrenics is typically low voltage grouped bilateral spikes and waves with paroxysmal slow waves (Hill & Parr 1963). Changes in the spectral profile of the EEG are also seen as has been recently reviewed by Fenton, Fenwick and colleagues (1980). Heath (1977) has studied groups of patients with schizophrenic and psychotic illnesses in whom both implanted and scalp EEGs were recorded. He found that during the psychotic episodes spikes and slow waves were recorded from the septal region. If the patient had a non-specific psychosis then the abnormal activity was found in a different brain area but one usually connected directly to the septum. Stevens (1977) has chemically induced epileptic spiking in the nucleus accumbens, in the septal region, in cats. The cats with spikes in this area show behaviour changes akin to catatonia in man with episodes of immobility or staring. If psychotic episodes in man are accompanied by septal spiking then it is not surprising that from time to time this will be reflected in cortical sharp wave activity. The presence of spike activity in the scalp EEG thus probably reflects the occurrence of septal spikes and does not carry any special significance apart from this. It must also, however, be remembered that many of the drugs used in the treatment of schizophrenia are epileptogenic and so some of the paroxsymal EEG changes seen may be drug-induced.

Depression

Betts (1976) has found that depression was the commonest formal diagnosis made on the admission of epileptic patients to psychiatric care. Depressed patients who do not have epilepsy have also been shown to have abnormal EEGs. An excellent review is given by Struve and colleagues (1977) on this subject although it is slanted towards patients with suicidal ideas. Many authors have reported EEG changes associated with depression. These are mainly a normal record with increased alpha activity or, less frequently, paroxysmal activity. Low voltage spike activity is also reported. Heath (1977) has shown via intra-cerebral electrode studies that during painful emotional states high amplitude fast spindling focal in the hippocampus and amygdala arises; at the same time activity of the septal region decreases. It may well be that specific EEG patterns do relate to abnormal emotional states, particularly as abnormal central amine metabolism is known to be responsible for the affective changes seen in depression and to be related to epilepsy. Anti-depressant drugs could account for some of the changes in the EEG as they are known to cause paroxysmal activity but many authors have taken this into account with matched control groups and the differences between the control groups and those with depression still remain.

Recent advances

Long-term monitoring

Routine electroencephalography samples the patient's EEG for only 20–40 minutes. This is a short time and it is not unusual for paroxysmal discharges to be missed during the recording. Some authors claim that only 30–70 per cent of patients, depending on the type of epilepsy, show paroxysmal EEGs during routine EEG recording (Kooi 1971). Hopkins & Scrambler (1977) reported that only 39 out of 77 patients in the community who had epilepsy and had had EEGs recorded showed abnormal activity. To overcome this disadvantage, many of the larger centres now have 24 hour observation units, where the patients' EEGs and behaviour can be monitored for hours or days. Both the EEG and television pictures of the patient are recorded on video-tape. If a seizure occurs, then the tapes can be replayed and the episode examined (Penry 1973, Woods et al 1973).

A second method made possible by the miniaturisation of tape recorders and EEG amplifiers is the use of a small portable tape recorder, which is carried throughout the 24 hours by the patient. The EEG electrodes are well hidden in the hair and the whole package is well tolerated by the patients. A marker switch allows the patient to mark the tape when a significant event occurs. The tapes may be examined later for epileptic activity. This method is known as ambulatory monitoring (Ives et al 1973, Sato et al 1976, Stores 1980).

Figures for the intensive method of EEG recording are still incomplete, but they appear to show a definite advance. The unit in the National Hospital, Queen Square, London, reported (personal communication) that the detection rate of abnormality in 300 minute recordings rose to 80 per cent of the patients, while in 20 minute records it was only just over half. Kellaway & Cavrice (1977) reported a marked increase in detection rate for spike and wave epilepsy with 24 hour recording. There was also an increase in detection rate for focal abnormalities as this activity varied almost as much throughout the 24 hours as spike and wave activity did. They report the percentage change from smallest to largest number of abnormal events recorded per hour in five subjects was 1231 per cent. Rowan et al (1980) report a 'success rate' for long-term monitoring of 65–70 per cent which is in agreement with previous authors.

Long-term monitoring has been used to record both scalp and implanted depth electrode activity. The response to anticonvulsant medication is also usefully followed by continuous monitoring. Browne et al (1974) compared the rating by long-term monitoring of spike and wave activity in a patient's EEG over 12 hours with those of the ward staff and the patient's relatives who noted the patient's clinical seizures. There was a poor correlation as many more seizures than were reported were seen on the 12 hour tape. Rowan et al (1975) have reported two cases where the analysis of the recorded seizure data was used to treat the patients.

Penry & Porter (1977) suggest that long-term monitoring is essential in patients with intractable epilepsy. They studied 25 such patients. Two thirds were improved as regards seizure control and one third showed improvement in terms of social adjustment. However, it is difficult to know whether or not these figures would have been achieved anyway without the monitoring as the authors did not use a control group.

In summary, long-term monitoring is of definite advantage in detecting, treating and monitoring the effects of treatment on abnormal epileptic activity. The case for ambulatory monitoring is as strong, since the patient's EEG activity can be recorded during their daily activity and correlations between EEG abnormality, task and social situations investigated.

SUMMARY

This chapter presents evidence that certain concepts that we accept might now be disregarded and others viewed with suspicion. Landolt's theory of forced normalisation could well be dropped, as it appears to be of little help in either the diagnosis, prognosis, treatment or explanation of interictal psychotic episodes.

The term centrencephalic should not be used as it clearly does not mean what its originators had hoped it would indicate; that is, a control system situated in the brain midline structures from which synchronous spike and wave activity arises to involve the whole cortex. There is now evidence for a cortical genesis of spike and wave activity so the retention of the term centrencephalic can only confuse, as it assumes a method of generation of spike and wave activity which is no longer thought to be true. The term primary subcortical epilepsy, which makes use of the same electrophysiological concepts, is also best avoided and the term primary generalised epilepsy, which is a clinical term, used instead.

Finally, Stevens' suggestion that the spike is a normal method of CNS transmission and the speculation that the spike is involved in normal sexual functioning raises the question of abnormalities of sexual functioning in epilepsy, particularly among adolescent girls. Her model of normal spikes confined to the central amine system of the brain should stimulate further research in this area.

References

Abraham K, Ajmone-Marsan C 1958 Patterns of cortical discharges and their relation to routine scalp electroencephalography. Electroenceph. Clin. Neurological 10:447–461
Andersen P, Andersson S A 1968 Physiological basis of the alpha rhythm. Appleton, New York
Andersen, P Andersson S A 1974 Thalamic origin of cortical rhythmical activity. In: Handbook of electroencephalography and clinical neurophysiology. Elsevier, Amsterdam, p 90–114
Andersen P, Sears T A 1964 The role of inhibition in the phasing of spontaneous thalamo-cortical discharge. J Physiol (London) 173:459–480
Angeleri F, Scorpino O, Mauro A M, Giuliani G 1980 Computerised processing of interictal spike rate and morphology in human focal epilepsy. 11th epilepsy international symposium: Advances in epileptology, p 155–157
Bancaud J, Telairach J, Morel P, Bresson M, Bonis A, Grier S, Hemon E, Buser P 1974 'Generalised' epileptic seizures elicited by electrical stimulation of the frontal lobes in man. Electroenceph Clin Neurophysiol 37:275–282
Baird H W, John E R, Ahn H, Maisel E 1980 Neurometric evaluation of epileptic children who do well and poorly in school. Electroenceph Clin Neurophysiol 48:683–693
Bear D, Fedio P 1977 Quantitative analysis of interictal behavior in temporal lobe epilepsy. Arch Neurol 34:454–467
Betts T A, Merskey H, Pond D A 1976 Psychiatry. In: Laidlaw J, Richens A (eds) A textbook of epilepsy. Churchill Livingstone, Edinburgh.
Bray P F, Wiser W C 1965 Hereditary characteristics of familial temporal-cortical focal epilepsy. Pediatrics 36:207–211

Brazier M A B 1955 Neuronal structures, brain potentials and epileptic discharge. Epilepsia 4:9

Brazier M A B 1973 In: Brazier M A B (ed) Epilepsy, its phenomena in man. Academic Press, New York and London, p 155–167

Browne T R, Penry J K, Porter R J, Dreifuss F E 1974 The comparison of clinical estimates of absence seizure frequency with estimates based on prolonged telemetered EEGs. Neurology 24:381–382

Bruens J H 1974 Psychosis in epilepsy. In: Vinken P J, Bruyn G W (eds) Handbook of Clinical Neurology, vol 15 The epilepsies. North Holland, Amsterdam

Calvet J, Calvet M C, Scherrer T 1964. A cortical stratigraphic study of spontaneous EEG activity. Electroenceph Clin Neurophysiol 17:109–125

Cobb W 1975 Paper presented at the British Epilepsy Association Meeting. Present address of authors: EEG Dept., National Hospital, Queen Square, London WC2, England

Cooper R, Wintter A L, Crow H J, Walter W G 1965 Comparison of subcortical and scalp activity using chronically indwelling electrodes in man. Electroenceph Clin Neurophysiol 18:217–228

Corbin H P F, Bickford R G 1955 Studies of the electroencephalogram of normal children. Comparison of visual and automatic frequency analysis. Electroenceph Clin Neurophysiol 7:15–28

Creutzfeldt O D, Watanabe S, Lasc H D 1966 Relations between EEG phenomena and potentials of single cortical cells. Electroenceph Clin Neurophysiol 20:19–36

De Lucchi M R, Garoutte B, Aird R B 1962 The scalp as an electro-encephalographic averager. Electroenceph Clin Neurophysiol 14:191–196

Dongier S 1959 Statistical study of clinical and electroencephalographic manifestations of 536 psychotic episodes occurring in 516 epileptics between clinical seizures. Epilepsia 1:117–142

Dummermouth G 1968 Variance spectra of electroencephalograms in twins—a contribution to the problem of quantification of EEG background activity in childhood. In: Kellaway P, Peterssen I (eds) Clinical encephalography of children. Grune and Stratton, New York, p 119–154

Eccles J C 1974 Facing reality. Longmans, London and New York

Elul R 1972 'Randomness and synchrony in the generation of the electroencephalogram'. In: Petsche H, Brazier M A B (eds) Synchronization of EEG activity in epileptics. Springer-Verlag, New York and Vienna

Falconer M, Taylor D C 1970 In: Price J H (ed) Modern trends in psychological medicine. Butterworths, London

Fedio P, Mirsky A F 1969 Selective intellectual defects in children with temporal lobe or centrencephalic epilepsy. Neuropsychologia 7: 287–300

Fenton G W 1972 Epilepsy and automatism. Br J Hosp Med 7:57–64

Fenton G W, Tennent T G, Fenwick P B C, Rattray N, 1974 The EEG in antisocial behaviour: a study of posterior temporal slow activity in special hospital patients. Psychol. med. 4:181–186

Fenton G W, Fenwick P B C, Dollimore J, Dun L, Hirsh S 1980 EEG spectral analysis in schizophrenia. Br J Psychiat 136:445–455

Gestaut H 1953 So-called 'psychomotor' and 'temporal' epilepsy: a critical study. Epilepsia 2:59–96

Gestaut H, Fischer-Williams M 1959 The physiopathology of epileptic seizures. In: The handbook of physiology. Section 1: Neurophysiology. American Physiological Society, Washington D.C., Vol 1, p 329

Glaser G H 1964 The problem of psychosis in psychomotor temporal lobe epileptics. Epilepsia 5:271–278

Gloor P 1968 Generalized cortico-reticular epilepsies. Epilepsia 9:249–263

Goode D J, Penry J K, Dreifuss F E 1970 Effects of paroxysmal spike-wave on continuous visual motor performance. Epilepsia 11:241–254

Halliday A M 1967 The electrophysiological study of myoclonus in man. Brain 90:241–284

Heath R G 1977 Subcortical brain function correlates of psychopathology and epilepsy. In: Shagass C, Gershon S, Friedhoff A J (eds) Psychopathology and brain dysfunction. Raven Press, New York

Hill D, Parr G 1963 Electroencephalography, 2nd edn. A symposium of its various aspects. Macdonald, London

Hopkins A, Scambler G 1977 How doctors deal with epilepsy. Lancet 1:183–186

Ives J R, Thompson C J, Woods J P 1973 Acquisition by telemetry and computer analysis of 4 channel long-term EEG recordings from patients subject to 'petit-mal' absence attacks. Electroenceph Clin Neurophysiol 34:665–668

Ives J R, Woods J F 1975 4-channel 24-hour cassette recorder for long-term EEG monitoring of ambulatory patients. Electroenceph & Clin Neurophysiol 39:88–92

Jasper H H, Fitzpatrick C P, Solomon P 1939 Analogies and opposites in schizophrenia and epilepsy. Electroencephalographic and clinical studies. Amer J Psychiat 95:835

Jus A, Jus K 1962 Retrograde amnesia in petit mal. Arch Gen Psychiat 6:71–75

Kellaway P, Carrie J R G 1977 Relationship between quantitative EEG measurements and clinical states in epileptic patients. In: Penry J K (ed) Advances in epileptology. Eighth International Epilepsy Symposium, p 153–158

Kooi K A 1971 Fundamentals of electroencephalography. Harper and Row, New York

Lairy G C 1967 L'EEG comme moyen d'investigation des modalités individuelles d'adaptation aux situations de stress. In: Recent advances in clinical neurophysiology. Electroenceph Clin Neurophysiol Suppl 25:282–298

Landolt H 1953 Proceedings Electroenceph Clin Neurophysiol 5:121

Landolt H 1955 Uber verstimmungen dammerzostande und schizophrene zustanbidder bei epilepsie. Schweiz Arch Neurol Psychiat 76:313

Landolt H 1956 L'électroencephalographio dans les psychoses épileptiques et les épisodes schizophreniques. Rev Neurol 95:597–599

Landolt H 1958 Serial EEG investigations during psychotic episodes in epileptic patients during schizophrenic attacks. In: Lorentz de Haas A M (ed) Lectures on epilepsy. Elsevier, Amsterdam, p 91–133

Landolt H 1960 Die Temporall appenepilepsie und ihre psychopathologie. Basel Karger

Landsell H, Mirsky A F 1964 Attention in focal and centrencephalic epilepsy. Expl Neurol 9:463–469

Lennox W G, Gibbs F A, Gibbs E L 1942 Twins, brain waves and epilepsy. Arch Neurol Psychiat (Chicago) 47:702

Lindsley D A 1939 A longitudinal study of the occipital alpha rhythms in normal children. J Genet Psychol 55:197

Lockard J S 1980 A primate model of clinical epilepsy: mechanisms of action through quantification of therapeutic effects. In: Lockard J S, Ward A A (eds) Epilepsy: a window to brain mechanisms. Ravens Press, New York

Lockard J S 1981 Social primate model of epilepsy. In: Lockhard J S, Ward A A (eds) Epilepsy: a window to brain mechanisms. Raven Press, New York

Marcus E M, Watson C W 1968 Symmetrical epileptogenic foci in monkey cerebral cortex. Arch Neurol Psychiat (Chicago) 19:99–116

Metrakos K, Metrakos J D 1974 The genetics of epilepsy In: Vinken P J, Bruyn G W (eds) The handbook of neurology, Vol 15, ch. 24

Mirsky A F, Primac D W, Ajmone-Marsan C, Rosvold H E, Stevens J R 1960 A comparison of the psychological test performance of patients with focal and non-focal epilepsy. Expl Neurol 2:75–89

Mirsky A F, Van Buren J M 1965 On the nature of the 'absence' in centrencephalic epilepsy: a study of some behavioural electroencephalographic and autonomic factors. Electroenceph Clin Neurophysiol 18:334–48

Morell F 1960 Secondary epileptogenic lesions. Epilepsia 1:538–560

Musgrave J, Gloor P 1980 The role of the corpus callosum in bilateral interhemispheric synchrony of spike and wave discharge in feline generalized penicillin epilepsy. Epilepsia 21:369–378

Mutani R, Berganini L, Fariello R, Quattrocola G 1973 Bilateral synchrony of epileptic discharge associated with chronic asymmetrical cortical foci. Electroenceph Clin Neurophysiol 34:53–59

Niedermeyer E, Khalifeh R 1965 Petit mal status ('spike wave stupor'): an electro-clinical appraisal. Epilepsia 6:250–62

Nuffield E J 1961 Neurophysiology and behaviour disorders in epileptic children. J Ment Sci 107:438–458

Ounstead K, Hutt S J, Lee D 1963 The retrograde amnesia of petit mal. Lancet 1:671

Penfield W 1938 The cerebral cortex and consciousness. Arch Neurol Psychiat 40:417–442

Penfield W, Jasper H H 1954 Epilepsy and the functional anatomy of the human brain. Little Brown, Boston

Penry J K 1973 In: Brazier M A B (ed) Epilepsy, its phenomena in man. Academic Press, New York and London, p 172

Penry J K, Porter R J, Dreifuss G E 1975 Simultaneous recording of absence seizures with video tape and electroencephalography: a study of 374 seizures in 48 patients Brain 98:427–440

Penry J K, Porter R J 1977 In: Penry J K (ed) Epilepsy: The eighth international symposium. Raven Press, New York, p 95–101

Peronnet F, Sindon M, Lariron A, Quoex F, Gevin P 1972 Human cortical electrogenesis: statigraphy and spectral analysis. In: Petche H, Brazier M A B (eds) Synchronization of EEG in epilepsies. Springer-Verlag, New York and Vienna

Petersen I 1980 Poster display. 12th international epilepsy symposium, Copenhagen

Petsche H, Rappelsberger P 1973 The problems of synchronization of epileptic discharge leading to seizures in man. In: Brazier M A B Epilepsy, its phenomena in man. Academic Press, New York and London

Rodin E, Gonzales S 1966 Hereditary components in epileptic patients. Electroencephalogram family studies. J Am med Ass 198:221–225

Rowan A J, Binnie C D, Overweg J, de Vives J, Kamp A 1980 The value of prolonged EEG/video monitoring as a routine diagnostic procedure in epilepsy. In: Canger R, Angeleri F, Penry J K (eds) Advances in epileptology, eleventh epilepsy international symposium. Raven Press, New York, p 139–142

Rowan A J, Pippenger C E, MacGregor P A, French J H 1975 Seizure activity and anticonvulsant drug concentration. Arch. Neurol. 32:281–288

Sannit T 1963 The ten-twenty system: footnotes to measuring technique. Am J EEG Technol 3:23

Sato S, Penry J K, Dreifuss F E 1976 In: Kellaway P, Petersen I (eds) Quantitative analytic studies in epilepsy. Raven Press, New York, p 237–251

Schwab R S 1939 Method of measuring consciousness in attacks of petit mal epilepsy. Arch Neurol Psychiat 41:215–217

Schwartz M S, Scott D F 1971 Isolated petit-mal status presenting de novo in middle age. Lancet 2:1399–1401

Smith J R 1937 Electroencephalogram during infancy and childhood. Proc Soc Exp Biol (New York) 36:384–386

Smith J R 1941 The frequency growth of the human alpha rhythms during normal infancy and childhood. J Psychiat 11:177–198

Stevens J R 1977 All that spikes is not fits. In: Shagass C, Gershon S, Friedhoff A J Psychopathology and brain dysfunction. Raven Press, New York

Stores G, Hart J A 1976 Proceedings: reading skills of children with generalized and focal epilepsy attending ordinary school. Electroenceph Clin Neurophysiol 39(4):429–430

Stores G, Hart J, Piron N 1978 Inattentiveness in school-children with epilepsy. Epilepsia 19:169–175

Stores G 1980 Ambulatory EEG monitoring in the diagnosis of attacks of uncertain origin. In: Advances in epileptology: the XIth epilepsy international symposium, Florence, Italy. Raven Press, New York

Storm van Leeuwen W, et al 1966 Proposal for an EEG terminology. Electroenceph Clin Neurophysiol 20:306. Reprinted in Am J EEG Technol 1967 7:41

Struve F A, Kishore R S, Arko R S, Klein D F, Becka D 1977 Relationship between paroxysmal electroencephalographic dysrhythmia and suicide ideation and attempts in psychiatric patients. In: Shagass C, Gershon S, Friedhoff A J (eds) Psychopathology and brain dysfunction. Raven Press, New York

Symposium on the spike and wave discharge 1968 Epilepsia 9:173–353

Taylor D C 1972 Mental state and temporal lobe epilepsy. A correlative account of 100 patients treated surgically. Epilepsia 13:727–765

Tecce J J 1972 Contingent negative variation and psychological processes in man. Psychol Bull 77:73–108

Tizzard B, Margerison J H 1963 The relationship between EEG paroxysmal discharges and various test situations in two epileptic patients. J Neurol Neurosurg Psychiat 26:308–313

Tizzard B, Marjerison J H 1964 Psychological functions during wave-spike discharge. Br J Soc Clin Psychol 3:6–15

Walter W G, Cooper R, Aldridge V J, McCallum W C, Winter A L 1964 Contingent negative variation: an electric sign of sensori-motor association and expectancy in the human brain. Nature 203:380

Williams D 1941 The significance of an abnormal electroencephalogram. J Neurol Psychiat 4:257–268

Williams D 1944 The nature of transient outbursts in the electro-encephalogram of epileptics. Brain 67:10–36

Williams D 1969 Neural factors related to habitual aggression. Brain 92:503

Williams D 1975 Studies of persons confined for crimes of violence. In: Fields W S, Sweet W H (eds) Neural bases of violence and aggression. W H Green, St. Louis, p 285–291

Woods J F, Ives J R, Robb J P 1973 The application of telemetric recordings of the electroencephalogram to the clinical management of epilepsy. Electroenceph. Clin. Neurophysiol. 39:88–92

Biological factors in psychological disorders associated with epilepsy

'Epilepsy, the great teacher.' — Wilder Penfield (1967)

INTRODUCTION

One approach to the understanding of psychiatric disorders is the increasingly precise delineation of clearly recognised syndromes whose causative factors are then studied in detail. Another approach is to begin with possible aetiological factors and observe their relationship to various syndromes in which they may play a role. The first approach is covered in many chapters in this book, based as they are on the separation of certain well-known clinical categories. In this chapter I will adopt the alternative approach. This may have particular advantages in the study of the psychiatric disorders associated with epilepsy as there are clearly several possible adverse influences which merit special attention.

Table 19.1 includes the more important factors which many authors agree

Table 19.1 Factors affecting mental function in epilepsy

Seizures
Brain damage
Heredity
Psychosocial
Anticonvulsant drugs

should be considered in the development of the cognitive, personality and psychiatric disorders associated with epilepsy (e.g. Lennox & Lennox 1960, Pond 1961, Guerrant et al 1962, Lishman 1978). However it is clear from the literature that there has been much less agreement as to the *relative* importance of seizures, brain damage, genetic factors, psychosocial influences and drugs, either in groups of epileptic subjects or in individuals. The varying opinions throughout this century on this subject have been well reviewed by Guerrant et al (1962) and summarised in Table 19.2. The older view that epilepsy was frequently, and perhaps inevitably, associated with mental deterioration, gradually gave way to the concept of specific personality traits. The latter concept in turn was succeeded by the view dominant at the time of the review by Guerrant et al, and still to a large extent with us, that most epileptic patients are psychologically normal but that psychomotor epileptics may be particularly vulnerable to psychiatric disturbance.

Table 19.2A Historical evolution of concepts of mental
changes in epilepsy (Guerrant et al 1962)

The period of epileptic deterioration	−1900
The period of the epileptic character	1900–1930
The period of normality	1930–
The period of psychomotor peculiarity	1948–

Table 19.2B Summary of the periods of normality and psychomotor peculiarity (Guerrant et al 1962)

1. Most epileptics are normal in intellect and personality; there is no specific epileptic character, nor are there any physical stigmata of epilepsy
2. Defects of personality or intellect, *except in psychomotor epileptics*, are due to one or more of the following:
a. Structural brain disease
b. Uncontrolled seizures
c. Anticonvulsant drugs
d. Psychological reaction to familial and social isolation and rejection
3. Half or more of psychomotor epileptics have severe psychiatric disturbances of various sorts

In this chapter I will review the biological factors which contribute to the psychological disorders associated with epilepsy, which will include all the factors listed in Table 19.1 with the exception of psychosocial influences which are covered by Pond in Chapter 20.

EPIDEMIOLOGICAL STUDIES OF BIOLOGICAL FACTORS

Epidemiological studies may provide important clues to biological factors, and certainly help to place known factors in a clearer perspective. The epidemiology of psychiatric disorders associated with epilepsy is reviewed in Chapter 3 but certain findings are relevant to the present discussion.

Pond & Bidwell (1960), in a pioneering study, surveyed 14 general practices in the south-east of England and found 29 per cent of 245 patients had psychological difficulties. In patients with temporal lobe epilepsy however the figure rose to 52 per cent, and the proportion who had previously had psychiatric admissions was at least twice that for other types of epilepsy. However it should be noted that only 39 (16 per cent) of the epileptic patients were thought to have temporal lobe epilepsy. This may be an underestimate of the true incidence as the diagnosis was based on the general practitioner and social worker's report, very often without ancillary investigations. Further, admission to hospital, for whatever reason, might be expected to increase the possibility of the diagnosis of temporal lobe epilepsy because of access to such investigations.

Gudmundsson (1966) reviewed 987 patients who were considered to have epilepsy in Iceland on January 1st 1960. 52 per cent had various personality changes, and these were more frequent: in patients with epilepsy of known or 'probably known' aetiology than in those of unknown aetiology; in the presence of focal EEG abnormalities; in those on anticonvulsant drugs compared to those on no drugs (perhaps reflecting more severe epilepsy); and in those with the earliest onset of epilepsy. Even patients with a history of only one or two seizures have more personality changes than in the general population. He concluded that mental changes were the result of various factors of which the most important was the extent of the brain injury.

In a survey of schoolchildren between the ages of 5 and 15 on the Isle of Wight Graham & Rutter (1968) were able to compare the psychological disorders associated with epilepsy, with other chronic neurological and non-neurological handicaps, and in the general population. Table 19.3 shows that in epilepsy

Table 19.3   Prevalence of psychiatric disorder in neuro-epileptic children aged 5–14 years attending school (Graham & Rutter 1968)

	With psychiatric disorder		Total
	No.	%	
General population (10- and 11-year-old children)	144	6.6	2189
Physical disorders not involving brain	16	11.5	139
Blind only	1	16.6	6
Deaf only	2	15.4	13
Lesion at or below brain stem	2	13.3	15
Miscellaneous other physical disorders★	11	10.3	107
Brain disorder	34	34.3	99
Uncomplicated epilepsy	18	28.6	63
Lesion above brain stem (but no fits)	9	37.5	24
Lesion above brain stem (with fits)	7	58.3	12

★This group includes two children who also have lesions below the brain stem

uncomplicated by evidence of a brain lesion as many as 29 per cent had psychiatric disorders. The latter figure rose to 58 per cent in the presence of a brain lesion. The corresponding figures for the general population were 6.6 per cent, for non-neurological chronic diseases (e.g. asthma, diabetes, etc.) 11.5 per cent, and for cerebral disorders without fits 39 per cent. The remarkably high prevalence of psychiatric disorders in the epileptic children compared with other chronic diseases suggested that chronic handicap per se was unlikely to be a major factor, and that even adverse influences such as community prejudice or disturbed family background might be less important than the disturbance of cerebral function associated with epilepsy. This view was reinforced by the high prevalence of psychiatric disorder in children with brain disorders without epilepsy, such as cerebral palsy, who would not be expected to face so much prejudice. The authors also observed a significantly higher incidence of psychiatric disorders in association with psychomotor seizures compared with other seizure types, but it should be noted that this analysis is based only on the clinical description of seizure type, without reference to, or indeed, investigation for temporal lobe epilepsy. Further, the number of patients involved were small, only six having both psychomotor seizures and psychiatric disorder. The major conclusion from this study of a close association between psychiatric problems and a disorder of cerebral function left open the question of the nature of the cerebral disorder, which could of course include seizures, brain damage, or drug effects, each of which I will consider separately in more detail.

One final point to emerge from these community studies is that there was little evidence that the type of psychiatric or personality disorder associated with epilepsy differed to any major degree from those in the general or other handicapped populations, although the amount of such disorder was significantly higher.

SEIZURE ACTIVITY

I am principally concerned in this chapter with the biological mechanisms underlying *inter-seizure* cognitive, personality and psychiatric disorder. It is clearly important however to consider what role, if any, the seizure activity itself may play in these more prolonged psychological disturbances, as has long been of great interest, if uncertainty, to psychiatrists. A major impetus to such enquiry comes from the well-known fact that a wide range of affective, perceptual and cognitive symptoms or experiences can form the main or even the only components of some epileptic attacks, especially, but not exclusively, those arising in the temporal lobe (see Chapter 2). Such symptoms may be combined with sometimes complex motor behaviour to comprise so-called 'psychomotor seizures'. Such attacks are usually of abrupt onset, relatively short duration (minutes), and fairly clear-cut termination, and are accompanied by an alteration in the electrical activity of the brain throughout the duration of the episode. In essence they are the complex behavioural and experiential manifestations of ongoing epileptic discharge (Lishman 1978).

In general the clinical and electrical distinction between these brief ictal episodes and prolonged interictal psychological disturbances is clear enough. However there is a grey, borderland area in which psychomotor episodes of a rather more prolonged kind (hours, days, weeks) are a source of confusion, not only to the patient experiencing such 'attacks', but also to the psychiatrist and neurologist trying to understand them. The confusion for the observer is compounded by a bewildering array of terms which have been applied to such phenomena, which include automatisms, petit mal status, temporal lobe status, fugues, twilight states, psychoses, postictal disorders and epileptic or psychic equivalents. The interrelations and the clinical difficulties in distinguishing between the various syndromes embraced by these terms has been well discussed by Lishman (1978). For most episodes however certain clinical features, especially clouding of consciousness, but also less commonly, the onset or termination with a more clear-cut seizure (e.g. grand mal), together with EEG evidence of an ongoing electrical disturbance of various kinds, clarifies the ictal or postictal nature of the disturbance. Most difficulty arises if there is no clouding of consciousness, if there is no change in the electrical activity on the EEG, or rarely if the EEG actually shows less abnormal activity ('forced normalisation' of Landolt) during the period of psychological disturbance.

Dongier (1959) summarised the combined experience of several collaborators who had examined electro-clinical correlations in the 536 'acute psychotic episodes' in 516 epileptic patients. Clinical features which were rated included conscious level, affect, anxiety, delusions, hallucinations and behaviour. Clouding of consciousness was present in two-thirds. The episodes lasted hours or more commonly days, but in 32 per cent for weeks; they were preceded by seizures in 25 per cent, and terminated by a seizure in 10 per cent. In the remainder a relationship to seizures was absent or unclear. Certain recurring themes emerged, with a trend towards some differences between 'centrencephalic' epilepsy and temporal lobe epilepsy. Amongst the former, episodes were more often characterised by clouding of consciousness and confusion. The two main EEG correlates were: bisynchronous spike/wave discharges, seen more often in children, and corresponding to reports of petit mal status; and diffuse delta dysrhythmia, seen more often in adults following a seizure, and suggestive of a postictal disorder. In patients with temporal lobe epilepsy the episodes were more often longer with less frequent or severe disturbances in consciousness. Relationships to seizures were less clear but some episodes terminated in a seizure. The EEG was more variable. Sometimes enhancement of the temporal focal discharges (presumably temporal lobe status) was seen, but in others there were no changes, and in some 'forced normalisation' occurred. Dongier tentatively concluded that many such episodes in the temporal lobe group might be considered 'pre-' or 'subictal' phenomena.

Dongier however emphasised that the above synthesis is by no means clear-cut, nor based on statistically significant differences between the groups. He stressed that there was considerable variability between the groups and it was not possible to prognosticate what sort of 'psychotic' episode would characterise a given type of epilepsy, nor could the EEG give any sure guide as to the likely development of mental symptoms. Finally, it was clearly not possible to give a precise explanation of the pathophysiology of these mental episodes. To which I would add that it is also uncertain to what extent the episodes reviewed by Dongier are representative of the problem as a whole.

'Subclinical' epilepsy

Many authors in attempting to explain interictal psychiatric disorders, especially psychosis, have invoked the hypothesis of 'subictal' or 'subclinical' epilepsy, as illustrated for example by Dongier (1959) above. This concept has become more fashionable since the discovery of the EEG, and the term has to some extent replaced the much older concept of 'epileptic equivalent', the history of which is discussed by Hill in Chapter 1. As knowledge has grown about surface electrical discharges during epileptic attacks it has perhaps been inevitable that in contemplating interictal phenomena some, indeed many, would propose an 'epileptic' mechanism in deep (most recently limbic) structures, undetectable by scalp EEG recordings. Similar mechanisms have been invoked by many psychiatrists to explain some psychiatric disorders in non-epileptic patients in whom 'epileptic' type abnormalities have been discovered, mainly in temporal areas, on the EEG (see Chapter 18).

The concept of subclinical epilepsy however, while perhaps superficially attractive, is on closer examination a difficult notion or, at the very least, a hazardous one. Its proof would seem to depend on depth electrode studies not only in epileptic and psychiatric patients but also in large numbers of normal subjects, all of which seems unlikely for ethical reasons. Further, our concept of what constitutes an 'epileptic discharge' is based on relating certain surface EEG features, such as spikes or spike/wave activity, to well recognised clinical attacks which have been called 'seizures' or 'epilepsy'. As electrodes penetrate deeper into the nervous system the electrical phenomena that are met are limited in kind, much of it having a superficial resemblance to 'epileptic' phenomena, and indeed some structures such as the amygdala and hippocampus seem to respond normally to almost all stimuli by 'epileptic' spike discharges (e.g. Freedman et al 1979). It should not be forgotten that 'spikes' are a fundamental feature of all neuronal activity. At the neurophysiological level the distinction between 'non-epileptic activity' and the aggregation and propagation of spike activity in association with a clinical epileptic attack is never likely to be an easy one. The problem is in part a semantic one. The word 'epilepsy' having been applied initially to certain clinical phenomena and later associated with certain electrical disturbances, clumsy attempts have then been made to associate the word with other clinical phenomena in which similar or related electrical discharges have been noted or hypothesised. However, even the attempt to link undoubted clinical epileptic attacks with electrical activity have not been as straightforward as is sometimes supposed. It is reasonably well known that discharges of the sort associated with epileptic attacks may be found in scalp EEG recordings in up to 5 per cent or more of the normal population, with a higher incidence in patients with a variety of neuropsychiatric disorders, none of whom have had seizures. Even the assumption that such subjects will be particularly vulnerable to epilepsy in the future is open to question. Cavazzutti et al (1980) followed up for 9 years 100 normal children with epileptic EEG discharges. Only seven developed epileptic attacks, and in the majority the EEG abnormality disappeared. If so many problems undermine the attempt to link epileptic attacks to electrical phenomena how many times will these difficulties be multiplied in attempting to define 'subclinical epilepsy'?

The concept of subclinical epilepsy is a slippery slope at the end of which it can be and has been argued that many forms of mental illness, behavioural disorder and neurological disease are embraced by this term, based, as they might be, on evidence of imbalance between excitatory and inhibitory processes, or disorders of neurotransmitter function. This might return us to the last century with the re-introduction of 'epilepsy per se' (in the form of 'subclinical epilepsy per se') as a variety of mental illness in national and international classifications (see Chapter 1), with all the social repercussions for the epileptic patient which only now are being gradually eroded.

Kindling

Having cast some doubt on it, or at least pointed out its enormous problems, the concept of subclinical epilepsy may well linger with us for some time as it has been given a boost recently by the discovery of the phenomenon of kindling (Goddard et al 1969). The essence of this phenomenon is that repeated subthreshold electrical stimulations, each of which on its own would have no clinical effect, may in series be accompanied by increasingly prolonged after discharges, culminating eventually in a clinical event such as a seizure. Furthermore, once a seizure has been kindled it can be repeatedly induced by the same subthreshold stimulus even weeks or months later. Eventually a state of spontaneous recurrent seizures may occur, something that has always been difficult to induce in animals. Undoubtedly this phenomenon which has been demonstrated in different brain areas (especially the limbic system) in many species, provides a very interesting experimental model for studying many aspects of epilepsy (Wada 1976). I am here concerned, however, with the problem of interictal psychiatric disorders. It seems that the kindling phenomenon is not limited to seizures and that it is also possible to kindle behavioural changes, especially in the mesolimbic dopamine systems, as discussed by Stevens & Livermore (1978), who themselves induced fear, hiding and withdrawal behaviour in cats kindled in the ventral tegmental area. Trimble proposes in Chapter 16 that some of the interictal behavioural or psychiatric disorders in patients with temporal lobe epilepsy may perhaps be kindled by persisting electrical activity in the limbic circuits. Whether it is appropriate or even desirable to refer to the putative persisting electrical disturbance as 'subictal' or 'subclinical epilepsy' is open to question, as discussed above, but the possibility of kindled behaviour or mental disturbance, by whatever mechanism, is an interesting one.

For the series of subthreshold stimuli to kindle a seizure there must be at least a certain interval between each one, which varies with both site and species. The need for this interval may perhaps be related to another phenomenon which is the temporary elevation of seizure threshold, or resistance to further seizures, following a convulsion (Herberg et al 1969). Pharmacological and metabolic studies have so far failed to identify the mechanism of this effect, which may perhaps represent an adaptation of the brain to diminish or prevent the spread of further seizure activity (Green et al 1981). Clinically it reminds one of the group of epileptic subjects who, following a seizure or bout of seizures, can be reasonably confident that they will not have another attack for a certain interval, which varies between patients, but is usually consistent in the individual.

The Gowers phenomenon

I suspect that Gowers would have been interested in the phenomenon of kindling because he described in 1881 in his book, the centenary of which is celebrated here, a possibly related phenomenon, as follows: 'The effect of a convulsion on the nerve centres is such as to render the occurrence of another more easy, to intensify the predisposition that already exists. Thus every fit may be said to be, in part, the result of those which have preceded it, the cause of those which follow it.'

Clearly Gowers was very attracted to this hypothesis as it is the second paragraph in his opening chapter. Curiously, notwithstanding his widely acknowledged contributions to neurology, this particular concept, based on his clinical observations, has been largely ignored. More recent clinical studies may be quoted in support of his view. Rodin (1968) has summarised the evidence that the longer the history of epilepsy prior to effective treatment the more difficult it is to control. Studies of the drug treatment of new referrals with epilepsy also bear this out, as it has proved easier to suppress seizures in such patients than in chronic patients (Reynolds & Shorvon 1981). The occasional patient who presents with the onset of epilepsy after a course of ECT, also suggests that there may be some substance in Gowers' proposal, although I am not aware that the incidence of post-ECT seizures has been assessed rigorously.

There are distinct parallels between the clinical phenomenon described by Gowers and the more recent experimental phenomenon of kindling. As discussed above the kindling model may be relevant to behavioural and other psychiatric disorders. One wonders therefore, whether the clinical concept concerning the recurrence of seizures, expounded by Gowers, might also be extrapolated to other neuropsychiatric disorders? In other words the longer abnormal behaviour or disturbed mental function continues the more likely it is to persist, and the more difficult it is to reverse with treatment. As in the case of chronic epilepsy, there is at least a strong suspicion that chronic psychiatric disorders are very resistant to treatment.

Brain damage due to seizures

An obviously potentially important mechanism as a result of which seizure activity might lead to mental symptoms is due to brain damage. Here there is particular interest in hippocampal or Ammon's horn sclerosis (or the more extensive lesion referred to as 'mesial temporal sclerosis') especially in view of a widely held suspicion of a special association between temporal lobe epilepsy and personality or psychiatric disorders, which will be discussed later in this chapter. The relationship between epilepsy and brain damage is a complex one and has been well reviewed by Meldrum (1981). A great variety of cerebral pathology may of course be responsible for seizures, the more so the later the onset of epilepsy. In some patients brain pathology and seizures may be unrelated. I am here however concerned with brain damage consequent upon seizure activity, excluding those indirect causes, such as contrecoup lesions due to head trauma in an attack, or the more uncertain pathology which may result from chronic drug intoxiation (see below — mechanisms of anticonvulsant effects on mental function). Amongst chronic epileptic patients dying in institutions or hospitals a high proportion show evidence of focal or diffuse atrophy of the cerebral cortex, symmetrical lobular atrophy of the cerebellum, and most commonly, predominantly asymmetrical atrophy of the hippocampus, as reviewed by Margerison & Corsellis (1966) and Meldrum (1981), who also describe the histological details. Hippocampal sclerosis, which when present is unilateral in 80 per cent, may involve the amygdala and uncus with lateral spread to the parahippocampal gyrus and other parts of the temporal lobe, leading to the term mesial temporal sclerosis (MTS). MTS is present in some 50 per cent of resected specimens in patients undergoing neurosurgical treatment for temporal lobe epilepsy (Falconer 1974), but how common such lesions would be in unselected epileptic populations is of course unknown.

A more acute but related type of brain pathology is found in both children and adults dying in, or shortly after, status epilepticus, although the relative distribution of the lesions may be different. The duration of status that produces brain damage in children is less than that in adults and the suspicion has grown recently that prolonged febrile convulsions in early childhood may lead to varying degrees of brain damage such as MTS, which is then responsible for the development of temporal lobe epilepsy later in childhood or adolescence (Ounsted et al 1966, Falconer 1974). However, the picture is complicated by the fact that children with pre-existing brain damage are both more vulnerable to febrile convulsions and to the subsequent development of epilepsy following such convulsions. Further, perinatal asphyxia may also cause generalised brain damage, which can include MTS.

While it has not been possible to demonstrate in man correlations between physiological changes during prolonged seizure activity and subsequent brain damage, studies in animals have provided important insights with practical implications for the management of recurrent seizures or status (Meldrum 1975, 1981). Adverse systemic factors include hypoxia, arterial hypotension, hyperpyrexia and hypoglycaemia. Rises in cerebral venous pressure, focal venous thrombosis and cerebral oedema may also sometimes play a part. However, even when such systemic changes are controlled, experimental pathological changes, mainly in the hippocampus, can be produced by repeated brief generalised seizures or sustained seizures in the limbic system, and are thought to be a direct result of the seizure activity, perhaps due to failure of oxidative energy metabolism.

The possible relationship of seizure induced brain damage to psychiatric and cognitive problems in some epileptic patients is discussed later in this chapter and also in Chapter 12.

Neuropsychological deficits during seizures

Another possible mechanism as a result of which ongoing seizure activity might contribute to subsequent interictal cognitive or other psychological disturbances is through repeated disruption of conscious or even subconscious neuropsychological processes. Particular interest has focussed on the relationship between impairment of attention and EEG spike/wave paroxysms (Penry 1973, Stores 1973; see also Chapter 4 and 18). As might be predicted simple relationships are not readily detected. To begin with both the concept of attention and the recording and classification of spike/wave paroxysms are complex matters. Different or interchangeable meanings may be embraced by terms such as attention, alertness, arousal, vigilance, selection, concentration; and almost certainly several different components of a sensory, integretive, selective and motor nature are involved in this or these concepts (Stores 1973). The analysis of the spike/wave paroxysms has to take into account such features as symmetry, rate of build-up of voltage, duration, and background rhythms. Studies of spike/wave bursts in epileptic subjects have utilised, for example, a continuous performance task (Mirsky & Van Buren 1965), a pursuit rotor task (Goode et al 1970) and auditory reaction times (Browne et al 1974). Although these test procedures are not strictly comparable they all tended to show a greater percentage of errors during paroxysms than between them. The time course relationships with the EEG data have varied for different tasks. Although some have tended to show a trough-like impairment in the middle or early part of the spike/wave burst (Penry 1973), others have shown an interrupted or intermittent impairment, and some may begin concurrently with (Browne et al 1974), or before (Mirsky & Van Buren 1965) the paroxysms. It is clear however, as emphasised by Mirsky & Van Buren (1965), that despite some correlation between them the behavioural and electrical data must be considered as separable events, as impaired performance can be detected between and before spike/wave paroxysms in some patients, and in others there is no impairment during such paroxysms.

The question to what extent such interruptions of neuropsychological function are 'subclinical' is difficult to answer at the present time, but it is interesting that in a careful study of the relationship between clinically observed absence attacks and telemetered spike/wave bursts there was a reasonable correlation with bursts of 3 or more seconds, which is also the time during which errors in attention tasks are most likely to appear (Penry 1973). However Browne et al (1974) reported that impairment of reaction time is unrelated to the duration of the paroxysms, and they therefore advocated a vigorous onslaught on all spike/wave activity with anticonvulsant therapy irrespective of recognisable clinical expression. This latter advice however is open to question until a clearer picture of spike/wave and neuropsychological relations emerges. It is by no means certain that all spikes and spike/wave activity are clinically harmful, as will be discussed below. Furthermore anticonvulsant drugs themselves have adverse neuropsychological effects as will also be discussed. Further studies in this area can be expected especially with the development of more intensive and sophisticated clinical, EEG and psychometric monitoring techniques. Inevitably depth electrode studies will be reported (Rausch et al 1978) but the results are likely to be difficult to interpret at least for some time for the reasons already discussed under the heading 'subclinical epilepsy'.

The relationship of repeated interruption of neuropsychological function to cognitive, personality and psychiatric disorders remains conjectural at the present time. Cognitive disorders are considered in more detail in Chapter 12 but it is remarkable how relatively little long-term impairment may occur in children with petit mal, even with quite frequent attacks (Lennox & Lennox 1960, Metrakos & Metrakos 1960, Pond 1961). However impairment of attention whether due to seizures or other causes may well be important in the persistent impression of educational under-achievement in relation to formal intelligence testing in epileptic children (Stores 1973; Chapter 4). Some studies have shown differences in personality and behaviour between children with petit mal and other, especially temporal lobe, types of epilepsy (Pond 1961, Nuffield 1961). On the whole personality disorders are less obtrusive with petit mal, and Nuffield (1961) showed a tendency to more neurotic and less aggressive symptoms. Whether such differences, however, are related to the seizure type or to other factors such as brain damage, or disturbed family background, which are also more common for example, in temporal lobe epilepsy, is again open to question (Pond 1961).

Beneficial effects of seizure activity on mental function

I have so far discussed several different mechanisms through which seizure activity per se might contribute to psychological disorders. However there are reasons to suspect that not all the effects of seizure activity on mental function are adverse ones. We are in fact presented with a distinct paradox. Although there is an increased prevalence of mental disorders in epileptic subjects, electro-convulsive therapy (ECT) is widely regarded as a useful treatment for some psychiatric disorders, especially depression, and its effectiveness is thought to depend on the production of generalised seizure activity. Indeed, amongst other reasons, it was the improvement in the mental state of some patients with catatonic schizophrenia following spontaneous seizures that led Meduna (1937) to introduce convulsive therapy. Hill (1952), in his study of the EEG in episodic behaviour disorders, also comments that besides catatonic schizophrenics, in whom paroxysmal EEG activity may be found in up to 25 per cent, other occasional patients with behaviour or psychopathic disorders with paroxysmal EEG findings may benefit psychologically from the occurrence of epileptic seizures. Hill proposed that the paroxysmal spike or spike/wave activity in the catatonic schizophrenic may represent a 'homeostatic' response on the part of the organism, with the EEG changes disappearing with psychological recovery. Stevens (1975, 1977) has also commented that all that spikes is not necessarily epilepsy, and that such spike activity might have 'restitutive' functions. The phenomenon of resistance to seizures following a seizure, discussed above, may perhaps be relevant to these concepts.

A number of observations in epileptic patients support the view that generalised seizure activity may sometimes have psychologically beneficial effects. Special interest has centred on a group of patients in whom psychotic episodes seem to alternate with seizures, as for example described by Landolt (1958) who also described the 'forced normalisation' of the EEG in which epileptic activity may disappear as seizures cease and the patient becomes psychotic. I have pointed out elsewhere (Reynolds 1968a) that Landolt's 'forced normalisation' observations are the inverse of Hill's 'homeostatic' proposals. The subject of the relationship between epilepsy and schizophrenia is a complex one which is also discussed by Toone in Chapter 10. The subgroup of patients with alternating epilepsy and psychosis may perhaps be different from the more chronic schizophrenia-like psychoses, but it is interesting that there is at least some evidence that the latter psychoses also tend to occur as seizures, usually psychomotor, come under better control (Reynolds 1968a, Flor-Henry 1969, Kristensen & Sindrup 1978). It is of interest in this context that psychoses occurred in nine out of 74 patients following temporal lobectomy, usually in association with good control of the seizures (Jensen & Larsen 1979).

Davison & Bagley (1969) reviewed three apparently contradictory theories concerning the relationship between epilepsy and schizophrenia. One theory, the affinity concept, suggests an increased association between these two disorders. A second suggests that any association is by chance. The third is Meduna's (1937) theory of biological antagonism between the two disorders which led him to try convulsive therapy. Although convulsive therapy has been widely utilised, especially in depression, Meduna's theory has largely been forgotten or ignored mainly because psychiatrists are well aware that epilepsy and schizophrenia-like illness can and do occur together. However, in supporting and restating Meduna's hypothesis I have argued (Reynolds 1968a) that the co-existence of these two disorders does not exclude some antagonism, which is readily apparent in a few patients, as discussed above. Further the situation is complicated by the influence of the drug treatment of one condition in the precipitation of the other i.e. the precipitation of seizures in schizophrenia by phenothiazines, or psychoses in epilepsy by anticonvulsant drugs. The influence of anticonvulsant drugs on mental function will be discussed in more detail below.

There is also a surprising amount of biochemical data which tends to support the cononcept of antagonism, which is summarised in Table 19.4 (Reynolds

Table 19.4   Evidence of biological antagonism between epilepsy and schizophrenia from Reynolds (1968a)

Agent	Epilepsy	Schizophrenia
Anticonvulsant drugs, barbiturates	Therapeutic	?Aggravation
Phenothiazines	Convulsant	Therapeutic
Methionine	?Therapeutic	Aggravation
Methionine-sulfoximine	Convulsant	?Therapeutic
EEG	'Forced normalisation' (Landolt)	'Homeostatic' (Hill)
Folic acid	?Aggravation	??

? implies need for more substantial evidence

1968a) and Figure 19.1 (Trimble & Meldrum 1979). It is well documented that methionine may aggravate schizophrenia and that its antagonist methionine-sulfoximine is a convulsant. Less well substantiated is a possible therapeutic effect

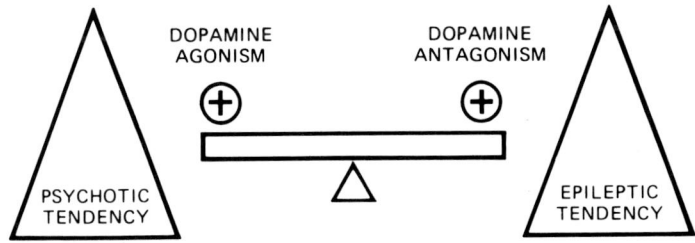

AGONISTS *eg. L.DOPA, PIRIBEDIL, APOMORPHINE, NOMIFENSINE*

ANTAGONISTS *eg. PHENOTHIAZINES, HALOPERIDOL, PIMOZIDE*

Fig. 19.1   Relationship between epilepsy, psychosis and dopamine (from Trimble & Meldrum 1979)

of the former in epilepsy and the latter in schizophrenia. The excitatory properties of folic acid and its derivatives are now well established (Hommes et al 1979) and there is growing evidence that deficiency of the vitamin can lead to a variety of neuropsychiatric complications, especially affective disorder and dementia, but including psychoses (Botez & Reynolds 1979, Shorvon et al 1980). Further evidence is derived from the study of monoamine (especially catecholamine) metabolism as has been reviewed by Trimble (1977) and Trimble & Meldrum (1979) who point out that dopamine antagonists, such as phenothiazines, are therapeutic in psychoses and reduce seizure threshold, while dopamine agonists like L-dopa and amphetamines have the reverse effects, elevating seizure threshold but aggravating or precipitating psychoses.

Although the preceding discussion has been concerned with the subject of epilepsy and psychoses, there are hints that the concept of biological antagonism may not be quite so specific. For example, the occasional improvement in mood following a grand mal seizure is familiar to epileptologists, and it may also be true that depression in some epileptic patients occurs at times of better seizure control (Betts 1974; Chapter 6). Also convulsive therapy is more widely used for depression than it is for psychosis. The main point however is that seizure activity of a generalised kind is not always detrimental to the mental health of epileptic or non-epileptic subjects, and this has to be borne in mind in evaluating the biological factors underlying mental illness associated with epilepsy.

BRAIN LESIONS

It is well known that epilepsy may be associated with a wide range of cerebral pathology. Indeed almost any type of cerebral pathology can be responsible for seizures in otherwise predisposed individuals. There are many reviews of such pathology, most recently those of Marsden & Reynolds (1981) and Meldrum (1981). I have already discussed in this chapter the subject of brain damage resulting from seizures.

The most recent new insight into the brain lesions associated with epilepsy is derived from the CAT scan. Gastaut (1976) has summarised the CAT scan findings in 1702 epileptic patients of all ages combined from seven research groups. Overall the number of abnormalities varied from 34 to 51 per cent with a mean of 46 per cent. Amongst these lesions 56 per cent were atrophic in character. Tumours were found in 8–11 per cent, and this figure rose to 16 per cent in patients over the age of 20, and to 22 per cent when only partial seizures were considered. Patients with primary generalised seizures had a relatively low incidence of abnormalities (11 per cent) compared with a much higher percentage (60–80 per cent) in relation to other seizure types (Gastaut & Gastaut 1976).

These observations have been extended by Yang et al (1979) who scanned 256 children between the ages of a few days and 17 years (mean 4 years) and found abnormalities in 33 per cent. They were able to distinguish a low yield group (2.5–8 per cent) with idiopathic generalised seizures, or normal neurological examination, or focal slowing but not focal spiking on the EEG (Table 19.5). The highest incidence was seen in neonatal seizures or with a history of seizures beginning in the neonatal period. Amongst children with mental retardation 45 per cent had abnormal scans. Only 2 per cent of the series had tumours. It must be borne in mind that milder degrees of cerebral pathology may be undetected by present CAT scan techniques.

It has long been suspected that brain lesions, whether responsible for or the result of seizures, must be one of the contributing factors for the interictal psychological disorders associated with epilepsy (Tables 19.1 and 19.2; see also Vislie & Henricksen 1958). Their relative importance however has never been clear, mainly for lack of adequate study. The epidemiological studies should provide some of the most relevant data, and seem to imply an important role. I have already mentioned Gudmundsson's (1966) conclusion, based on his survey of Iceland, that the extent of brain pathology is the most important of the various factors which contribute to mental change. In Graham & Rutter's (1968) study of children in the Isle of Wight, it was also striking how the incidence of psychiatric disorder rose when brain damage was added to uncomplicated epilepsy. The influence of cerebral pathology was again emphasised in their control group of

Table 19.5   CAT findings in children with epilepsy (Yang et al 1979)

A. *Classification of CAT findings*
1. Normal
2. Bilateral atrophy
   Central atrophy: dilation of lateral ventricles only
   Cortical atrophy: dilation of sulci, lateral ventricles normal
   Generalized atrophy: dilation of sulci and lateral ventricles
3. Focal findings
   Atrophy
   Hemiatrophy
   Porencephalic cysts
   Tumours
4. Other findings
   Pathological calcifications
   Congenital abnormalities of brain
   Evidence of intracranial bleeding

B. *Results of CAT findings*	*Abnormal CAT* (%)
Low yield groups	
1. Idiopathic generalised seizures	8
2. Neurologic examination and EEG normal	5
3. Generalized seizures (idiopathic or known aetiology with normal neurologic examination and normal EEG)	2.5
High yield groups	
1. Partial seizures with elementary symptomatology	52
2. Partial seizures with complex symptomatology	30
3. Generalised seizures (known aetiology)	40
4. Neonates with seizures	68
5. Children whose seizures began as neonates	100
6. Focal slowing on EEG	65
7. Abnormal neurologic examination	64

children with brain disorders without epilepsy, who also had a high incidence of mental problems.

Indirect support for the importance of brain lesions may perhaps be derived from the valuable study of Lishman (1968) of the psychiatric sequelae of penetrating head injuries. Here there were some interesting correlations between the amount and type of psychiatric disorder and the degree and location of the brain damage. For example, intellectual disorders were more commonly associated with left hemisphere damage, especially of the parietal and temporal lobes. Affective disorders, behavioural disorders and somatic complaints were more frequent with right hemisphere damage, especially to the frontal lobe. Further, the addition of post-traumatic epilepsy to the brain damage, especially in the first year, significantly increased the amount of psychiatric disability.

The importance of cerebral pathology in the cognitive disorders associated with epilepsy is discussed in Chapter 12. There has been relatively little study of the psychiatric associations of brain pathology in epilepsy, apart from the interest in the psychological disorders accompanying temporal lobe epilepsy.

Temporal lobe epilepsy
As emphasised in the introduction and reviewed, for example by Guerrant et al 1962 (Table 19.2) and Lishman (1978), amongst many others, there has been a widespread conviction, especially amongst psychiatrists, of a special association

between temporal lobe epilepsy and personality, psychiatric and cognitive disorders. The literature on this subject is enormous and will not be reviewed by me especially as most of it is covered in several other chapters in this book. The basis for this conviction is understandable. As discussed by Trimble (Chapter 16) the limbic system is thought to play a central role in the affective and behavioural life of the individual, as evidenced by animal and clinical studies. Furthermore there is no doubt that psychiatrists and neurologists find that psychiatric disorders are frequently associated with epilepsy of the temporal lobe variety. However, the literature on this subject is by no means conclusive and many studies have also failed to confirm any particular association between personality traits or mental symptoms and temporal lobe epilepsy.

The epidemiological evidence is equivocal. As I have already indicated the observation of more psychological disorders associated with temporal lobe epilepsy in the general practice survey of Pond & Bidwell (1960) is at least open to question because of the lack of diagnostic precision with regard to the epilepsy. The association noted by Graham & Rutter (1968) was between psychological disorder and psychomotor seizures (which are not always temporal lobe in origin), and the numbers were small.

With regard to many reports from psychiatric hospitals or epilepsy centres supporting the concept of a particular association between mental disorder and temporal lobe epilepsy, Stevens (1966, 1975) has consistently pointed out the selected nature of the material and the lack of adequate control for a number of variables. It is frequently overlooked that temporal lobe epilepsy is by far the commonest form of seizure disorder over the age of 15, at least in hospital clinics where it may account for some 60–70 per cent of patients (Alving 1978). Therefore amongst patients of the same age with psychological disorders temporal lobe epilepsy is also likely to be common. In neurological clinics several studies have failed to confirm a special association of temporal lobe epilepsy and mental disorder (Stevens 1975) and indeed the incidence of psychiatric disorders in temporal lobe epilepsy may not be excessive (Currie et al 1971).

Trimble & Perez (1980) have reviewed those studies which have attempted to quantitate psychopathology with rating scales in different types of epilepsy. Although some results suggest personality differences between different subgroups of epilepsy, including those with complex partial seizures, no consistent picture emerges. Bear & Fedio (1977) have criticised these studies for using questionnaires standardised on psychiatric rather than the relevant epileptic patients. They developed their own scale which showed differences in personality traits between patients with right and left temporal epileptic foci, but they did not examine patients with non-temporal epilepsy.

The difficulties in controlling for all the variables is illustrated in the careful study of Rodin et al (1976) who compared 78 temporal lobe epileptic patients with a similar number with other seizure types, matched for age, sex and IQ. Although significantly more psychological problems emerged in the temporal lobe patients, Table 19.6 also shows that two of the biggest differences between the groups were (1) the greater number of anticonvulsant drugs used, and (2) the more common occurrence of more than one seizure type, in the temporal lobe group. Indeed, the authors go on to show that temporal lobe patients with one seizure

Table 19.6 Differences between patients with temporal lobe epilepsy and other seizure types matched for age, sex and IQ (Rodin et al 1976)

Temporal lobe seizure patients had	T	P<
Greater number of anticonvulsants used in treatment	3.3	0.01
More commonly more than one seizure type	3.2	0.01
More clusters of major seizures	3.0	0.01
More common history of meningitis	2.7	0.01
Less common hereditary cause for illness only	2.5	0.01
More frequent occurrence of sleep after minor seizures	2.3	0.05
More common bleeding or threatened abortion during pregnancy	2.3	0.05
More random circadian distribution	2.2	0.05
More common mixed hereditary and external etiologic factors	2.1	0.05
More frequent major seizures	2.0	0.05
Longer history of major seizures	2.0	0.05
More decreased overall psychomotor activity	2.0	0.05
More impaired peer relations	3.3	0.05
More personality disturbance on psychological tests	2.8	0.01
Poorer performance on information subtest on WAIS	2.7	0.01
More psychotic tendencies during psychiatric interview	2.4	0.05
Higher elevation on depression scale on MMPI	2.3	0.05
Higher elevation on paranoia scale on MMPI	2.1	0.05
More psychotic tendencies on psychological test results	2.1	0.05
More organic disturbances on psychological test results	2.0	0.05

type do not differ psychologically from non-temporal lobe patients with one seizure type. They therefore attribute much of the increased psychopathology in temporal lobe epilepsy to the occurrence of more than one seizure type. However, I would add that it is well known that patients with temporal lobe epilepsy, especially with more than one seizure type, have a generally poorer prognosis for seizure control (Rodin 1968), and it is understandable therefore that they tend to be treated with more drugs, which may also contribute to the suspected increased psychopathology (see below).

Another difficulty in evaluating reports of the relationship of temporal lobe epilepsy and psychological disorder is variation in the criteria for the diagnosis of temporal lobe epilepsy, and uncertainty as to whether it is the electrical disturbance, the seizures or the underlying pathology that is actually responsible for the mental changes. These problems are illustrated by some of the conflicting reports concerning the chronic schizophrenia-like psychoses associated with temporal lobe epilepsy. The diagnosis of temporal lobe epilepsy was made clinically (complex partial seizures) by Kristensen & Sindrup (1978), clinically and electrically by Flor Henry (1969) and either clinically or electrically by Slater et al (1963). Flor Henry and Kristensen & Sindrup agree that psychomotor seizure frequency is reduced in association with the psychoses, but Slater et al found no particular relationship with seizure frequency. The latter, however, emphasised the mean interval of 14 years between the onset of epilepsy and the onset of psychosis. Kristensen & Sindrup found a median of 21 years, but Flor Henry doubted the aetiological relevance of such an interval based on the evidence of his control material. Flor Henry concluded that the psychosis was fundamentally related to the epileptic process ('antithetical manifestation of the same underlying disturbance of function') rather than any underlying structural brain damage. Kristensen & Sindrup concluded that the psychoses were truly organic, caused by structural damage to the deep limbic parts of the temporal lobe, responsible for both epilepsy and psychoses. Slater et al (1963), although finding a high incidence of organic features and structural lesions underlying the seizures, left open the question of a physiogenic or pathogenic basis for the psychoses. This open-minded attitude still seems appropriate today, both for the schizophrenia-like psychoses, and for many of the other possible psycho-pathological relationships with temporal lobe epilepsy.

Mention should be made here of the very careful study of the neuropsychiatric associations of the pathology found in the resected specimens of the patients undergoing temporal lobectomy at the Guys/Maudsley Neurosurgical Unit (Taylor 1972, 1975; Chapter 17). Taylor discusses in Chapter 17 how psychological variables may be influenced by the laterality of the lesion, the sex and the handedness of the patient, and the nature of the pathology (in this instance mesial temporal sclerosis compared with 'alien tissue' lesions). Further he points out how the psychological effects of the pathological lesion must be viewed in an ontogenetic context. Extension of this approach to include other cerebral pathology, perhaps with CAT scanning, in less selected populations would be valuable.

Flor Henry (1969) first suggested the importance of laterality of the lesion or EEG focus in relation to psychological disorders associated with epilepsy, when he implicated the dominant hemisphere in schizophrenia-like psychoses of epilepsy. The growing literature on this subject is reviewed by Toone in Chapter 10. Stores in Chapter 4 also discusses the influence of sex in relation to the behavioural disorders associated with childhood epilepsy.

ANTICONVULSANT DRUGS

Until recently the chronic administration of anticonvulsant drugs has only rarely been suspected as a cause of mental illness in epilepsy. If referred to at all anticonvulsants have usually appeared at the bottom of the list of aetiological factors (Table 19.1). Most authors have regarded the drugs as relatively harmless to the mental state, apart from the sedative effects of phenobarbitone, irritability and hyperkinetic problems associated with the same drug, mainly in children, and the more florid psychological symptoms associated with acute drug intoxication. In their review of the sparse literature Trimble & Reynolds (1976) found there had been little systematic investigation of the influence of the drugs on mental performance. Lennox (1942) included anticonvulsant drugs among his five possible causes of mental 'decay' in epileptic patients. He incriminated the drugs (at that time phenobarbitone and bromide) in 15 per cent of cases, but, in a later review, (Lennox & Lennox 1960) this was revised downwards to 5 per cent. These figures seem however to have been based on clinical impression. Lennox commented in 1942 that 'many physicians, in attempting to extinguish seizures, only succeeded in drowning the finer intellectual processes of their patient', but added 'that the intelligent and individualistic use of anticonvulsant drugs should not and does not impair the patient's mind.' He also noted that 'strangely enough, properly controlled observations of the side effects of drug therapy seem to be lacking . . . . the careful study of the effect of anticonvulsant drugs on the intellectual processes of normal and epileptic persons is long overdue'. Little or no notice was taken of Lennox's remarks until the last few years, when interest has been stimulated by growing awareness of the chronic toxic effects of the drugs on many tissues, including the nervous system (Reynolds 1975), and by new insight into the more effective use of the drugs following the development of techniques for monitoring them in blood (see Chapter 23). The literature has most recently been reviewed by Trimble (1979).

Subacute or chronic phenytoin encephalopathy

An encephalopathy ('delirium' or 'psychosis') has long been recognised due to intoxication with phenytoin, in association with other physical signs of toxicity, such as nystagmus or ataxia. More recently blood level monitoring of this drug has revealed the occasional more insidious encephalopathy (Trimble & Reynolds 1976). In this syndrome reversible impairment of intellectual function and memory evolve subacutely or chronically, usually in association with a toxic blood level, but in the absence of nystagmus or ataxia. Occasionally unusual neurological signs such as involuntary movements (dyskinesia) have been noted (Chadwick et al 1976). There may be a modest rise in CSF protein and an excess of slow activity on the EEG. This encephalopathy can occur in adults but has been noted particularly in children, especially those with pre-existing mental retardation or brain damage in whom further deterioration in intellectutal function, in the absence of more classical signs of toxicity, may be overlooked or mistakenly regarded as part of an underlying progressive neurological disease (Logan & Freeman 1969).

Mental impairment with non-toxic levels
of anticonvulsant drugs

Although impairment of mental function with toxic levels of phenytoin or other drugs is perhaps understandable, slightly more disconcerting is the possibility that subtle impairment of cognitive function and behaviour leading eventually to mental illness may occur with more modest or 'therapeutic' levels of some anticonvulsants. In a study of 57 epileptic outpatients Reynolds & Travers (1974) found that after exclusion of overt drug toxicity, gross cerebral lesions or mental illness preceding the onset of epilepsy, patients with intellectual deterioration, psychiatric illness, personality change or psychomotor slowing had significantly higher levels of phenytoin or phenobarbitone than those without such changes (Table 19.7). Furthermore the mean blood levels of the two drugs in the patients with mental changes were within the optimum or therapeutic range. These observations were not simply the reflection of higher anticonvulsant prescribing for more severe epilepsy, as similar differences were noted in those patients with infrequent seizures. Similar findings were reported by Trimble & Corbett, cited by Trimble et al (1980), in a study of 312 epileptic children in a residential hospital school. Those children with a fall in IQ of between 10 and 40 points in at least one year had significantly higher levels of phenytoin and primidone, with a similar trend for phenobarbitone. Again the mean blood drug values were within the

Table 19.7   Drug concentrations in relation to psychomotor slowing, intellectual deterioration, psychiatric illness or personality change (from Reynolds & Travers 1974)

		Number	Diphenylhydantoin concentration mean (μg/ml)	P	Phenobarbitone concentration mean (μg/ml)	P
Psychomotor slowing	Present	19	14.5	0.07	16.8	N.S.
	Absent	35	9.1		13.7	
Intellectual deterioration	Present	8	18.0	0.01	19.0	0.07
	Absent	35	7.7		12.6	
Psychiatric illness or personality change	Present	20	15.7		21.0	
	Absent	24	7.0	0.01	12.0	0.01

optimum range. Carbamazepine was also included in this study and no differences in blood level were found between mentally impaired and non-impaired groups.

The suspicion that there may be a causal relationship between relatively higher drug levels and psychological impairment is strengthened by the reported change in mental state that can occur following reduction or cessation of hydantoin or barbiturate drugs (Rosen 1968, Reynolds 1970, Shorvon & Reynolds 1979). Particular improvement has been noted in alertness, concentration, drive, mood and sociability. Further, many patients may be unaware of the adverse effects of the drugs until they are withdrawn, particularly if they have been on the drugs from early life and thus have no concept of how they would feel without drug therapy.

Further support for the view that some drugs subtly affect mental function is now being derived from psychometric investigations. Studies in normal volunteers have shown that phenobarbitone may impair sustained attention and various measures of perceptual-motor performance with low or 'therapeutic' blood levels (Hutt et al 1968), and that low levels of phenytoin can impair some aspects of psychomotor performance (Ideström et al 1972). In a double blind crossover study with placebo, Trimble et al (1980) showed that two weeks administration of phenytoin or carbamazepine could impair some measures of immediate or delayed visual or verbal memory or decision making. In general the differences from placebo were significant for phenytoin but not for carbamazepine (Table 19.8). There were also significant correlations between impaired performance and phenytoin blood levels. Similar studies are now being undertaken on epileptic patients. The need to develop suitably sensitive techniques and the difficulties in controlling for all the many variables in epileptic patients are discussed by Thompson & Huppert (1980), and Tomlinson & Stores (1980).

Although most of the evidence has so far incriminated barbiturate and hydantoin drugs it is also true that these are the most widely used anticonvulsants. Carbamazepine does seem to be relatively free of the adverse effects discussed above, and it may be particularly useful in the treatment of epilepsy associated with psychiatric disorders (see Chapter 23). Comparative psychometric studies of phenytoin and carbamazepine in epileptic patients (Dodrill & Troupin 1977) or normal volunteers (Trimble et al 1980; Table 19.8) certainly suggest that the

Table 19.8 Mean number of correct responses on tests of
memory in normal subjects on phenytoin, carbamazepine or
placebo for two weeks (Thompson et al 1980)

	DPH	Placebo	CBZ	Placebo
Pictures				
Immediate recall	10.9	12.3*	12.1	12.9
Delayed recall	10.1	12.3***	11.1	12.3
Recognition	39.4	39.8	38.6	39.8
Words				
Immediate recall	6.6	8.8**	7.4	8.8
Delayed recall	3.4	6.0*	5.3	6.3
Recognition	30.6	32.4*	31.5	31.6

*P < 0.05;   **P < 0.025;   ***P < 0.01
DPH = phenytoin, CBZ = carbamazepine

latter drug has less adverse effects. However suggestions that carbamazepine has positive psychotropic properties, especially in view of its structural relationship to tricyclic antidepressants, are as yet unproven (Dalby 1975, Parnas et al 1979). The newest drug, sodium valproate, has been less studied. Claims that it, too, is free from harmful psychological effects have been premature. It is certainly capable occasionally of causing an encephalopathy and is frequently responsible for drowsiness, especially in combination with other drugs (Corbett et al 1981). It should also be stressed that the adverse psychological complications of anticonvulsant drugs may often stem as much from the traditional, but largely unnecessary, use of polytherapy, as from the effects of any individual drug (Reynolds & Shorvon 1981). Nevertheless there is a clear need to define more carefully and on a long-term basis the relative impact of the various major anticonvulsants, utilised on their own with blood level monitoring, in both new and chronic patients with epilepsy.

Mechanisms of anticonvulsant effects on mental function
If, as the above evidence suggests, anticonvulsant drugs can impair mental performance, ultimately contributing (along with many other factors discussed in this chapter) to cognitive, psychiatric or personality change, how may these effects by mediated? Adverse effects of barbiturates and hydantoin drugs on many tissues and several metabolic systems have been detected in recent years (Reynolds 1975), and at least some may be relevant to drug-induced mental impairment, although no doubt there are others about which we are ignorant.

1. *Neuropathological damage*
There is clinical and electrical evidence that chronic anticonvulsant therapy may lead to irreversible damage to peripheral nerves, mainly due to polytherapy or perhaps repeated exposure to acute intoxication with phenytoin or barbiturates (Shorvon 1979). If this can occur in the peripheral nervous system one may wonder if neuronal damage can occur in the central nervous system? Clinical and experimental neuropathological studies of the effect of phenytoin on the cerebellum have however been conflicting (Reynolds 1975, Dam 1977).

2. *Folate deficiency*

It is now well established that chronic barbiturate or phenytoin therapy can depress serum, red cell or CSF folate levels in a high proportion of patients (Reynolds 1976). The mechanism of this effect, which is partly related to the blood levels of the drugs, remains uncertain. It has been suggested that prolonged drug-induced folate deficiency may, as with folate deficiency in other clinical situations, sometimes lead to neuropsychiatric complications (Reynolds 1968b, 1976). The deficiency is rarely severe enough to produce megaloblastic anaemia, but it is interesting that when this does occur it is usually associated with various neuropsychiatric disorders, which may also improve on treatment of the anaemia. Several studies have demonstrated a higher incidence of low folate levels in serum, red cells or CSF in adult epileptic patients with mental symptoms than in epileptic subjects with normal mental states (Reynolds 1976). No particular psychiatric diagnosis has been incriminated but the highest incidence of deficiency is associated with depression, psychoses, or especially dementia. However the statistical association between folate deficiency and mental illness does not imply that all epileptic patients with psychological disorders have low folate levels, nor that low folate levels are invariably associated with neuropsychiatric problems. These observations have been extended recently by Trimble et al (1980) studying epileptic children resident in a hospital school. Children with a fall of IQ between 10 and 40 points in at least one year, as well as those with depression and neurotic disturbances had significantly more folate deficiency than children without these problems.

Uncontrolled reports of improvement in the mental state of non-anaemic epileptic patients with folic acid therapy have not been confirmed in controlled trials, but I have argued elsewhere that, for several reasons, the negative trials in these very heterogenous groups do not exclude an effect of the vitamin in some patients (Reynolds 1981).

Many studies of non-epileptic patients (neurological, psychiatric, geriatric), as well as inborn errors of folate metabolism associated with mental retardation, support the concept of neuropsychiatric disease due to folate deficiency (Botez & Reynolds 1979). The subject is however complex, and it is sometimes difficult to distinguish cause, effect or coincidence. A comparative investigation of megaloblastic anaemia due to vitamin B_{12} or folic acid deficiency suggests that, although there is considerable overlap, the former deficiency has a greater impact on spinal cord and peripheral nerve and the latter on cerebral function (Shorvon et al 1980). Further, even in the presence of deficiency of either vitamin severe enough to produce megaloblastic anaemia as many as one third had no neuropsychiatric complications. This is likely to apply to a much higher proportion in the milder drug-induced deficiency associated with epilepsy. It seems probable that it is the interaction of the deficiency with other factors that may lead to neuropsychiatric sequelae in some.

3. *Monoamine metabolism*

It is widely believed that disturbances in cerebral monoamine metabolism may underlie or contribute to a variety of psychiatric, especially affective disorders. It has been known for some years that many anticonvulsant drugs influence brain levels of indoleamines, especially serotonin (Bonnycastle et al 1957, Chadwick et al 1977). Recently it has been reported in epileptic subjects that phenobarbitone and phenytoin may elevate CSF levels of tryptophan, 5-hydroxyindole acetic acid (5-HIAA) and homovanillic acid (HVA), and by implication influence indoleamine and catecholamine metabolism (Chadwick et al 1977). A more recent study (Young et al 1980) found no significant differences in CSF indices of indoleamine metabolism between treated and untreated epileptics except for a slight lowering of CSF 5-HIAA in the latter. However, it should be noted that the 'untreated' group in this study were chronic epileptic patients in whom the drugs had been withdrawn a week earlier.

The effect of the drugs on monoamine metabolism is again highly complex and several different mechanisms may be operating, one of which is that the drugs may reduce the activity of the serotonergic system (Chadwick et al 1978). Again the possibility has to be considered that such effects may contribute to psychological, especially mood, disorders in epileptic subjects (Trimble et al 1975), but this has yet to be investigated. There are also interesting possible relationships between folate and monoamine metabolism (Reynolds 1976, Botez et al 1979, Turner 1980).

4. *Hormone metabolism*

Another possible area with implications for mental function is the growing evidence of subtle effects of several anticonvulsants on endocrine function (Reynolds 1975, London 1980). The study of the clinical implications will probably have to await clarification of the nature, mechanisms and individual drug contributions to these hormonal changes.

HEREDITY

Although genetic factors have been investigated to a limited extent in relation to cognitive function in epilepsy (see Chapter 12), there is an extraordinary lack of information in relation to personality and psychiatric disorders. This is all the more remarkable in view of the widespread view in the 19th century that psychological deterioration of various kinds was a frequent and perhaps inevitable accompaniment of epilepsy on a *genetic* basis (see Chapters 1 and 12). Although such views have rightly been discarded it seems the pendulum may have swung very far in the opposite direction. A recent book on the genetics of epilepsy (Newmark & Penry 1979) does not mention psychiatric aspects. A comprehensive textbook of organic psychiatry (Lishman 1978) includes in the section on epilepsy, reference only to the absence of a genetic background to schizophrenia-like psychoses, based on the study of Slater et al (1963). As genetic factors have been shown to be important in many psychiatric disorders outside the field of epilepsy it would seem likely that they have some role to play also within this field. There would appear to be a need to investigate the role of genetics in the psychiatry of epilepsy with modern methods.

CONCLUSIONS

I have reviewed the contribution of several biological factors — seizures, brain damage, drugs and heredity — to the psychological disorders that frequently accompany epilepsy. It is clear that our knowledge of the role of each varies from inadequate to, in the case of heredity, almost non-existent. Brain damage is perhaps the most widely accepted of these factors but has been the subject of very little systematic investigation. Its role in the psychiatric disorders associated for example with temporal lobe epilepsy, and the influence of localised or diffuse pathology elsewhere, remains uncertain. The contribution of the seizures themselves is complex and controversial. I have discussed a number of mechanisms as a result of which seizure activity might exert an adverse influence on mental function (in addition to the obvious psychosocial ones, see Chapter 20), but the issues are sometimes confounded by potentially beneficial effects of generalised seizures (cf. convulsive therapy) in a few instances, and by the introduction of EEG data! The role of anticonvulsant therapy has been greatly underestimated in the past, but with the advent of blood level monitoring, leading to more rational prescribing (see Chapter 23), and a greater knowledge of the metabolic consequences of prolonged treatment, a relatively greater influence of the drugs on psychological function is beginning to emerge.

It is an understatement to say that the study of each of these factors is a complex matter in its own right. I have illustrated how even one aspect of one factor i.e. drug-induced folate deficiency, is a highly complex subject. There is clearly a need to explore all the factors in much more detail. Several techniques such as CAT scanning, blood drug and other metabolic measurements, more sophisticated EEG monitoring and more precise analysis of seizures and psychopathology are all available now to facilitate this process. The importance of simultaneously examining or controlling for all the variables discussed needs stressing. The widely varying opinions about biological and psychosocial factors in the past literature have stemmed in large measure from the examination of individual factors e.g. brain damage or temporal lobe foci, while ignoring so many of the other factors, especially drugs or heredity. Ultimately I suspect that it is the interaction between these many factors which will prove to be crucial in the genesis of many of the psychiatric disorders associated with epilepsy. Further, as stressed by Taylor (Chapter 17) both epilepsy and associated psychological disorders are often long-term problems beginning in childhood, and must be viewed ontogenetically.

Encouragement for a more intensive exploration of the psychiatric aspects of epilepsy may be derived not only from the size of the problem but also from the potential light it may shed on biological and psychosocial mechanisms in other psychiatric disorders. The study of epilepsy has greatly illuminated neurology from the time of Jackson and Gowers a century ago. There are many reasons to suspect that it can do the same for psychiatry. In no other psychiatric disorder can the simultaneous operation of such overt metabolic/pharmacological, physiological, pathological, genetic and psychosocial factors be so readily studied together. Despite the complexity of this challenge the isolation and interaction of these processes is surely relevant to our understanding of other psychiatric disorders, as well as to more basic issues such as the mode of action of convulsive therapy.

References

Alving, J 1978 Classification of the epilepsies. An investigation of 1508 consecutive adult patients. Acta neurol scand 58:205–212

Bear D M, Fedio E 1977 Quantitative analysis of interictal behaviour in temporal lobe epilepsy. Arch neurol 34:454–467

Betts T A 1974 A follow-up study of a cohort of patients with epilepsy admitted to psychiatric care in an English city. In: Harris P, Mawdsley C (eds) Epilepsy: proceedings of the Hans Berger centenary symposium. Churchill Livingstone, Edinburgh, p 326–336

Bonnycastle D D, Giarman N J, Paasonen M K 1957 Anticonvulsant compounds and 5-hydroxytryptamine in rat brain. Br J Pharmac 12:228–231

Botez M I, Reynolds E H (eds) 1979 Folic acid in neurology, psychiatry and internal medicine. Raven Press, New York.

Botez M I, Young S N, Bachevalier J, Gauthier S 1979 Folate deficiency and decreased brain 5-hydroxytryptamine synthesis in man and rat. Nature 278:182–183

Browne T R, Penry J K, Porter R J, Dreifuss F E 1974 Responsiveness before, during and after spike-wave paroxysm. Neurology 24:659–665

Cavazzuti G B, Cappella L, Nalin A 1980 Longitudinal study of epileptiform EEG patterns in normal children. Epilepsia 21:43–55

Chadwick D, Reynolds E H, Marsden C D 1976 Anticonvulsant-induced dyskinesias: a comparison with dyskinesias induced by neuroleptics. J Neurol Neurosurg Psychiat 39:1210–1218

Chadwick D, Jenner P, Reynolds E H 1977 Serotonin metabolism in human epilepsy. Ann Neurol 1:218–224

Chadwick D, Gorrod J W, Jenner P, Marsden C D, Reynolds E H 1978 Functional changes in cerebral 5-hydroxytryptamine metabolism in the mouse induced by anticonvulsant drugs. Br J Pharmac 62:115–124

Corbett J, Driver M, Reynolds E H 1981 Valproate encephalopathy. Communication to British branch of the International League against Epilepsy, April 1980 (in preparation)

Currie S, Heathfield W G, Henson R A, Scott D F 1971 Clinical course and prognosis of temporal lobe epilepsy. A survey of 666 patients. Brain 94:173–190

Dalby M A 1975 Behavioural effects of carbamazepine. In: Penry J K, Daly D D (eds) Complex partial seizures and their treatment. Raven Press, New York, p 331–344

Dam M 1977 Chronic toxicity of antiepileptic drugs. In: Meinardi H, Rowan A J (eds) Advances in epileptology. Swets and Zietlinger B V Lisse, p 330–339

Davison K, Bagley C R 1969 Schizophrenia-like psychoses associated with organic disorders of the central nervous system: a review of the literature. In: Herrington R N (ed) Current problems in neuropsychiatry Br J Psychiat Special publication no 4. Headley Brothers, Ashford

Dodrill C E, Troupin A S 1977 Psychotropic effect of carbamazepine in epilepsy: a double blind comparison with phenytoin. Neurology 27:1023–1028

Dongier S 1959 Statistical study of clinical and electroencephalographic manifestations of 536 psychotic episodes occurring in 516 epileptics between clinical seizures. Epilepsia 1:117–142

Falconer M A 1974 Mesial temporal (Ammon's horn) sclerosis as a common cause of epilepsy: aetiology, treatment and prevention. Lancet 2:767–770

Flor-Henry P 1969 Psychosis and temporal lobe epilepsy. A controlled investigation. Epilepsia 10:363–398

Freedman R, Taylor D A, Seiger A, Olson L, Hoffer B J 1979 Seizures and related epileptiform activity in hippocampus transplanted to the anterior chamber of the eye: modulation by cholinergic and adrenergic input. Ann Neurol 6:281–295

Gastaut H 1976 Conclusions: computerized transverse axial tomography in epilepsy. Epilepsia 17:337–338

Gastaut H, Gastaut J L 1976 Computerized transverse axial tomography in epilepsy. Epilepsia 17:325–335

Goddard G V, McIntyre D C, Leech C K 1969 A permanent change in brain function resulting from daily electrical stimulation. Exper Neurol 25:296–330

Goode D J, Penry J K, Dreifus F E 1970 Effects of paroxysmal spike/wave on continuous visual motor performance. Epilepsia 11:241–254

Gowers W R 1881 Epilepsy and other chronic convulsive disorders. Churchill, London

Graham P, Rutter M 1968 Organic brain dysfunction and child psychiatric disorder. Br med J 3:695–700

Green A R, Nutt D J, Cowen P J 1981 The increased seizure threshold following convulsion. In: Sandler M (ed) The psychopharmacology of anticonvulsants. A British Association of Psychopharmacology monograph. Oxford University Press

Gudmundsson G 1966 Epilepsy in Iceland. A clinical and epidemiological investigation. Acta neurol scand supplement 25

Guerrant J, Anderson W W, Fischer A, Weinstein M R, Jaros R M, Deskins A 1962 Personality in epilepsy. Thomas, Springfield

Herberg L J, Tress K H, Blundell J E 1969 Raising the threshold in experimental epilepsy by hypothalamic and septal stimulation and by audiogenic seizures. Brain 92:313–328

Hill D 1952 EEG in episodic psychotic and psychopathic behaviour. Electroenceph Neurophysiol 4:419–442

Hommes O R, Hollinger J L, Jansen N J T, Schoofs M, van der Weil Th, Kok J C N 1979 Convulsant properties of folate compounds: some considerations and speculations. In: Botez M I, Reynolds E H (eds) Folic acid in neurology, psychiatry, and internal medicine. Raven Press, New York, p 285–316

Hutt S J, Jackson P M, Belsham A N, Higgins G 1968 Perceptual motor behaviour in relation to blood phenobarbitone level. Develop Med Child Neurol 10:626–632

Ideström C M, Schalling D, Carlquist U, Sjöquist F 1972 Behavioural and psychophysiological studies: acute effects of diphenylhydantoin in relation to plasma levels. Psychol Med 2:111–120

Jensen I, Larsen, J K 1979 Mental aspects of temporal lobe epilepsy. J Neurol Neurosurg Psychiat 42:256–265

Kristensen O, Sindrup E H 1978 Psychomotor epilepsy and psychosis. 1. Physical aspects. Acta neurol scand 57:361–369

Landolt H 1958 Serial electroencephalographic investigations during psychotic episodes in epileptic patients and during schizophrenic attacks. In: Lorentz de Haas A M (ed) Lectures on epilepsy. Elsevier, Amsterdam, p 91–133

Lennox W G 1942 Brain injury, drugs and environment as causes of mental decay in epilepsy. Am J Psychiat 99:174–180

Lennox W G Lennox M A 1960 Epilepsy and related disorders vol 1 & 2. Little Brown, Boston

Lishman W A 1968 Brain damage in relation to psychiatric disability after head injury. Br J Psychiat 114:373–410

Lishman W A 1978 Organic psychiatry Blackwell Scientific Publications, Oxford

London D R 1980 Hormonal effects of anticonvulsant drugs. In Canger R, Angeleri F, Penry J K (eds). Advances in epileptology. Raven Press, New York, p 399–405

Logan W J, Freeman J M 1969 Pseudodegenerative disease due to diphenylhydantoin intoxication. Arch Neurol 21:631–637

Margerison J H, Corsellis J A N 1966 Epilepsy and the temporal lobes—a clinical, electroencephalographic and neuropathological study of the brain in epilepsy with particular reference to the temporal lobes. Brain 89:499–530

Marsden C D, Reynolds E H 1981 Neurology. In: Laidlaw J, Richens A (eds) A textbook of epilepsy. Churchill Livingstone, Edinburgh

Meduna L 1937 Die Konvulsionstherapie der Schizophrenie. Halle

Meldrum B S 1975 Present views of hippocampal sclerosis and epilepsy. In: Williams D (ed) Modern trends in neurology no. 6 Butterworths, London p 223–239

Meldrum B S 1981 Neuropathology and pathophysiology. In: Laidlaw J, Richens A (eds) A textbook of epilepsy. Churchill Livingstone, Edinburgh

Metrakos J D, Metrakos K 1960 Genetics of convulsive disorders. 1. Problems, methods and baselines. Neurology 10:228–240

Mirsky A F, van Buren J M 1965 On the nature of the 'absence' in centrencephalic epilepsy: a study of some behavioral, electroencephalographic and autonomic factors. Electroenceph Neurophysiol 18:334–348

Newmark M E, Penry J K 1979 Photosensitivity and epilepsy: a review. Raven Press, New York

Nuffield E J A 1961 Neuro-physiology and behaviour disorders in epileptic children. J Ment Sci 107:438–458

Ounsted C, Lindsay J, Norman R 1966 Biological factors in temporal lobe epilepsy. Heinemann, London

Parnas J, Flachs H, Gram L 1979 Psychotropic effect of antiepileptic drugs. Acta neurol scand 16:329–343

Penfield W 1967 Epilepsy, the great teacher. Acta neurol scand 43:1–10

Penry J K 1973 Behaviour correlates of generalised spike-wave discharge in the electroencephalogram. In: Brazier M A B (ed) Epilepsy: its phenomenon in man. Academic Press, London, p 171–188

Pond D A 1961 Psychiatric aspects of epileptic and brain-damaged children. Br med J 2:1377–1382

Pond D A, Bidwell B H 1960 A survey of epilepsy in 14 general practices 2. social and psychological aspects. Epilepsia 1:285–299

Rausch R, Lieb J P, Crandall P H 1978 Neuropsychologic correlates of depth spike activity in epileptic patients. Arch neurol 35:699–705

Reynolds E H 1968a Epilepsy and schizophrenia. Relationship and biochemistry. Lancet 1:398–401

Reynolds E H 1968b Mental effects of anticonvulsants and folic acid metabolism. Brain 91:197–294

Reynolds E H 1970 Iatrogenic disorders in epilepsy. In: Williams D (ed) Modern trends in neurology. No. 5. Butterworths, London, p 271–286

Reynolds E H 1975 Chronic antiepileptic toxicity: a review. Epilepsia 16:319–352

Reynolds E H 1976 Neurological aspects of folate and vitamin B_{12} metabolism. In: Hoffbrand A V (ed) Clinics in Haematology 5. W. B. Saunders, Philadelphia, p 661–696

Reynolds E H 1981 Anticonvulsant drugs, folate metabolism and mental symptoms. In: Proceedings of the 12th epilepsy international symposium, Copenhagen. Raven Press, New York

Reynolds E H, Travers R D 1974 Serum anticonvulsant concentrations in epileptic patients with mental symptoms. Br J Psychiat 124:440–445

Reynolds E H, Shorvon S D 1981 Monotherapy or polytherapy for epilepsy? Epilepsia 22:1–10

Rodin E A 1968 The prognosis of patients with epilepsy. Thomas, Springfield

Rodin E A, Katz M, Lennox K 1976 Differences between patients with temporal lobe seizures and those with other forms of epileptic attacks. Epilepsia 17:313–320

Rosen J A 1968 Dilantin dementia. Transactions of the American Neurological Association 93:273

Shorvon S D 1979 Anticonvulsant therapy and peripheral neuropathy. In: Botez M I, Reynolds E H (eds) Folic acid in neurology, psychiatry and internal medicine. Raven Press, New York p 335–347

Shorvon S D, Reynolds E H 1979 Reduction of polypharmacy for epilepsy. Br med J 2:1023–1025

Shorvon S D, Carney M W P, Chanarin I, Reynolds E H 1980 The neuropsychiatry of megaloblastic anaemia. Br med J 281:1036–1043

Slater E, Beard A W, Glithero E 1963 The schizophrenia-like psychoses of epilepsy. Br J Psychiat 109:95–150

Stevens J R 1966 Psychiatric implications of psychomotor epilepsy. Arch Gen Psychiat 14:461–471

Stevens J R 1975 Interictal clinical manifestations of complex partial seizures. In: Penry J K, Daly D D (eds) Complex partial seizures and their treatment. Raven Press, New York, p 85–112

Stevens J R 1977 All that spikes is not fits. In: Shagass C, Gershon S, Friedhoff A J (eds) Psychopathology and brain dysfunction. Raven Press, New York

Stevens J R, Livermore A 1978 Kindling of the mesolimbic dopamine system: animal model of psychosis. Neurology 28:36–46

Stores G 1973 Studies of attention and seizure disorders. Devel med child neurol 15:376–382

Taylor D C 1972 Mental state and temporal lobe epilepsy. A correlative account of 100 patients treated surgically. Epilepsia 13:727–765

Taylor D C 1975 Factors influencing the occurrence of schizophrenia-like psychosis in patients with temporal lobe epilepsy. Psychol Med 5:249–254

Thompson P J, Huppert F 1980 Problems in the development of measures to test cognitive performance in adult epileptic patients. In: Kulig B, Meinardi H, Stores G (eds) Epilepsy and behaviour '79. Swets & Zeitlinger B.V. Lisse, p 37–42

Tomlinson L, Stores G 1980 The choice of measures in drug studies of people with epilepsy. In: Kulig B, Meinardi H, Stores G (eds) Epilepsy and behaviour '79. Swets and Zeitlinger B.V. Lisse, p 67–75

Trimble M 1977 The relationship between epilepsy and schizophrenia: a biochemical hypothesis. Biol Psychiat 12:299–304

Trimble M 1979 The effect of anti-convulsant drugs on cognitive abilities. Pharmac Ther 4:677–685

Trimble M, Reynolds E H 1976 Anticonvulsant drugs and mental symptoms. A review. Psychol Med 6:169–178

Trimble M R, Meldrum B S 1979 Monoamines, epilepsy and schizophrenia. In: Obiols J, Ballus E, Gonzales M, Pujol J (eds) Biological psychiatry today Elsevier, Amsterdam, p 470–475

Trimble M R, Chadwick D, Reynolds E H, Marsden C D 1975 L-5-hydroxytryptophan and mood. Lancet 1:583

Trimble M R, Perez M M 1980 Quantification of psychopathology in adult patients with epilepsy. In: Kulig B, Meinardi H, Stores G (eds) Epilepsy and behaviour '79. Swets and Zeitlinger B.V. Lisse, p 118–126

Trimble M R, Thompson P J, Huppert F 1980 Anticonvulsant drugs and cognitive abilities. In: Canger R, Angeleri F, Penry J K (eds) Advances in epileptology. Raven Press, New York, p 199–204

Trimble M R, Corbett J, Donaldson 1980 Folic acid and mental symptoms in children with epilepsy. J Neurol Neurosurg Psychiat 43:1030–1034.

Turner A J 1980 Folate/amine relationships. In: Parsonage M J (ed) Aspects of epilepsy. MCS Consultants, Tunbridge Wells, p 103–107

Vislie H, Henriksen G F 1958 Psychic disturbances in epilepsy In: Lorentz de Haas A M (ed) Lectures on epilepsy. Elsevier, Amsterdam, p 327–331

Wada J A (ed) 1976 Kindling. Raven Press, New York

Yang P J, Berger P E, Cohen M E, Duffner P K 1979 Computed tomography and childhood seizure disorders. Neurology 29:1084–1088

Young S N, Gauthier S, Anderson G M, Purdy W C 1980 Tryptophan, 5-hydroxyindole acetic acid and indoleacetic acid in human cerebrospinal fluid: interrelationships and the influence of age, sex, epilepsy and anticonvulsant drugs. J Neurol Neurosurg Psychiat 43:438–445

Psycho-social aspects of epilepsy — the family

This chapter will deal mainly with the impact on the sufferer and his or her family of 'being epileptic', a term formerly as emotive as being a leper or consumptive. The approach is similar to that of Dr Helen Pond who has been concerned for a number of years with the care of diabetic children who suffer, as epileptic patients do, from a life-time condition that requires daily treatment and is also punctuated by the threat of attacks with loss or impairment of consciousness.

In recent years Talcott Parsons and other medical sociologists have elaborated the concept of the *sick-rôle* which, as Marinker (1969) has well described, must be distinguished from the *disease* (the doctors' shorthand for the medical condition) and the *illness*, which is what the patient suffers from and complains about. The *sick-rôle* is largely determined by the pattern of family interaction in response to the threat of an illness. As far as we know this has little or nothing to do with whatever caused the epilepsy. The social class distribution of epilepsy is certainly affected by a 'drift-down' from disability, but the families of origin are probably normally distributed, though such occasional causes of epilepsy as severe non-accidental injury introduce a slight bias towards disturbed families.

The family responses may conveniently be considered under the following headings (Pond 1979):

1. Attitude to aetiology and hereditary factors
2. Attitudes of parents to their sick child
3. Attitudes of parents to treatment
4. Attitudes of parents to doctors and other members of the medical team
5. Attitudes of parents to each other, and the siblings, if any.

The moment of first diagnosis is disturbing as the word 'epilepsy' still often conjures up the idea of an hereditary degenerative stigma. There may be denial, sometimes in collusion with the doctor — 'It's just a convulsion, not epilepsy' — with the vital final word, 'yet', omitted. If, unusually, the cause is known, fears of heredity can commonly be laid and the prognosis discussed. More often 'idiopathic' is used to cover ignorance and the parents are left to speculate on whether they might have caused it by, for example, some minor accidental bang on the head. 'Battering' is in a different class and needs its own special approach by the paediatric team who has to be alert to its possibility when the epilepsy develops months or years after the non-accidental injury. Some guilt-ridden families think the condition is caused by psychological trauma to the child arising from their own inter-personal difficulties. It is important to make clear that epilepsy is an 'organic' condition, however much the frequency and timing of attacks is influenced by 'stress'. Denial, projection and introjection may thus all be seen in family responses to the diagnosis and later in the treatment of the afflicted child.

The fear of attacks occurring in potentially dangerous situations is very powerful—and understandably so in some children with frequent seizures. If he is 5 minutes late from school, perhaps he is under a bus; the bedroom door ought to be left open so that nocturnal fits can be heard and attended to, or the child can be watched unobtrusively and regularly in case he is suffocating; teachers may reinforce parents' anxiety over the dangers of physical exercise, especially gym and swimming. The child's response to these restrictions is variable; some rebel (especially in adolescence) and tantrums and violence may result: these are not to be regarded as epileptic equivalents or some such idea which allows them to be treated by more anticonvulsants or the addition of other drugs. Others acquiesce more or less reluctantly and this may go on to contribute to the passivity or withdrawal that characterises some chronic epileptics.

As regards the treatment, patient compliance (or adherence, to use the now-preferred term) is variable. Sometimes it is meticulous with parents imposing a complicated and unnecessary distribution of the pills over the whole day. This often goes with elaborate notes on the frequency and timing of seizures and demands for changes every time another fit occurs. Other parents are quite vague about dosage or are happy to leave it to the child which in one way is a good thing as it encourages self-reliance, but it may be difficult for him to appreciate the necessity of carrying on long after he is fit-free and apparently perfectly well. Side effects of anticonvulsants are now well known to parents and others who may gratuitously offer advice to stop taking dangerous poisons. Doctors are now better aware than they were that some of these complaints may have substance, so each case needs judging on its own merits, balancing fit-control with undesirable side effects. At the same time, the family doctor should assess whether complaints of slowness or behaviour disturbance may be projected onto the drugs or the fits by parents or child whereas in fact they may be due to family tensions that may have little or nothing to do with the epilepsy. To be effective, such advice on this (and other) matters should come from a known and trusted doctor, usually the general practitioner. Unfortunately hospital follow-up clinics for 'old patients' are often staffed by rapidly rotating inexperienced junior doctors who may be less well-equipped than the general practitioner who turns to them for consultant advice.

As the condition continues so family attitudes tend to harden, but a variety of reactions may be seen. At one extreme, often as a continuation of early denial, the child will be expected to be 'normal' in every way. This is often a good thing as regards encouraging self-reliance and responsibility for managing their own treatment, but can be disastrous as regards intelligence and school performance, if, as often happens, the child cannot compete equally with non-handicapped peers. At the other extreme the patient may be so watched over as to feel 'smothered' not mothered. At times even the diagnosis may be kept from the sufferer—I once saw an intelligent man in his 30s whose ageing middle-class parents still looked after his drugs telling him that he was a lifelong sufferer from migraine, not epilepsy! Extreme reactions always imply intense anxiety on the part of the parents for whom the epilepsy must mean something other than the realities of the condition. Sometimes a fancied connection with some irrelevant family skeleton is made.

Instead of denial, some parents may use the rather opposite mechanism of rejection. It can be of the disease itself (an example above is given) but more often it is of the unfortunate sufferer who may in some way be extruded by the family, for example to a special residential school; or he or she may be written off as untrainable or ineducable, not worth wasting time on. The long-term consequences of the condition begin to come home in adolescence, and Goffmann's concept of stigma is of use in understanding what may happen. Hodgman et al (1979), testing a small group of epileptic adolescents, found (paradoxically, they thought) that those least disabled had the most communication difficulties with peers and parents. One third of their group had IQs below 80 and were thus educationally subnormal. This finding suggests to me that the level of aspiration of the more severely disabled was much lower than the others, with acceptance by both schools and parents that they were unlikely to lead a normal, wholly independent social life. In contrast, the less disabled aimed to pass for normal socially and in employment. They had a fear of failure, even of shameful discovery of the stigma, similar to those blacks who try to 'make white' in an apartheid society. Ryan et al (1980) showed that the extent to which persons with epilepsy feel stigmatized by the disorder does not bear any close relationship to the severity of the individual seizures. It is much more closely related to psychosocial factors, such as the person's perception of employment discrimination and social limitations, and the number of years of schooling the person has had.

Epilepsy beginning in adult life does not usually pose as many problems as the sufferer probably has a stable home and job. The position is of course different if the fits are part of a serious progressive neurological disorder, but in these cases the other symptoms usually cause more difficulty than the fits. Stable adults starting the disorder are usually well accepted at work, their mates or colleagues often 'carrying' them and making every allowance for the occasional disruption from a fit. Chapter 21 deals in more detail with these general social topics.

The management of the psychosocial problems of persons with epilepsy should be an integral part of the medical treatment. This implies that relatively few cases need referral to a psychiatrist, though of course they have an important role with the more serious non-ictal disorders, especially the psychoses. In a busy clinic dealing with many patients a specially experienced social worker or similar paramedical is useful as counsellor. He or she is often more likely to be relatively permanent in contrast to constantly changing trainee doctors, and so represent the stability and continuity of personal care that patients with long-term disabilities crave for and deserve. Many years ago Mrs Bidwell and I thought that an average of about five consultations spread over weeks or months enabled most patients (and families) to have not only the correct drug treatment but also adequate opportunities to talk over the associated problems of 'coming to terms' with the condition.

The common problems seen in many families have mostly already been described but are worth enumerating again. There are problems about parental and family roles in the cause, such as genetic influences; the role of physical damage, real or feared; and the influence of psychological tensions and stresses. There may be worries over management — especially possible side-effects of drugs, how to manage non-compliance and discipline generally, and what sort of restriction to place on physical activity. Longer-term fears concern employability, the chances of marriage and the risks of parenthood, and, if the patient is seriously disabled (usually because of associated handicaps, especially subnormality), who will look after him when the care-givers (parents usually) can no longer cope. So common are most of these worries that it is sometimes helpful for the doctor or social worker to raise them before the parents themselves formulate their own fears and worries. It is often a relief to them to discover that 'you have been there before' and can anticipate their predicaments. Needless to say, there are no pat answers, and it is essential for the counsellor to know as much as possible about the medical facts and prognosis of the individual person under discussion. The ever present risk of suicide (see Chapter 7) perhaps years later must be borne in mind, especially by the general practitioner.

There are a few comments to be made on the specific roles of the psychiatrist both for children and adults. A few of us who have taken a special interest in epilepsy may be of particular help in the awkward problems of the differential diagnosis of attacks. Even if having proven epilepsy, patients may also have psychogenic seizures, and their diagnosis requires a full psychiatric assessment. Then there is the more general problem of behaviour disorders associated with epilepsy but not obviously directly related in timing to seizures. How much they may be due to 'organic' factors and how much to psychosocial stresses is discussed elsewhere in this book, and the psychiatrist may be of particular help in sorting this out. Williams et al (1979) discuss this matter in relation to uncontrolled seizures, but do not specifically say that epileptic fits as opposed to psychogenic seizures were diminished after psychiatric intervention.

There are plenty of anecdotes and personal experiences of patients' fit frequency being dramatically reduced by psychotherapy, but a proper controlled trial is so far lacking and would indeed be difficult to mount. As a general rule one may say that the prime task of psychiatric treatment in difficult cases with much obvious psychological disturbance in the patient (and usually in the family) is to try and isolate the epilepsy from the psychiatric disorder and treat both more or less separately and appropriately. This may take some time, but once the family accept that there is a psychological problem existing in its own right, as it were, from the dynamics of the situation, perhaps exacerbated or precipitated by the epilepsy but not mainly caused by it, then the way is clear to treat it by individual or other psychotherapy as appropriate.

References

Hodgman C M, McAnamey E R, Myers G J, Iker H 1979 Emotional complications of adolescent grand mal epilepsy. Journal of Pediatrics 95:309–312

Marinker M 1969 The general practitioner as family doctor. Journal of the Royal College of General Practitioners 17:227–236

Pond H 1979 Parental attitudes toward children with a chronic medical disorder: special reference to diabetes mellitus. Diabetes Care 2:425–431

Ryan R, Kempner K, Emlen A C 1980 The stigma of epilepsy as a self-concept. Epilepsia 21, 4:433–435

Williams D T et al 1979 Impact of psychiatric intervention on patients with uncontrolled seizures. Journal of Nervous and Mental Diseases 167:626–631

Social aspects

INTRODUCTION

The purpose of this chapter is to review the part played by epilepsy in affecting the choices open to the individual in developing his life-style. It will conclude by examining the social consequences for someone who has epilepsy accompanied by a psychiatric disorder or by a mental deficit, and also by discussing the role of the social worker in the management of these situations.

Before discussing the social aspects of epilepsy and what it means to the individual to have epileptic fits, it is desirable to restate a few very simple principles. First, that there are many different types of epilepsy in many different people and that these are frequently due to many different causes. When discussing the aetiology of epilepsy, classifying seizures or selecting appropriate therapy the importance of this fact is readily accepted by the physician. However, it is frequently forgotten when considering the social outlook for someone who is diagnosed as suffering from epilepsy. Time and time again those of us who are concerned in the care and treatment of people with epilepsy fall into the error of thinking that 'an epileptic' cannot follow a particular way of living, should not be permitted to pursue certain occupations or take part in some leisure activity or another.

It is very much open to question whether it is ever justifiable to label someone as an epileptic. It may be argued that someone who is currently experiencing frequent epileptic fits or who requires institutional care may be considered to be an epileptic, but it is often difficult to know where one draws the line between epileptic and not epileptic. How many attacks and how frequently should they occur to justify the label? Do we accept that once an individual has experienced a series of attacks he or she should ever after be considered to be an epileptic? For example is it reasonable to apply this label to someone who had Rolandic epilepsy and has experienced no more fits since adolescence? My second principle is that so far as possible we should avoid labelling anyone 'an epileptic'. It is a label which is almost always socially damaging and once it is attached to an individual it is very difficult to have it detached. It is a label which is scientifically inaccurate unless we define how many fits in the past, now or in the future go to make up an epileptic.

Thirdly any consideration of social aspects demands a distinction between having epilepsy and having fits. Even when we have done so we are not always on safe ground. Rodin (1968) has shown that the presence or absence of epileptic fits does not correlate with employability. In the sample he studied for the Vocational Rehabilitation Service in Michigan he looked at 172 patients with epilepsy and found 88 were employed and 84 were unemployed. 44 patients had less than one fit a year, and of these 32 were employed and 12 were unemployed. 32 patients had several fits a week but of these 13 were employed and 19 unemployed. Other studies support his conclusion that one must look further than the occurrence of epileptic fits in an individual if one is to make some forecast of his success in life.

The several ways in which epileptic fits in early childhood may influence the individual's attitude towards himself and his condition have been discussed by Pond (Chapter 20). Some people seem to ride through childhood epilepsy with no obvious sign that this experience has made much difference to their lives. Others are not so fortunate, and may appear to go through a whole series of misfortunes — failure in school; inability to prepare for or follow employment; difficulties in making social adjustments; and broken marriages which are rightly or wrongly thought to be due to having epilepsy. It is this group who most frequently come within the purpose of this study and the scope of this volume.

Social aspects of epilepsy

Epilepsy is often a secondary handicap. It is not so much having fits which constitutes the problem for many people with epilepsy. The attitudes of people around them can be a great deal more important. The origins of prejudice about epilepsy are extremely debatable. Medical anthropologists have recorded some bizarre ideas which primitive people have about epilepsy. Aall-Jilek (1965), in her study of the Wapo Goro, reported that the people were ashamed to have a person with epilepsy in the family, and would prefer to hide the afflicted person in a hut away from strangers. They feared to touch someone in a seizure, believing that the evil spirits could leap over into someone near. They particularly feared excreta and saliva, and many people with epilepsy suffered from terrible burns because no one dared help them if they fell into the fire. Orley (1970) has reported in detail the social consequences for sufferers from epilepsy in Uganda, such as being compelled to live in a separate hut, eat out of separate bowls and have no contact with other members of the family. Primitive treatment is often based on the idea that if the patient can be made to vomit he will get rid of the cause of his fits, and this has led to some strange and unpleasant concoctions being recommended for the unfortunate patient. The attitudes of people who consider themselves far advanced in civilisation and education sometimes carry strange undertones of these primitive beliefs about epilepsy. What other explanation is there for the fact that some parents would not wish to have their children at school or at play with a child who has epilepsy?

Gunn (Chapter 13) has described the attempts to measure public attitudes. One is encouraged by the signs that there appears to be a steady improvement in the attitude towards epilepsy. Unfortunately a number of people continue to report experiences which suggest that all is not so well as opinion polls would have us believe. It is possible that when answering a questionnaire people give a more favourable reply in accord with their own self-esteem, but that their reaction is different when faced with a real-life situation. Thanks to advances in therapy few people see epileptic fits in public nowadays.

A recent assessment of family reactions to epilepsy was provided by Bower & Ward (1978) who studied the families of 81 children with epilepsy. All except four of the parents interviewed expressed fear or horror on seeing their child for the first time in an epileptic seizure. It is interesting to note that 21 parents had some professional knowledge of epilepsy (mainly as nurses), but this did not render them immune to the same reactions as other parents. Two out of three parents connected the diagnosis with some form of mental handicap or mental disorder. Anyone who has spoken to lay groups about epilepsy will not be surprised to know that one quarter of parents expressed fears about hereditary aspects. I have rarely addressed any meeting where the question 'Is it inherited?' has not been asked.

About the same time as the above study was carried out Harker (1977), a community physician, also in Oxford, was looking at the impact of febrile convulsions in children on mothers attending local clinics. He reported that the first thought of one half of the mothers seeing a child with febrile convulsions was that the child was dead or dying.

The child who has epilepsy goes to school with the awareness that he is different from other children. Strange things happen to him. He has to take tablets or some other regular medication which may not always be agreeable. He may be subject to a number of prohibitions. He will be aware that his parents are anxious about him. The attitude of the teachers in his school will often be coloured by their own anxiety, expecially about the likelihood of any action on their part liable to cause him to have a fit.

The progress of children with epilepsy has been studied in a number of ways by Rutter and colleagues (1970), Butler (1972) and by Holdsworth & Whitmore (1975). The Isle of Wight survey (Rutter et al 1970) gives some indication of the extent to which growing up with epilepsy may mark the child himself. Teachers were asked to assess the behaviour of children with epilepsy who were known to them. They considered that such children were more likely than the average child to be solitary, irritable, unresponsive and not much liked by other children.

The National Child Development study (Butler 1972) found that three out of five children with epilepsy were in normal schools and about one half of these were making good progress. The Isle of Wight study reported that children with epilepsy were, on average, 20 months behind their peers. Holdsworth & Whitmore (1975) surveyed children with epilepsy who were attending ordinary schools in Bedfordshire. They found that one third were making good progress, about one half were making poor progress and one sixth were noticeably behind other children of their age. The authors thought that there were four factors which contributed to children making poor progress, which were: medication, type of epilepsy, attitude of parents and attitude of teachers. It is possible that teachers may be over-protective and highly risk-conscious and that their concern for the physical welfare of the child with epilepsy might be a major factor in his poor progress.

In some instances teachers, and later on employers, may be unintentionally unhelpful to the young person with epilepsy because they have heard that stress can provoke epileptic fits. While there are undoubtedly some people in whom fits may appear to be caused by severely stressful experiences, it is important that we, for our part, do not overstress the significance of stress, nor do we fall into the error of suggesting that everyone with a diagnosis of epilepsy must be protected from every possible unpleasant experience, such as taking examinations or accepting a normal degree of responsibility.

Public attitudes towards epilepsy and misconceptions about this condition and the effect it may have on people who are liable to fits, probably, for the most part, account for the difficulties experienced in getting employment. Pond & Bidwell found in 1960 that nearly 40 per cent of the patients included in their survey of 14 general practices had experienced difficulties with employment. Bell's (1975) survey of patients admitted to the Special Centre for Epilepsy in York found that 54.9 per cent of these patients had problems with employment. The reasons for these difficulties are varied. Reference has already been made to the fear that stress may provoke a fit, and this sometimes accounts for someone with epilepsy being recommended for 'safe' or 'easy' or 'sheltered' employment. Promotion may be denied for the same reason and it is not always accepted that boredom, frustration and lack of opportunity may be just as likely to provoke epileptic attacks in some people. There are some words which appear to take on a double meaning, as for example 'reliable'. The employer may say that a worker is not reliable, meaning that one cannot depend on his regularity in coming to work or that he may have a fit at work and not be able to complete what he is doing. Serious problems can arise if he is working on a moving belt, and some essential part is missing from a number of appliances or from a car or whatever is under production. But there is also the implication that one cannot trust someone who is unreliable or on whom one cannot depend. The practical difficulty and the prejudice about the condition become mixed up in the employer's attitude. There are times when it is clear that lack of adequate information leads to the personnel officer, or whoever is taking the decision about employment, to be unduly pessimistic about the individual's liability to have fits at all times and in all places.

People still believe that someone with epilepsy should not be allowed to work near machinery. The fact that many people have complete or nearly complete control of their fits is not sufficiently well known. Nor is it generally realised that some people with epilepsy have fits while asleep or that others have fits on waking. Nor do people ask what happens during a fit. We hear a great deal about the danger of someone having a fit and falling on the machine he is operating, but an enquiry at the David Lewis Centre for Epilepsy, where the patients generally have severe epilepsy, revealed that the majority of those who had fits fall backwards when doing so and that it was unusual for someone to fall forward.

MacIntyre (1976) collected information from industrial medical officers in 29 industrial organisations where there were employees who had epilepsy. His report confirmed our impression that risk of accidents caused by epilepsy at work is greatly over-estimated. A wide variety of occupations was included in this survey, but a large number of the 150 000 people employed were in fairly 'heavy' industry. 177 employees had epilepsy and were engaged in many different occupations. Labourers, clerks and fitters formed the larger group, but there were also engineers, technicians and many different professional skills represented in the total number. The severity or frequency of their attacks was not stated but faints, vertigo and psychologically determined attacks were excluded from the survey. During the 10 years prior to this report 18 accidents attributable to epilepsy were noted. Accident frequency rate was defined as:

$$\frac{\text{Lost time accidents} \; x \; 10\,000}{\text{Man hours worked}}$$

In this situation an accident frequency rate of 0.06 was arrived at. MacIntyre commented that there may be a number of pitfalls in comparing the accident rates of different companies. He went on to say: 'if one looks at accident statistics from the British Chemical Industry (1972) it can be seen that the accident frequency rate of 29 companies employing over 1000 people varied from 0.09 to 4.64 with an average of 1.92. One cannot conclude that the way to reduce accidents is to employ only people with epilepsy, but certainly it is abundantly clear that those with epilepsy in this survey do not play any significant part in accident causation.'

Claims have been made by employers that employment cannot be offered to someone with epilepsy because the insurance company would not accept the risk. Usual experience is that group insurance, which is more often the practice in industry, will cover the employer for such accidents as do occur provided that the employee has not been asked to carry out tasks in particularly hazardous circumstances. Reference has already been made to Rodin's (1968) study in which he demonstrated that frequency of seizures alone does not always influence the individual's chances of obtaining or holding employment. The late Dr Robert Porter (1963) examined 100 patients with epilepsy who had been unemployed for more than 3 months or who were considered to be 'placement problems' by the Disablement Resettlement Officer of the Ministry of Labour. Of these he found that five did not have epilepsy at all and that 48 could be placed in employment after careful assessment, adjustment of medication and detailed attention to their needs and potential abilities. He concluded that more than half of the so-called 'unemployable' group could be placed given proper multi-disciplinary attention, and that those who could not be placed in employment were often additionally handicapped by poor intelligence, disturbed behaviour or other physical disability. He also concluded, like many other observers, that 'the controlled, stable epileptic is a good worker'.

In another study we have constructed an ABC of employment, from which it can be seen that very many occupations are open to people with epilepsy provided that their fits are well controlled. For example, while one may not be an airman or an ambulance driver, epilepsy need not prevent one from being an accountant, an architect or a shop assistant. It is easier to draw up a list of unsuitable occupations which would include heavy goods vehicle or public service driving, the armed services and work in one or two other particularly hazardous situations.

Misconceptions about employment are sometimes met where one least expects them, as is illustrated by the following experience:

A young lady in her early twenties had trained and qualified as a professional librarian. She obtained an appointment with a large local authority and made no secret about her epilepsy when interviewed. After working for some weeks she was suddenly suspended pending further medical examination, and then told she could not be employed in spite of representations on her behalf by her chief librarian. At the Industrial Tribunal a distinguished consultant physician testified that she could not be employed in a public library for two reasons. First, that there was a danger that when sitting on top of the ladder while putting books back on the shelves she might indulge in day-dreams, possibly about her boyfriend, and thereby have an epileptic fit. Secondly, that if she had a fit when she was alone in the library she might injure herself by falling against a radiator or in some other way, and there would be no one present to come to her aid. The British Epilepsy Association produced evidence from 149 public libraries, who reported that 35 had a total of 43 people with epilepsy in their employment. 30 were library assistants, six were librarians, one was a senior officer and the remainder were clerical assistants, a book-binder and a handyman. The young lady won her appeal to the tribunal, regrettably more on the grounds of the incorrect way her appointment and dismissal had been handled than on the question of suitability of employment in spite of the diagnosis. However she has since been employed as a librarian for more than two years by a more understanding local authority.

A brief reference is appropriate to the vexed question of epilepsy and driving. The Road Traffic Act (1930) expressly denied anyone suffering from epilepsy the right to hold a driving licence. There were many attempts during the following 40 years to define 'suffering from epilepsy', or to interpret the meaning of this statute. At one time licencing authorities favoured the ruling of the Lord Chief Justice in 1966 that anyone taking anticonvulsant medication, whether he had fits or not, must be 'suffering from epilepsy', and therefore required an applicant to have a period during which he was not taking medication. This unsatisfactory state of affairs was remedied in 1970 when regulations were introduced which permit the granting of a driving licence to an applicant suffering from epilepsy provided he shall have been free from any epileptic attack whilst awake for at least 3 years, or if he has attacks while asleep he shall only have had such attacks and for a period of longer than 3 years, or that there is no other way in which his holding a driving licence shall be a source of danger to the public. These regulations have had one or two minor amendments but remain basically the same 10 years later. From time to time there are cases in which the interpretations of the regulations causes special difficulty. At all times the officers of the Driver and Vehicles Licencing Centre will treat enquiries with sympathy and understanding. As mentioned earlier, licences to drive heavy goods vehicles and public service vehicles are not granted to anyone who has had any form of epileptic fit after reaching the age of 3 years. Most local authorities will not grant taxi driver licences in similar circumstances.

It is not unusual to come across cases where the parents of a young man or young woman have strong objections to their son or daughter having a lasting friendship with a view to marriage to someone who has epilepsy. At the beginning of this century several parts of the world had laws forbidding people with epilepsy to marry. In some states of America marriage was only permitted if the partners agreed to being sterilised. Fortunately these laws have mostly been abolished or allowed to lapse. In the U.K. it was possible until 1970 for either party to obtain annulment of a marriage within one year of the ceremony if the other party had not disclosed a history of epilepsy. This power was withdrawn under the Matrimonial Act of that date.

Another area in which prejudice and out-of-date information about epilepsy can cause serious difficulties for the individual or for the family where, for instance, a child has had epileptic fits, is when considering emigration. Some countries still have laws which bar anyone with a history of epilepsy from taking citizenship. One example is Australia where the Migration Act stipulates that would-be immigrants must not have a 'proscribed disease', one of which is epilepsy. This rule may apply to any member of the family of the person making the application. Several other countries take the health of any applicant into consideration and an earlier history of epileptic attacks may be just as detrimental as the present occurrence of these. Advice about individual cases can usually be obtained from the British Epilepsy Association.

'Epilepsy plus'

Having looked at the social aspects of epilepsy generally, it is appropriate to consider the situation of those people who have what Dr John Laidlaw, lately senior physician at the Chalfont Centre for Epilepsy, has called 'epilepsy plus'. By this he meant those patients whose epilepsy was rendered more complex and difficult to manage by the presence of psychiatric disorder, or when associated with some degree of mental retardation or other physical disorder. The reason why some people have difficulties, and others do not, is not always clear and, as noted, social adjustment is not only decided by frequency of fits. Infrequent seizures, well tolerated in one individual may be an intolerable hardship for another. For example, one lady had mild and infrequent fits of gelastic epilepsy. These caused her the minimum of inconvenience and she had learned how to pass them off if she was in the presence of other people, but they were sufficient to make it impossible for her to have a driving licence. Her husband relied on her to drive for the furtherance of their family business, and she became severely depressed through her inability to fulfil the role which her husband required of her for what seemed such a trivial reason.

A young man with absence seizures had qualified as a solicitor. He became increasingly frustrated when he had to give up appointments in the legal departments of local authorities because of his difficulty in not being able to drive to county courts where he was expected to appear on behalf of his authority. Was his frustration and rage due to his having epilepsy or would he have been an 'angry young man' in any case? One cannot say.

A young woman came to the clinic one day following a clumsy and ineffectual attempt at suicide. She had an IQ of less than 50 and a history of epileptic fits as a girl. She was happily married to a simple, tolerant and understanding husband. She had been working in a local bottle factory where she had been required to stick labels on bottles and apparently she had performed this simple task to the satisfaction of her employers. She was not a great mixer, but she got on well enough with other employees. A new forewoman was not so understanding, and was the cause of a number of distressing scenes. She worried about this and eventually gave up her job and stayed alone at home in her small flat. Her epileptic attacks recurred, and became more frequent, so that she felt useless and a burden to her husband and had nothing left to live for. Fortunately this was a situation which required very little more than social support and encouragement from an out-patient department.

More difficult and complex situations require the services of a special centre for epilepsy. Parsonage describes the function of a multi-disciplinary special centre (Chapter 26). We are indebted to Margaret Bell (1975), his social worker, for an assessment of the employment problems (as a measure of their social difficulties) among 182 in-patients at Parsonage's centre in York. She found that 31 per cent had problems due to frequent attacks: psychiatric disorder occurrred in 28 per cent: the type of attack, poor motivation and mental handicap each caused problems in just under 10 per cent, whereas choice of career, physical disorder, high local unemployment rate and sundry other factors made up the remaining 23 per cent. However, it is important to remember that this is a highly selected group. Employment is not always a good measure of social adjustment especially in times of economic difficulty in the community. Pond & Bidwell's survey included 157 patients of employable age. They concluded that although 65 (47 per cent) had had serious difficulties with employment at some time, only 17 (slightly less than 10 per cent) were unemployable.

There is no clear evidence whether epilepsy is a greater source of difficulty than the accompanying psychiatric illness or mental retardation. Some workers consider that mental retardation, cerebral palsy and psychiatric illness are greater problems, since they do not so readily respond to medical treatment as do epileptic fits. Way (1980) has observed that severely mentally retarded children who have epileptic fits appear to function at a much higher level as soon as their fits are brought under control, especially by some of the newer anticonvulsants. Cummings (Director of Education and Training for the National Society for Mentally Handicapped Children and Adults) confirms the view of Pond (1979) and Corbett (Chapter 11) that the lower the IQ the greater the possibility of the individual having epilepsy. In Cummings' experience, the young mentally handicapped person able to enter the labour market would, by and large, have a good chance of not having epilepsy, or at least not severely so. He concludes 'whether it be employment, residential care or fostering, one has to work twice as hard to persuade people to accept the dual handicapped person'. Certainly in working with the young person who is mentally retarded, and more so in the present economic situation, one has to think more in terms of a lifetime of learning, as Baranyay (1976) has entitled her survey, than look for any facile statistics of employment as a measure of social adaptation.

Management

There is no question that diagnosis and all decisions regarding medical therapy must be in the hands of the physician, but there is a great deal for the multi-disciplinary team to do. The role of the social worker is partly as therapist and partly as a bridge between the patient and the physician, and also the non-medical services available to the patient. In the first place it may be necessary to help the patient to come to terms with his condition, and to accept what it really means to him. Bell (1975) at York found that 53 per cent of the whole sample of patients experienced difficulty in fully accepting the fact of their epilepsy, and in nine cases out of the 97 the difficulty was serious. Relationships with parents, within marriage, with children and within the extended family caused problems in 83 cases (out of 182) and intensive casework helped to improve the situation in 24 cases. Problems concerned with education, employment, finance and housing require the services of the social worker as a bridge builder. The Disablement Resettlement Officer takes a much more hopeful attitude today when seeing an applicant with epilepsy than was the case 20 or 30 years ago. Even so, the patient may need encouragement to seek his advice and to persevere in following up his recommendations.

This writer's experience with parents is predominantly a demand from them for early information and counselling of how to manage their child's condition. There is a special need at the time of diagnosis, and the British Epilepsy Association has endeavoured to bring to the notice of physicians that literature, local support groups and experienced staff are available to help in this field. 10 per cent of applications to the Association's Advice Service are from people who have just learned of a diagnosis of epilepsy.

CONCLUSION

The problems of a condition which has so many facets cannot be answered by one discipline or in only one way. However if much more could be done in the way of bringing information at the right time to people who are experiencing difficulties, many of these would diminish in magnitude. The writer remains unrepentant in advocating more public education about what epilepsy is and what it is not.

References

Aall-Jilek L M 1965 Epilepsy in the Wapogoro tribe in Tanganyika. Acta psychiatrica scandinavica 41:57–86

Baranyay E 1976 A lifetime of learning. National Society for Mentally Handicapped Children and Adults

Bell M 1975 Social aspects of epilepsy. Report prepared for the North Yorkshire Social Services Department of work undertaken at the York Special Centre for Epilepsy. (Part of this report has appeared under the title of Some social problems of adults with epilepsy. Epilepsy 79:93–98, British Epilepsy Association)

Bower B, Ward F 1978 A study of certain social aspects of epilepsy in childhood. Spastics International Medical Publications and William Heinemann, London

Burden G, Schurr P H 1980 Understanding epilepsy, 2nd edn. Granada Publishing, London

Butler N 1972 Kenneth Gibson memorial lecture. The Candle, Journal of the British Epilepsy Association, Autumn 1972

Cummings J National Society for Mentally Handicapped Children and Adults, 117–123 Golden Lane, London EC1Y ORT (personal communication)

Harker P 1977 Primary immunisation and febrile convulsions in Oxford 1972–75. British Medical Journal 2:490–493

Holdsworth L, Whitmore K 1975 A study of children with epilepsy attending ordinary schools. II Information and attitudes held by teachers. Developmental Medicine and Child Neurology 16:759–765

MacIntyre I 1976 Epilepsy and employment. Community Health vol 7, 4:195–204

Orley J H 1970 Culture and mental illness. East African studies 36. Makerere Institute of Social Research, East African Publishing House, Nairobi

Pond D A, Bidwell B H 1960 A survey of epilepsy in fourteen general practices. II Social and psychological aspects. Epilepsia 1:285–299

Pond D A 1979 Epilepsy and mental retardation. In: Treadgold R H (ed) Mental retardation, 12th edn. Baillière Tindall

Porter R 1963 Unemployable? Epilepsy and employment. Social Studies in Epilepsy 1. British Epilepsy Association and the International Bureau for Epilepsy

Rodin E A 1968 The prognosis of patients with epilepsy. Charles C Thomas, Springfield, Illinois

Rutter M, Graham P, Yule W 1970 A neuropsychiatric study in childhood. Clinics in developmental medicine. Spastics International Medical Publications and William Heinemann, London

Way M 1980 Consultant Psychiatrist, Earls House Hospital, Durham (personal communication)

Precipitation and inhibition of seizures

INTRODUCTION

Ever since epilepsy has been recognised as a disease, so has folk lore suggested methods for stopping and starting the attacks. As long ago as Roman times in the slave markets when buying slaves it is said that: 'the rotation of the potter's wheel before his eyes would make the epileptic feel giddy and might be the cause of seizures' (Temkin 1945). This, together with the burning of fat or horn so that the fumes could be inhaled (Lennox & Lennox 1960), were ways of attempting to precipitate seizures so that epileptic slaves could be detected before being bought. Most modern patients have their own private theories as to how to control their own seizures and a smaller group describe what they have to do in order to precipitate an attack. Theories range from control of diet or the avoidance of upsetting circumstances to the wearing of bar magnets to alter the magnetic field around the patient's head. Despite these rather fanciful methods, there are many cases reported in the literature of specific stimuli which can trigger seizures. The avoiding of these triggers reduces the patients' seizure frequency.

The aim of this chapter is not to review the field of specific precipitants of seizures in detail, but to direct the emphasis firstly to current thinking on how specific stimuli may cause seizures and, secondly, towards those behavioural and conditioning techniques that are available for stopping seizures and which do not involve the taking of anticonvulsant medication.

Nomenclature

The precipitation of seizures by specific stimuli has been called 'reflex epilepsy'. This term has a long tradition, and an excellent review of the whole subject is given by Merlis (1974). The term reflex epilepsy is thought to have been applied by Marshall Hall in the last century, and to have found support in the work of Brown-Séquard (1857), who produced seizures in guinea pigs by peripheral stimulation of animals with spinal cord lesions. Gowers (1881) described the precipitation of seizures by external stimuli and formalised the idea of reflex epilepsy in 1901. Hughlings Jackson (1925) also recognised the term. Since then, with the advance of physiology, the term reflex epilepsy has fallen into disrepute. A review is given by Allen (1945). 'Evoked seizures' was the term preferred by Symonds (1959), while Penfield & Erickson (1941) preferred the term 'sensory precipitation epilepsy'. However, as Merlis points out, the term 'sensory' would exclude many seizures that may be triggered by an emotional or other non-sensory component. The term 'evoked seizures', used by Symonds, will be used in this chapter for all those epilepsies which have a specific external precipitant. The term psychogenic seizures will be used in the correct sense, for those epileptic attacks which can be generated by an act of will or by the mind (psyche) *without* an external stimulus; e.g. seizures which can be triggered by an act of attention, or by a particular emotion, or by thinking or calculating. Thus, the thinking epilepsies would be included in the term psychogenic seizures. Frequently, the term psychogenic has been misapplied to simulated seizures or hysterical pseudo-seizures (see Chapter 9). This is unfortunate as this has left the word psychogenic with a pejorative flavour that it should not rightly have.

Incidence

This is very difficult to determine, as only single case studies are usually mentioned in the literature. However, since there is now a greater awareness of the possibility of both evoked and psychogenic seizures occuring, the incidence is likely to be much higher than given in the previous studies. Gowers (1881) mentioned only about six to 10 cases in his series of 1450 cases, or an incidence of approximately 0.5–1 per cent. Symonds (1959) reported an incidence of 6.5 per cent in a series of 1000 cases, while Servit et al (1962) reported evoked seizures in 5.1 per cent of their 895 epileptics. The incidence will vary with the population studied, probably being higher in those units that have a greater number of psychiatric disorders. At the Maudsley Hospital, the incidence of evoked seizures is probably very similar to that of Symonds and Servit et al. However, psychogenic seizures are considerably more common, with the incidence rising to nearly three times the other figures.

EVOKED SEIZURES

Since the main thrust of this chapter is towards psychogenic seizures and their possible mechanism, only a brief review of evoked seizures will be given. Very good reviews already exist as mentioned above i.e. those of Allen (1945) and Merlis (1974). Any sensory stimulus, providing it is specific, may be the cause of evoked seizures, and seizures have been triggered by stimuli in all sensory modalities.

Hearing– or auditory–induced seizures

Seizures can be induced in a number of patients with epilepsy by a sudden loud noise. Equally effective in a few cases is a monotonous continuous noise, such as machinery, humming or a kettle boiling (Critchley 1937). Symonds (1959) described patients whose seizures were triggered by the continual croaking of a frog or the mewing of a kitten. He also reported one case where the sudden cessation of a continuous noise precipitated seizures.

An increase in epileptic discharges in the EEG has been reported by Arrellano et al (1950), in response to continuous pure tones. Prechtl (1959) mentioned three patients whose temporal lobe seizures were triggered by clicks sounded at the rate of two a second, while many others had an increase in the number of abnormal EEG discharges.

Click stimulation, like photic stimulation, has been tried by several authors with only limited success, but Stevens (1962) has reported an increased incidence of abnormality in the EEGs of patients with both generalised and temporal lobe epilepsy. Of considerable interest, as it is against prediction, is the finding that the induced incidence of abnormality was over four times higher in the patients with generalised epilepsies, compared to those with temporal lobe epilepsies.

Musicogenic epilepsy

It is not surprising if pure tones and clicks can induce seizures that patterned tones, e.g. music, are able to do the same. Almost any musical sound can act as a stimulus, patients being reported who respond to either classical or other music. Also, almost every musical instrument has been involved. Some patients have a very specific trigger, such as the case mentioned by Poskanzer et al (1962), whose seizures were triggered by the sounding of a bell. These authors point out that there are two groups of patients, those whose seizures are generated by the specific sound itself and those whose seizures are generated by the affective changes produced on hearing the music. These latter attacks are not true evoked seizures, but probably fit better into the class of psychogenic seizures as music is only one of many stimuli that can trigger the attacks. An example of this latter category is given by Shaw & Hill (1947). Fuller reviews are given by Titeca (1965) and Servit et al (1962), dating back to Critchley's 1937 paper, in which he described 20 cases whose seizures were triggered by music. Interestingly, both Critchley, and Forster et al (1969), have identified a sub-group of patients whose seizures are precipitated by speaking. Many of the above reports show that the induced seizures are located in the temporal lobe and probably arise from foci in the auditory cortex.

Somatosensory evoked seizures

It is perfectly possible for any sensory stimulus, providing it is of sufficient intensity, to trigger a seizure in susceptible individuals. Symonds reported a case where the wearing of an artificial leg stimulated the stump and induced seizures, due to a meningioma over the appropriate motor centre. Dawson (1947) reported a case of seizures induced by tapping a tendon. The literature contains many other exotic tactile stimuli. Pressure on the left gum (Penfield & Jasper 1954) or on the testicles and pricking of the palms of the hand (André-Thomas et al 1942) were all effective; as was touching and tapping of the skin (Scollo-Lavizzori & Hess 1967, Forster et al 1949, Calderon-Gonzalez et al 1966). Sudden stimuli are usually more effective than those that the patient is expecting, although this is not true in every case. The seizures are frequently focal, as in the case Symonds described above, although the EEG may show bilateral or even generalised changes. Parsonage (1975) describes three patients whose seizures were precipitated on getting into a hot bath.

Movement evoked seizures

Seizures due to sudden movements have been described by several authors. Gowers (1881) reported several cases. In one, 'any passive movement of the spine at once brought on an attack of general tonic spasm. . . . During the attack, which lasted only 10 or 15 seconds, there was a complete unconsciousness.' Gowers reported in other cases that movement after rest was particularly effective, such as getting out of a chair quickly or turning over in bed.

This article will not describe in detail a group of paroxysmal involuntary movements which are precipitated in susceptible subjects by sudden movement and without loss of consciousness. These were first described by Mount & Redback in 1940. For adequate reviews, see Merlis (1972) and Laidlaw & Richens (1976). There is some dispute as to whether or not the syndrome is due to epileptic seizure discharges.

Passive movement can occasionally trigger both seizures and focal discharges in the EEG (Asseni et al 1967), although repeated and continuous movement has also been described as being effective (Pitha 1938). However, the general feeling still follows that of Gowers, that it is the suddenness of the movement, the startle response, that is effective (Stevens 1966, Kertez 1967).

Visceral evoked seizures

Symonds (1959) suggested that these seizures are much more common than most writers recognise, although Merlis (1974) felt that they form only a minor group. Certainly, not very many have been reported in the literature. Symonds mentioned the case of a man whose attacks were precipitated by gastric distension after eating a heavy meal quickly and were temporal lobe in character. A second patient of Symonds' never had his minor attack 'if I eat slowly and read . . .' Allen (1945) reported a similar case. Boudouresques & Gastaut (1954) described four patients who had temporal lobe foci and whose seizures were precipitated by gastric distension due to eating. Gastaut et al (1956) reported an unusual case of seizures precipitated by colonic distension due to enemas.

Visual evoked seizures

Photic stimulation—flash
Although light had been known for many years to precipitate seizures, its formal demonstration was shown by Cobb (1947) when he published a paper on three patients whose seizures could be induced by flickering light. Since that time, the effects of flashes of light have been widely studied. Three excellent reviews are available for those readers interested in the subject: Jeavons & Harding (1975), Newmark & Penry (1979) and Wilkins et al (1980).

Intermittent flashes from a gas discharge tube with a range of 1 to 30 flashes per second are commonly used to evoke the abnormal photoconvulsive potentials. 15–20 per cent of patients with seizure disorders show a photoconvulsive response, which consists of irregular, slow waves with a frequency of about 3 Hz, mixed with spikes, and seen predominantly in the fronto-central leads. Some authors give the incidence of this abnormal response as being as high as 40 per cent in patients with primary generalised epilepsy (Melsen 1959). 1.6–4.0 per cent of normal adults can also show this response (Kooi et al 1960), while the incidence amongst children below the age of 15 is around 14 per cent (Brandt et al 1961), although Watson & Marcus (1962) have shown that this is dependent on age, with the maximum sensitivity occurring at the age of about 16 years. The precise flash frequency varies from patient to patient, but Jeavons & Harding have shown that the most evocative frequencies are from 18–22 flashes per second.

Several other potentials may be evoked by the flashes which are not true photoconvulsive responses.

1. 'Following' evoked potentials seen over the occipital area, which are a harmonic or subharmonic of the flash frequency.

2. Photomyoclonic responses, demonstrable in 50 per cent of normal adults. These are rhythmic contractions of the muscles of the head, but mainly the frontalis muscle, and so they are seen maximally frontally (Bickford et al 1952 and Gastaut et al 1958).

3. Occipital spikes, which are abnormal components of the visual evoked response.

Certain stimulus parameters are important. Fixation of the light source should be on the macula as eccentric fixation may eliminate the response (Jeavons & Harding 1975, Newmark & Penry 1979, Wilkins et al 1980). Colour is not important, with the possible exception of blue (Newmark & Penry 1979). Open or closed eyes can produce marked differences. Most people are more sensitive with the eyes open while a few only show photoconvulsive responses with the eyes closed. Greatest sensitivity is obtained when both eyes are stimulated, and this is markedly attenuated with monocular stimulation in 90 per cent of cases (Jeavons & Harding 1975).

Pattern stimulation

Viewing an evenly illuminated pattern has been found to be an effective stimulus for precipitating seizures. The incidence varies from 0.25 per cent in a series of 40 000 epileptic patients, to 60–70 per cent of patients who show photoconvulsive responses. It is important if all sensitive subjects are to be detected that the pattern is oscillated in a direction orthogonal to the stimulus lines, and as Wilkins et al (1979) mentions, the incidence will thus vary according to the effectiveness of the stimulus used.

Effective stimulus parameters are black and white stripes of equal width, with a spatial frequency of 1 to 4 cycles per degree. Binocular viewing is more effective than monocular, and luminance has to be changed by more than 1 log unit of change if the evoked activity is to occur (Wilkins et al 1980).

Reading epilepsies

Bickford et al (1956) drew attention to two groups of patients who developed epilepsy on reading. The primary group on reading had a clicking in the jaw which preceded a grand mal seizure. During reading, the EEG slowed, with bilateral and synchronous 3–6 Hz activity which appeared maximal in the occipital and parietal areas. The secondary group had seizures sometimes precipitated by reading, but also by other activities as well. Many other authors have added unusual cases (see Merlis 1974 for a review). The seizures may be triggered by reading aloud or reading silently, reading nonsense or reading emotional material. Critchley (1962) has suggested that several factors may be important: photic stimulation, jaw movement, intellectual content, concentration and the emotion evoked by the text.

PSYCHOGENIC SEIZURES

In this group will be included all those seizures which are triggered by an act of will, in addition to those which are triggered by a specific mental activity. It is however useful to divide this group into two, primary and secondary.

a. Primary

The primary group would be those in which a direct act of will could precipitate a seizure. Three examples from the Maudsley clinic may help:

1. A 44 year old woman with mild generalised brain damage had generalised seizures with a focal onset since the age of 12. The commencement of the attack was a classical aversive seizure with head and eyes turning to the left. She discovered when in her teens, that she could trigger a seizure if she attended very hard to a point in her visual field and then slowly swung her head and eyes to the left, mimicking the seizure onset. She then noticed that the movement became automatic and a generalised seizure followed. She also reported that the converse was true, and that attempting to inhibit the movement of her head and eyes once a spontaneous seizure had commenced, providing the process had not gone too far, would prevent the generalisation of the seizure.

2. A young man of 21 had generalized seizures since the age of 10. These seizures were probably due to mild generalised brain damage caused by a difficult birth. He discovered in his teens that if he lay down on his bed and made his mind a blank and continued to make his mind blank, then he could induce a generalised seizure.

3. The third case is that of a young man of 30, who has had petit mal attacks since early childhood, with typical spike and wave discharges in the EEG. He found that he could precipitate a petit mal seizure by what he called splitting his attention. He said that if he suddenly swung his attention to something peripheral to his attentional field, an attack would be triggered. He frequently used this mechanism, when a child and adolescent, to defend himself from his mother's anger, precipitating a shower of seizures while she was scolding him.

These three patients illustrate three different types of mechanism employed by patients to produce psychogenic seizures. First, the genesis of normal activity in those structures which are involved in the focal onset of the seizure. Secondly, the non-specific manipulation of attention. Thirdly, the direct use of attention.

A further type of seizure precipitation that should be included in the primary category are those seizures which are initiated by an act of will, the activity so generated appears to be independent of the epileptic focus and only spreads to it indirectly. For example, a patient of 30 years had left-sided temporal lobe epilepsy from childhood, probably due to mesial temporal sclerosis following febrile convulsions. He suffered from both partial and generalised seizures. His auras were either visual field changes or a feeling of thinking a most interesting thought which he could not subsequently remember, after which his seizures would frequently generalise. When in his teens, he learnt that if he felt sad and concentrated on the emotion of the unfairness of life and how unhappy he was, a seizure could be triggered. He used this mechanism deliberately at school, when unhappy, to solve his personal problems and he has continued with this into adult life; although he now does it less frequently. After a recent break-up with his girlfriend, he went home, put on the gramophone to create the correct atmosphere and deliberately induced serial seizures to blank out his unhappiness. It would appear in this case that the induced discharges generated by his feelings of sadness spread into those structures which were epileptogenic and a seizure was triggered.

The incidence of true primary psychogenic seizures is much commoner than the literature suggests. An incidence of three in ten to one in seven patients has been found at the Maudsley Hospital epilepsy clinic. However, patients are only likely to admit to a voluntary mechanism when the questioning physician has their confidence!

b. Secondary

Seizures in this category are those which are precipitated by a specific function of the mind, without a deliberate intention on the part of the patient to precipitate a seizure and without a clear evoking peripheral stimulus. Into this category fall the thinking epilepsies of Ingram & Ryman (1962). The latter authors described a patient whose seizures were precipitated by simple calculation. At this time, his EEG showed a spike and wave discharge and he had blurring of consciousness. Wilkins et al (1981) reports a patient whose seizures could be precipitated by mental arithmetic, and it was found after intensive investigation that a variety of psychological tasks requiring parietal lobe functioning, such as block design or Brooks' letter copying test, were also effective. Other authors who have reported seizures specifically related to mental activity are Bingel (1957), Symonds (1959), Gomez & Escueta (1977), Ch'en et al (1965), Forster (1975, 1977) and Cirignotta et al (1980).

A hypothesis put forward to explain the mechanism of the psychogenic seizures, both primary and secondary, is simply an extension of that used to explain the evoked epilepsies. In the case of the evoked epilepsies, it is now accepted that the sensory inputs initiate normal activity in those areas which are epileptogenic and thus trigger a seizure discharge. For the psychogenic epilepsies, the argument is similar, in that specific forms of mental activity, whether voluntary or involuntary, are associated with the activation of specific neural circuits, which, if epileptogenic, will precipitate seizures. It is suggested that in some patients, the areas are well localised and thus very specific activities are required to trigger a seizure.

Considerable evidence for this hypothesis has already been accumulated, and it has recently been extended by Wilkins et al (1980) in his suggested mechanism for photogenic seizures and in his model of thinking epilepsies. In summary, his two-stage model is as follows: 'When normal physiological excitations exceed some (slightly variable) limit, paroxysmal disturbance is triggered. When the disturbance exceeds some topographic limit, complete generalisation occurs.' In the case of both primary and secondary psychogenic seizures, this model implies areas of cortex which are damaged and so epileptogenic. Mental activity in these areas will first of all evoke abnormal activity and then, if the threshold is exceeded, generalise to a seizure.

METHODS USED TO INHIBIT SEIZURES

The range of techniques which have been tried in the last three decades to inhibit seizures, and which do not involve anticonvulsant medication, is still very limited. Only a few centres have taken up the study of methods for the inhibition of seizures by non-pharmacological methods in a large way. The literature contains mainly case reports. Part of the reason for this is undoubtedly the difficulty in designing an effective study for a condition, the precipitating causes of which are poorly understood physiologically and which may be influenced by many events outside the experimenters' control. Other factors are the unpopularity of epilepsy as a research subject, and the conservative attitudes of many patients with epilepsy who do not wish to enter a study which may not be effective. In an excellent article reviewing the literature relating to what the authors call the 'psychobiological control of seizures', Mostofsky & Balaschak (1977) said that it 'makes it abundantly clear that it is extremely difficult, if not impossible, to examine any one procedure independently from the influences of other concurrent conditions . . . Treatment programmes are therefore designed to attack more than a single objective.' It is this confusion of procedures which has led to such slow progress in the behavioural treatment of patients with seizures.

The following are the main techniques that have been used:

a. 'Spontaneous methods' discovered and used by patients
b. Conditioning procedures:
   (i) Extinction and habituation
   (ii) Conditioning the seizures to an inhibitory stimulus
c. Behavioural modification programmes
   (i) Reward and punishment
   (ii) Relaxation
   (iii) Desensitization
d. Biofeedback measures
   (i) the 'conditioning' of rhythms which are said to have an anticonvulsant effect
   (ii) the conditioning of rhythms the production of which is likely to produce a mental state antagonistic to seizure activity, or the production of which may act in a non-specific way to inhibit seizures.
   (iii) the deliberate reduction of abnormal electrical discharges which are thought to be related to seizure occurrence, e.g. the reduction of spike activity from an epileptogenic focus or the inhibition of paroxysmal activity.
e. Miscellaneous methods
   (i) Diets
   (ii) Life-style changes
   (iii) Others

Spontaneous methods

Many patients in the clinic will describe techniques which they have evolved to inhibit seizure activity. These range from the specific, usually those patients whose epilepsy has a focal onset, to the non-specific, those patients whose seizures are generalised. Examples of specific techniques are the clasping of a limb involved in the onset of either a focal sensory or motor seizure or the prevention of a movement occurring at the start of a seizure. Non-specific examples are the patient who deliberately relaxes when tense as he knows tension is likely to produce a seizure. Symonds (1959) suggested in his series that 5.3 per cent of his patients could inhibit their seizures, although how they did this was not always obvious. Laidlaw & Richens (1976) felt that inhibition is commoner than reported at present. They also report that many patients are unwilling to inhibit their seizures because they feel unwell afterwards, the seizure having the effect of 'clearing the air'. There is no doubt that inhibition of seizures is practised by many patients with epilepsy; the ability to stop seizures was commoner than the ability to start seizures in the Maudsley series (personal communication) Mostofsky & Balaschak (1977) agree with this, and add several cases of their own to illustrate the point. It is surprising that there is as yet no comprehensive survey of mechanisms used by patients to inhibit their seizures.

Conditioning procedures

Classical conditioning procedures have been tried by many authors in an attempt to reduce the seizure frequency. Forster et al (1969, 1972) is the major author in the field of applying the classical method of habituation and extinction to the control of epilepsy. The aim of this method is to extinguish the abnormal cortical discharges which are evoked by a specific stimulus, by continually exposing the subject to the stimulus until habituation occurs. Habituation has been tried with stimuli which may cause seizures in the visual, auditory and sensory modalities.

Booker et al (1965) described the case of a 10 year old boy whose myoclonic jerks, precipitated by sudden auditory stimuli, were attenuated by recurrent sounding of the stimulus. Forster, in his review, mentioned cases of musicogenic epilepsy which were improved after habituation by repeated exposure to the precipitating stimulus. Not only has Forster attempted to extinguish abnormal responses in the auditory modality, but also in the visual system. Several studies are reported modifying the photoconvulsive responses in the EEGs of patients evoked by flashing lights. The paradigm varies from study to study but in essence the aim is to determine the frequency of light stimulation to which the subject is most sensitive and then by repeated exposure to attenuate the abnormal responses. This has had varied success, although in certain cases there was a limited improvement (Forster & Campos 1964, Forster et al 1964). An interesting case report, also by Forster et al (1965), used both auditory and visual stimuli in the desensitization procedure, auditory clicks being generated when the surrounding light intensity reached a given threshold. Other authors have applied the principle of habituation to pattern evoked seizures, somatosensory evoked seizures and voice induced epilepsy (see Forster's (1977) review article or Mostofsky & Balaschak (1977)).

An extension of the principle of extinction is the competing response paradigm or the direct conditioning of an inhibitory stimulus to prevent seizures. A case has been reported by Efron (1956), who described a patient with uncinate seizures who, by the inhalation of a strong and unpleasant stimulus, was able to arrest the seizure or to prevent its spread. Finally, after repeated trials, the patient was able simply to think about the unpleasant odour and thus prevent the attacks.

Other authors have applied the principle in the reading epilepsies. Tap your knee whenever you see a certain word or letter (Forster et al 1969), or in the language epilepsies, whenever you hear a certain word (de Weerdt & van Rijn 1975).

These studies using classical methods of extinction and habituation are of interest as they make use of internally induced cerebral inhibition to prevent seizure spread.

Behavioural methods

The aim of these methods is to treat the occurrence of seizures as an element of behaviour which can be modified by behaviour therapy techniques. The first of these techniques is the use of positive and negative reinforcement, or rewarding the absence of seizures and the punishment of their occurrence. Punishment may be given in two ways, either by the denial of reward or by punishing the occurrence of the seizures, and both methods have been used. Gardner (1967) used denial of reward by instructing the parents of a 10 year old girl with seizures to ignore their daughter's attacks and reward her good behaviour. He reported that she became seizure free. Daniels (1975) has also tried the method with some success, as have Iwata & Lorentzson (1976).

Wright (1973) used direct punishment, a mild electric shock, with a mentally retarded boy whenever he induced his seizures. In another study by the same author a boy with spontaneous seizures was studied, using a similar technique (Wright 1976) and in both cases a reduction in seizure frequency occurred. Zlutnick and co-workers (1972, 1975) used punishment in the form of shouting at or shaking children whose behaviour indicated they were about to have a seizure, again with some success.

Reward has been used by many authors [for a comprehensive review see the paper of Mostofsky & Balaschak (1977)]. The method consists of rewarding seizure absence either by the increased attention of nursing staff in hospital or by parents at home. Some studies have used such rewards as root beer or sweets and most studies report some success with these methods (Flannery & Cautela 1973, Balaschak 1976, Daniels 1975, Adams et al 1973).

Relaxation methods

These techniques depend on the observation that patients who are tense have frequent seizures so if the patient can be taught to relax then the seizure frequency should fall. The role of anxiety and psychic stress in the provocation and inhibition of seizures has been investigated by Mattson et al (1970). Psychic stress was shown to increase seizures, but not in a direct way, as none of the usual measures of anxiety directly correlated with the increased seizure frequency apart from involuntary hyperventilation. These findings suggest that the reduction of psychic stress in some patients should lead to a reduction in seizure frequency and several authors report some success with relaxation training (Ince 1976, Mostofsky 1975). A modification of simple relaxation training is desensitization. This makes use of the method originally suggested by Wolpe (1969): the patient relaxes while imagining the situation in which seizures are likely to occur. Standage (1972) employed this method of behaviour modification in a patient who was afraid of having seizures in social situations. The situations were rehearsed in imagination while the patient was relaxed. The patient's anxiety then lessened in the actual provocative situations, with a reduction in fit frequency. A study which was also successful is reported by Parrino (1971).

A further study which is worth mentioning is that of Feldman & Paul (1976). They studied a group of patients who had seizures, but were unable to identify the emotional trigger due to ictal amnesia. By video-taping the interview with the patient and replaying the tape, the patient was able to identify those emotional triggers which precipitated his seizures. There is very little doubt that showing these video tapes to the patients was a method of desensitizing them to their seizures and thus reducing their anxiety.

There is a report in the literature of desensitisation to a situation liable to provoke seizures by the method of 'flooding'. Pinto (1972) described a patient with agoraphobia, which was clearly related to movement epilepsy. He treated this by the behavioural technique of flooding, in which she was exposed to the phobic situation for long periods in the presence of the therapist. This procedure improved both her agoraphobia and her fits.

Biofeedback

a. *'Anticonvulsant' rhythms*
Sterman (1973), by a happy chance, found that cats who could be taught to increase a 12–16 Hz EEG rhythm over the sensorimotor cortex, the sensorimotor rhythm or SMR, were partially resistant, when compared to untrained cats, to the convulsant effects of the rocket fuel monomethylhydrazine. This led him to argue that this particular rhythm might have powerful anticonvulsant properties. To try out the conditioning procedure in man, Sterman's group trained four epileptic patients to enhance their SMR, using biofeedback techniques. To do this, they required a large number of sessions, ranging over eight to eighteen months. Sterman found that there was a reduction in both seizure frequency and in abnormal EEG activity. Other workers confirmed these findings. Lubar and co-workers obtained clinical improvement in eleven patients after SMR training, with some patients even becoming seizure free (Seifert & Lubar 1975, Lubar & Bahler 1976, Lubar 1977). Finley et al (1975) reported one patient in whom the number of atonic seizures was reduced nearly tenfold after seven months of SMR training.

These successes led to attempts to propose a model whereby the anticonvulsant effects of the SMR rhythms, to which seizure reduction was attributed, could be explained. After implanted electrode studies in cats, Sterman & MacDonald (1974) suggested that SMR training might 'activate' a hypothetical central inhibiting system. Seifert & Lubar (1975) felt the anticonvulsant effect was due to an enhancement of cortical idling, associated with inhibition of motor activity. Finley (1977) argued for a change in the balance of excitation and inhibition throughout the brain.

It has been pointed out by many observers since Sterman et al published their first paper that the evidence that it was an increase in the SMR which produced the reduction in seizure frequency was extremely tenuous. The epilepsy of the patients used by Sterman was severe and drug-resistant. The biofeedback treatment was intensive and daily and extended over many months. The most likely explanation for the reduction in seizures would thus be a placebo effect due to the new interest being taken in these patients and it was not necessary to implicate the SMR. Indeed, the evidence for there being a functionally discrete SMR in the EEGs of man is minimal. No group to date has yet shown a convincing correlation between SMR acquisition and seizure reduction. Finley et al (1975) claimed such a correlation, only to deny it later as being spurious (both SMR and seizure frequency correlated with trials) (Finley 1977). In a small trial with three patients, Kuhlman & Allison (1977) showed seizure reductions without an increase in SMR, thus confirming the lack of relationship between the two. Sterman (1977) reported that in patients undergoing SMR training there was frequently a reduction in seizure frequency without a corresponding change in the SMR. Finally, in a very thorough study of these patients, Quy et al (1979) could find no evidence that SMR enhancement was responsible for the reduction in seizure frequency of their group of patients. In summary, the issue remains open as to whether or not the augmentation of the SMR in man, if it exists, is responsible for the observed seizure reduction found in SMR training. On balance, the evidence to date is against this.

b. *Non-specific EEG biofeedback*
It was to be expected that once Sterman et al (1974) had shown that SMR biofeedback could apparently reduce seizure frequency, other investigators would try the effect of conditioning different rhythms. Cabral & Scott (1976) used conventional occipital alpha rhythm biofeedback, together with relaxation therapy. They treated three patients for six months with satisfactory results. All three showed seizure reduction and one became seizure free. Whyler et al (1976) used biofeedback training to increase fast low-voltage activity, and suppress slow wave activity surrounding an epileptic focus. Four patients showed a seizure reduction. Other workers, unconvinced about the presence of the SMR in man, attempted to enhance by biofeedback the naturally-occurring Mu rhythm (7–10 Hz), which is found over the central area in man and is blocked by limb movement. Kaplan (1975) and Kuhlman & Allison (1977) reported a reduction in seizure frequency of their patients when Mu activity was augmented by biofeedback.

Thus the conditioning of other EEG frequencies can be seen to reduce seizure frequency and there is evidence that biofeedback can reduce seizure activity; but whether this is a specific or non-specific effect is still being debated. However, Lockard et al (1977) have extended biofeedback techniques to the alumina-gel monkey model of epilepsy. Although some changes in the intensity of seizure activity were found, they concluded 'EEG operant conditioning...to decrease EMG, to increase 9 Hz or decrease 9 Hz and to increase 23 Hz (18 Hz with 26 Hz in two pilot monkeys) respectively was *not* consistently beneficial in reducing seizures'. There the matter stands at the present time. Interested readers should consult Quy et al's paper for a further discussion of possible mechanisms.

c. *Reduction of abnormal electrical discharges*
Much work still remains to be done with biofeedback training to suppress abnormal rhythms. However, the initial studies do not look very promising and

this may have discouraged many workers. Sterman (1977) taught three patients to suppress the 2–7 Hz frequency band with no clinical improvement. Cott et al (1977) had little success in seizure reduction in two patients who learned to reduce activity in the 4–7 Hz EEG frequency band. Quy et al in their paper sum up research to date by saying 'Hence it is evident that the suppression of pathological EEG activity is not in itself a sufficient tool for treating epilepsy'. The author and colleagues have studied two cases of temporal lobe epilepsy, using biofeedback to train the patients to reduce the frequency of abnormal spike activity. This pilot experiment was successful and it is planned to proceed to a full-scale study. It has yet to be shown whether or not biofeedback of abnormal cerebral rhythms will have a place in the future management of epilepsy.

In conclusion, there does appear to be a place for conditioning behavioural methods and biofeedback training in the treatment of epilepsy. However, its precise value and the mechanisms involved have still to be clearly defined.

References

Adams K, Klinge V, Keiser T W 1973 The extinction of a self-injurious behaviour in an epileptic child. Behaviour Research and Therapy 11:351–356

André-Thomas M, Mennau V, De Ajuriaguera V 1942 Crises d'épilepsie-tonique spontanées ou provoquées chez deux malades atteints d'une affection organique des centres nerveux. Rev Neurol (Paris) 74:171–172

Allen I M 1945 NZ Med J 44:135

Arrellano A P, Schwab R S, Casby T V 1950 Sonic activation. Electroenceph Clin Neurophysiol 2:217–219

Aroeni C, Stoica I, Serhànescu 1967 Electro-clinical investigations on the role of proprioceptive stimuli in the onset and arrest of convulsive epileptic paroxysms. Epilepsia 8:162–170

Balaschak B A 1976 Teacher-implemented behaviour modification in a case of organically based epilepsy. J Consult Clin Psychol 44:218–223

Bickford R G, Sem-Jacobsen C W, White P T, Daly D 1952 Some observations on the mechanism of photic and photometrazol activation. Electroenceph Clin Neurophysiol 4:275–282

Bickford R, Whelan J, Klass D, Corbin K 1956 Reading epilepsy. Trans Amer Neurol Ass 81:100–102

Bickford R G, Klass D W 1969 The EEG in seizures induced by visual patterns. Electroenceph Clin Neurophysiol 15:149–150

Bingel A 1957 Reading epilepsy. Neurology 7:752–756

Booker H E, Forster F M, Klove H 1965 Extinction factors in startle (acousticomotor) seizures. Neurology 15:1095–1103

Boudouresques J, Gastaut H 1954 Le 'mécanisme réflexe' de certaines épilepsies temporales. Rev Neurol 90:157–158

Brandt H, Brandt S, Vollmond K 1961 EEG response to photic stimulation in 120 normal children. Epilepsia (Amst) 2:313–317

Brown-Sequard E 1857 Researches on epilepsy: its artificial production in animals, and its etiology and treatment in man. David Clapp, Boston

Cabral, R J, Scott D F 1976 Effects of two desensitisation techniques, biofeedback and relaxation, on intractable epilepsy: follow-up study. J Neurol Neurosurg Psychiat 39:504–507

Calderon-Gonzalez R, Hopkins I, Mclean W T 1966 Tap seizures. A form of sensory precipitation epilepsy. J Am med Ass 198:521–523

Ch'en H P, Ch'in C, Ch'u C P 1965 Chess epilepsy and card epilepsy. Chinese med J 84:470–474

Cirignotta F, Cicogna P, Lugaresi E 1980 Epileptic seizures during card games and draughts. Epilepsia 21:137–140

Cobb S 1947 Photic driving as a cause of clinical seizures. Arch Neurol Psychiat (Chicago) 58:70–71

Cott A, Porloski R, Black A 1977 The role of sensorimotor rhythm feedback in the biofeedback treatment of epilepsy. A preliminary report. Proceedings of the International Meeting of biofeedback and self control, Tübingen

Critchley M 1935 Über reflex-Epilepsie. Schweiz Arch Neurol Psychiat 35:256–270

Critchley M 1937 Musicogenic epilepsy. Brain 60:13–27

Critchley M 1962 Reading epilepsy. Epilepsia (Amst) 3:402–406

Daniels L K 1975 The treatment of grand mal epilepsy by covert and operant conditioning techniques: a case study. Psychosomatics 16:65–67

Dawson G D 1947 Investigations on a patient subject to myoclonic seizures after sensory stimulation. J Neurol Neurosurg Psychiat 10:141–162

Efron R 1956 The effect of olfactory stimuli in arresting uncinate fits. Brain 79:267–281

de Weerdt C J, van Rijn A J 1975 Conditioning therapy in reading epilepsy. Electroenceph Clin Neurophysiol 39:417–420

Feldman R G, Paul N L 1976 Identity of emotional triggers in epilepsy. J Nerv Ment Dis 162:345

Finley W W, Smith H A, Etherton M D 1975 Reduction of seizures and normalisation of the EEG in a severe epileptic following sensorimotor biofeedback training: preliminary study. Biol Psychol 2:189–203

Finley W W 1977 Operant conditioning of the EEG in two patients with epilepsy. Methodologic and clinical considerations. Pavlovian Journal of Biological Science 12:93–11

Flannery R B Jr, Cautela J R 1973 Seizures: controlling the uncontrollable. J Rehab 39:34–36

Forster F M 1972 The classification and conditioning treatment of the reflex epilepsies. Int J of Neurol 9:73–86

Forster F M, Campos G B 1964 Conditioning factors in stroboscopic-induced seizures. Epilepsia 5:156–165

Forster F M, Hansotia P, Cleeland C S, Ludwig A 1969 A case of voice-induced epilepsy treated by conditioning. Neurology (Minneapolis) 19:325–331

Forster F M, Paulsen W, Baughman F 1969 Clinical therapeutic conditioning in reading epilepsy. Neurology 19:71–77

Forster F M, Penfield W, Jasper H, Madow L 1949 Focal epilepsy, sensory precipitation and evoked cortical potentials. Electroenceph Clin Neurophysiol. 1:349–356

Forster F M, Richards J F, Panitch H S, Huisman R E, Paulsen R E 1975 Reflex epilepsy evoked by decision making. Arch Neurol 32:54–56

Forster F M 1977 Reflex epilepsy. Behaviour therapy and conditional reflexes. Charles C Thomas, Springfield p 318

Forster F M, Ptacek L J, Peterson W G 1965 Auditory clicks in extinction of stroboscope-induced seizures. Epilepsia 6:217–225

Forster F M, Ptacek L J, Peterson W G, Chun R W, Bengzor A R A, Campos G B 1964 Stroboscopic-induced seizure discharges: modification by extinction techniques. Arch Neurol 11:603–608

Gardner J E 1967 Behaviour therapy treatment approach to a psychogenic seizure case. J of Consult Psychol 31:209–212

Gastaut H, Regis H, Dongier S, Roger A 1956 Conditionnement électroencéphalographique des décharges épileptiques et notion d'épilepsie réflexoconditionée. Rev. Neurol 94:829–835

Gastaut H, Trevisan C, Naquet R 1958 Diagnostic value of electroencephalographic abnormalities provoked by intermittent phobic stimulation. Electroenceph Clin Neurophysiol 10:194–195

Gomez G L, Escueta A V 1977 In: Forster F M (ed) Reflex epilepsy, behavioural therapy and conditional reflexes. Charles C Thomas, Springfield, p 318

Gowers W R 1881 Epilepsy and other chronic convulsive disease: their cause, symptoms and treatment. Churchill, London

Gowers W R 1901 Epilepsy and other chronic convulsive diseases, 2nd edn. J & A Churchill, London, p 320

Ince L P 1976 The use of relaxation training and a conditioned stimulus in the elimination of epileptic seizures in a child: a case study. Journal of Behaviour Therapy and Experimental Psychiatry 7:39–42

Ingram A, Ryman H 1962 Epilepsia arithmetics. Neurology (Minneapolis) 12:282–287

Iwata B A, Lorentzson A M 1976 Operant control of seizure-like behaviour in an institutionalised retarded adult. Behaviour Therapy 7: 247–251

Jackson J H 1925 Neurological fragments. London

Jeavons P M, Harding G F A 1975 Photosensitive epilepsy. A review of the literature and a study of 460 patients. William Heinemann, London

Joynt R J, Green D, Green R 1962 Musicogenic epilepsy. J Am Med Ass 179:501–504

Kaplan B J 1975 Biofeedback in epileptics: equivocal relationship of reinforced EEG frequency to seizure reduction. Epilepsia 16:477–485

Kertez A 1967 Paroxysmal kinesigenic choreoathetosis syndrome. Description of 10 cases, including one autopsical. Neurology (Minneapolis) 17:680–690

Kooi K A, Thomas M N, Mortenson F N 1960 Photoconvulsive and photomyoclonic responses in adults. Neurology (Minneapolis) 10:1051–1058

Kuhlman W M, Allison T 1977 EEG feedback training in the treatment of epilepsy: some questions and answers. Pavlovian Journal of Biological Science 12:112–122

Laidlaw J, Richens A 1976 A textbook of epilepsy. Churchill Livingstone, Edinburgh, p 164

Lennox W G, Lennox M 1960 Epilepsy and related disorders. Little, Brown and Co, Boston, p 25

Lockard J S, Wyler A R, Finch C A, Hulburt K E 1977 EEG operant conditioning in a monkey model. I Seizure data. Epilepsia 18(4):471–479

Lubar J F, Bahler J F 1976 Behavioural management of epileptic seizures following EEG biofeedback training of the sensori-motor rhythm. Biofeedback and Self-Regulation 1:77–104

Lubar J F 1977 Electroencephalographic methodology and the management of epilepsy. Pavlovian J of Biological Science 12:147–185

Mattson R H, Heninger G R, Gallagher B B, Glaser G H 1970 Psycho-physiological precipitants of seizures in epileptics. Neurology 20:407

Melsen S 1959 The value of photic stimulation in the diagnosis of epilepsy. J Nerv Ment Dis 128:508–519

Merlis J K 1974 Reflex epilepsy. In: Handbook of neurology vol 15 The epilepsies, ch 25

Mostofsky D I 1975 Teaching the nervous system. New York University Education Quarterly, Spring p 8–13

Mostofsky D I, Balaschak B A 1977 Psychobiological control of seizures. Psychol Bull 84 no 4:723–759

Mount L A, Redback S 1940 Familial paroxysmal choreoathetosis. Arch Neurol Psychiat (Chicago) 44:841–847

Newmark M E, Penry A K 1979 Photosensitivity and epilepsy. A review. Raven Press, New York

Parrino J J 1971 Reduction of seizures by desensitization. Journal of Behaviour Therapy and Experimental Psychiatry 2:215–218

Parsonage M J, Moran J H, Exley K A 1975 Epileptology proceedings of the 7th international symposium on epilepsy. Berlin (West)

Penfield W, Erickson T C 1941 Epilepsy and cerebral localization. Charles C Thomas, Springfield, Illinois, p 27–28

Penfield W, Jasper H 1954 Epilepsy and the functional anatomy of the human brain. Little, Brown and Co, Boston, p 364

Pinto R 1972 A case of movement epilepsy with agoraphobia treated successfully by flooding. Brit J Psychiat 121:287–288

Pitha V 1938 Épilepsie réflexe. Rev Neurol 70:178–181

Poskanzer D C, Brown A E, Miller H 1962 Musicogenic epilepsy caused only by a discrete frequency hand of church bells. Brain 85:77–92

Prechtl H F R 1959 Provocation of electroencephalographic changes in the temporal region by intermittent acoustic stimuli. Electroenceph Clin Neurophysiol 2:511–519

Quy R J, Hutt S J, Forrest S 1979 Sensorimotor rhythm feedback training and epilepsy. Biol Psychol 9:129–149

Scollo-Larizzori G, Hess R 1967 Sensory precipitation of epileptic seizures. Report on two unusual cases. Epilepsia 8:157–161

Seifert A R, Lubar T F 1975 Reduction of epileptic seizures through EEG biofeedback training. Biol. Psychol 3:156–184

Servit Z, Macher J, Štercova Á, Dudás D, Krištof M, Cervenková V 1962 Reflex influences in the pathogenesis of epilepsy in the light of clinical statistics. Epilepsia (Amsterdam) 3:315–322

Shaw D, Hill D 1947 A case of musicogenic epilepsy. J Neurol Neurosurg Psychiat 10:107–117

Standage K F 1972 Treatment of epilepsy by reciprocal inhibition of anxiety. Guy's Hospital Reports 121:217

Sterman M B 1973 Neurophysiologic and clinical studies of sensorimotor EEG biofeedback training: some effects of epilepsy. In: Birk L (ed) Biofeedback: behaviour medicine. Grune and Stratton, Boston, p 507–526

Sterman M B 1977 Effects of sensorimotor EEG feedback training on sleep and clinical manifestation of epilepsy. In: Beatty J, Legewie H (eds) Biofeedback and behaviour. Plenum Press, New York, p 167–200

Sterman M B MacDonald L R 1974 Alterations of seizure activity and EEG patterns in epileptics by sensorimotor cortex EEG biofeedback training. Electroencep Clin Neurophysiol 37:418

Stevens H 1966 Paroxysmal choreo-athetosis. A form of reflex epilepsy. Arch Neurol (Chicago) 14:415–420

Stevens J R 1962 Control and peripheral factors in epileptic discharge. Arch Neurol (Chicago) 7:330–338

Symonds C 1959 Excitation and inhibition in epilepsy Brain 82(2):133–146

Temkin O 1945 The falling sickness. The Johns Hopkins Press, Baltimore, p 42

Titeca J 1965 L'épilepsie musicogénique. Revue générale à propos d'un cas personnel suivi pendant quartorze ans. Acta neurol belg 65:598–648

Watson C S, Marcus E M 1962 The genetics and clinical significance of photogenic cerebral electrical abnormalities, myoclonus and seizures. Trans Am Neurol Ass 87:251–253

Whyler A R, Lockard J S, Ward A A, Finch C A 1976 Condition EEG desynchronization and seizure occurrence in patients. Electroenceph Clin Neurophysiol 41:501–512

Wilkins A J, Darby C E, Binnie C D, Stefansson S B, Jeavons P M, Harding G F A 1979 Television epilepsy, the role of pattern. J Electroenceph Clin Neurophysiol 47:163–171

Wilkins A J, Binnie C D, Darby C E 1980 Visually induced seizures. In: Progress in Neurobiology. Pergamon Press, UK, vol 15, p 1–33

Wilkins A J, Zifkin B, Anderman F, McGovern 1981 Seizures induced by thinking. Annals of Neurology (in preparation)

Wolpe J 1969 The practice of behaviour therapy. Pergamon Press, Elmsford, NY

Wright L 1973 Aversive conditioning of self-induced seizures. Behaviour Therapy 4:712–713

Zlutnick S I 1972 The control of seizures by the modification of pre-seizure behaviour: the punishment of behavioural chain components (doctoral dissertation Utah State College). Dissertation Abstracts International 33:6B University Microfilms no 72-31:182

Zlutnick S I, Mayville W J, Moffat S 1975 Behavioural control of seizure disorders: the interruption of chained behaviour. In: Katz R C, Zlutnick S I (eds) Behaviour therapy and health care: principles and applications. Pergamon Press, Elmsford, NY.

The management of seizures associated with psychological disorders

INTRODUCTION

A chapter or discussion devoted to the management of one aspect of a patient's problems, in this case the seizures but not the psychological disorders, may perhaps be accused of not treating the patient as a whole. The risks involved in such a myopic approach would be all the greater if there was any question of an epileptic basis for the psychological symptoms (see Chapter 19). Nevertheless in the great majority of patients the distinction between the seizures and the psychological disorder is sufficiently clear-cut, and the pharmacological and other aspects of management of each sufficiently different and complex in their own right, to justify this separate discussion of the treatment of the epilepsy, provided the risks are clearly stated. It is emphasised therefore that this chapter should be read in conjunction with those chapters which discuss the management of the associated psychological disorders. Furthermore, bearing in mind the interaction between seizures, emotional state, psychological and social stresses, (see Chapter 5) it is understood that the most effective management of the psychological and social problems of the epileptic patient is absolutely essential for the most effective control of seizures, especially in the more severe epileptic patient in whom pharmacological measures may be inadequate to suppress attacks.

The emphasis, then, in this chapter will be mainly on the pharmacological control of seizures in the context of psychiatric disorders.

PRINCIPLES OF PHARMACOLOGICAL MANAGEMENT

The first point to stress is that the principles of drug treatment of seizures in the presence of psychological diseases will differ little from those in the absence of such disorders. However particular problems in management do occur which justify special consideration.

The modern pharmacological management of epileptic patients has been greatly influenced by the rapid growth in our knowledge of the clinical pharmacology of the major anticonvulsants in the last decade. This in turn has resulted from the development of techniques to measure the drugs and their metabolites in biological fluids. Widespread experience has confirmed that blood level monitoring of many of the drugs can allow a more simple, rational and effective approach to drug treatment (Reynolds 1978). It is not necessary for me to review here the clinical pharmacological and pharmaco-kinetic knowledge on which such monitoring is based as the reader can be referred to several such reviews (e.g. Woodbury et al 1972, Richens 1976, Reynolds 1980, Eadie & Tyrer 1980). Rather it is my intention to provide practical advice on the application of such knowledge in the management of epileptic patients, especially those with psychological problems.

In discussing the management of epilepsy it is important to clearly distinguish between patients presenting for treatment for the first time, and the vast numbers of chronic patients already taking one or more anticonvulsants when first seen. The approach to treatment and prognosis is usually very different for these two groups (Reynolds 1980). The majority of patients with psychological disorders will of course fall into the latter group, but the former group deserve detailed consideration if only to prevent so many of the problems of chronicity, including some of their psychological complications (see Chapter 19), into which they might otherwise so readily drift.

NEW REFERRALS WITH EPILEPSY AND PSYCHOLOGICAL DISORDERS

1. The decision to treat

The question whether or not to institute anticonvulsant therapy in a patient (with or without psychological disorder) who has had one or more recent, or not so recent, seizures can be difficult. There can be no overall answer to the question and every case must be considered in the light of all the particular circumstances. Certain guiding principles however may be useful.

It has been widely accepted that a single first seizure does not usually justify institution of drug therapy, except in special situations in which the risk of recurrence may be high, e.g. in advancing cerebral lesions. In the event of recurrence of seizures the decision to treat will depend on the estimated risk of further attacks. Factors which might be thought to increase that risk will include several attacks in a short period of time, occurrence of major or partial attacks associated with cerebral pathology (usually non-progressive), a continuing high level of anxiety or stress, or the need to continue with psychotropic drugs (such as phenothiazines or tricyclic antidepressants) with mild epileptogenic properties. Factors which might indicate a decreased risk would be occurrence of attacks in unusual circumstances which could be avoided in the future, e.g. a stress situation which has passed, loss of sleep, alcohol or drug excess or abuse.

Other considerations that might enter into the decision may be that the recurrence of even a single seizure could be judged to be devastating to the morale or mental health of the patient, for example due to loss of a driving licence, or, alternatively, that one or more seizures might even have some advantage for the mental health of the patient, for example in a catatonic schizophrenic or in the alternating psychoses, as discussed in Chapter 19. It should also be borne in mind that there is some evidence that each seizure may to some extent facilitate the occurrence of another, as originally suggested by Gowers (1881) and discussed in Chapter 19. Therefore the more seizures occur, the greater perhaps the future risk. Further, the earlier the seizure disorder is suppressed, possibly the better will be the long-term seizure control (Rodin 1968, Reynolds 1980). On the other hand there is growing evidence that chronic therapy, especially with barbiturate or hydantoin drugs, may have long-term adverse effects on mental function (see Chapter 19).

If seizures present in a patient taking one of the more epileptogenic psychotropic drugs consideration should first be given to reduction of the dose of the latter, if high, or to switching to a less epileptogenic drug e.g. nomifensine instead of a tricyclic antidepressant (see Chapter 24). However, seizures in the context of drug abuse, alcohol withdrawal or the inadvertent or deliberate withdrawal from benzodiazepines, are not usually an indication for starting anticonvulsant therapy. It cannot be too strongly emphasized that a major factor in good seizure control is good compliance. A particular hazard with anticonvulsants is the occurrence of withdrawal seizures due to poor compliance. The patient may in fact be better off without any anticonvulsant therapy rather than to take it erratically. If there is any doubt about the willingness of the patient to comply with treatment, which is almost always the case with alcoholics and drug abusers, then antiepileptic therapy is best avoided, as the hazards of anticonvulsant withdrawal will be added to those of alcohol or other drug withdrawal. Unfortunately there is also some evidence that epileptic patients with psychosocial disorders comply less well with anticonvulsant therapy than patients without such complications, which may explain in part the generally poorer prognosis for seizure control in the presence of such additional handicaps (Rodin 1968, Reynolds 1980).

2. Choice of drug

One of the major problems associated with anticonvulsant therapy is the widespread practice of polytherapy (Reynolds & Shorvon 1981). This problem is compounded by the large number of drugs available and lack of agreement as to their relative merits. For example, according to Gastaut & Osuntokun (1976) Spain has 25 antiepileptic products in the form of 85 formulations, 23 of which are combinations of drugs! At present in Great Britain there are 21 formulations of 15 drugs. Although there might be general, but by no means universal, agreement about the shortlist of anticonvulsant drugs for generalised and partial seizures proposed in Table 23.1, there would be little agreement as to which of these drugs should be used first, which second, and so on. The main reason for these varying opinions is that there is very little scientific evidence on which to make a rational choice. This in turn reflects the poor quality of the trials which have accompanied the introduction of each new drug (Coatsworth 1971). Apart from the omission of basic clinical information, the absence of controlled design or appropriate statistical evaluation, a particular feature of such trials is that invariably they have been undertaken in chronic patients previously on one or usually more drugs, thus perpetuating the phenomenon of polytherapy. Furthermore, the major drugs have rarely been compared with each other in a satisfactory manner. What little evidence is available suggests there is little to choose between them for antiepileptic efficacy, although there are some clear differences in side effects and costs (Reynolds 1980).

Table 23.1   Shortlist of first-line anticonvulsants*

Type of epilepsy	Drug	Optimum serum levels (μg/ml)
Tonic-clonic (grand mal) or partial (focal) $\pm$ tonic-clonic	Phenobarbitone	15–40
	Phenytoin	10–20
	Primidone	as for phenobarbitone
	Carbamazepine	4–10
	Clonazepam‡	†
	Sodium valproate‡	50–100
Petit mal	Ethosuximide	40–80
	Clonazepam	†
	Sodium valproate	50–100

* In historical order of introduction, which does not imply any order of merit
† The value of monitoring clonazepam is not yet established
‡ Also useful for myoclonic epilepsy

Especially on a background of psychological disorder, certain adverse effects of some anticonvulsants may weigh heavily in the choice of first drug. For grand mal or partial seizures although there may be little to choose between phenobarbitone, phenytoin, primidone and carbamazepine for antiepileptic efficacy, the last drug almost certainly has less adverse effects on mental function (see Chapter 19), even if claims that it actually has positive psychotropic properties have not been substantiated (Parnas et al 1979). Phenobarbitone and primidone may cause drowsiness, depression, irritability and hyperkinetic behaviour; and phenytoin may also have subtle adverse effects on concentration, memory and psychomotor performance. Clonazepam also causes drowsiness, especially in the early stages. Although tolerance to this side effect may occur the same phenomenon may also apply to its antiepileptic properties, so that initially promising results may be followed later by some loss of seizure control. However this drug may be particularly useful for myoclonic forms of epilepsy, and also for other seizure disorders when anxiety forms a prominent part of the background. In the latter situation the tranquillising properties of the drug may be just as, if not more, important than the antiepileptic properties. The role of the most recent drug, sodium valproate, is less certain. It too may be very useful for myoclonic forms of epilepsy. Reports that it is as effective as the older major anticonvulsants for grand mal require confirmation. It is probably only of limited value for partial seizures. Claims that it is relatively free of side effects have probably been overstated. Apart from weight gain and occasional problems with platelet and liver function it can certainly cause drowsiness (especially in combination with other drugs) and may possibly cause or at least contribute to an encephalopathy (Corbett et al 1981).

For petit mal there is even less evidence on which to make a rational choice from the three drugs in Table 23.1. Until recently most physicians have started with ethosuximide. Sodium valproate is also undoubtedly effective, and there may be little to choose between the anti-petit mal effects of these two drugs. Occasional adverse effects of ethosuximide on mental function have been noted (Trimble & Reynolds 1976), as with sodium valproate (see above).

Although there are other drugs available for the treatment of different seizures there is no evidence that they are either as effective or superior to the drugs discussed and listed in Table 23.1. There would therefore seem to be little justification for using them as the first drug of choice in new referrals, although there may be a case for continuing them in chronic patients who have already taken them for some years.

In discussing the relative merits of the drugs in Table 23.1 I have emphasised there is little to choose between them with respect to their antiepileptic properties, partly for lack of adequate studies. The choice therefore may be influenced by the relative toxic effects of the drugs, of which there are undoubted differences. Bearing in mind the type of patient I am considering and the orientation of this book I have mainly discussed the effects of the drugs on mental function (see Chapter 19). There are of course many other subtle, chronic physical effects of the drugs which I have discussed elsewhere (Reynolds 1975), and which may also influence the choice of drug. Further there are considerable differences in the cost of the drugs which perhaps will be particularly relevant in underdeveloped countries, where there may be greater economic constraints on prescribing. However, a probably more important consideration than the actual choice of drug is the manner in which it is used. There is now much more scope for the effective utilisation of drugs, with the avoidance of so many of the pitfalls and problems which have characterised chronic anticonvulsant therapy in the past.

3. Utilisation of drugs: compliance and blood level monitoring

Once a decision to treat has been made, one of the drugs from Table 23.1, appropriate for the seizure type, should be started in a small dose (e.g. in adolescents or adults carbamazepine 100 mg b.d., phenytoin 100 mg b.d., phenobarbitone 30 mg b.d., primidone 125 mg b.d., clonazepam 0.5 mg b.d. or sodium valproate 200 mg b.d.). The reason for starting with a *small* dose is that the aim of treatment should be to control seizures with the minimum amount of medication necessary. There is evidence, at least in adolescents and adults, that for grand mal and/or partial seizures as many as one third may be controlled with the starting dose or at least with blood levels which fall below the so-called optimum ranges quoted in Table 23.1 (Reynolds 1980).

The results of treatment will be improved by emphasising to the patient the importance of good compliance and the hazards of withdrawal seizures in the event of inadvertent or deliberate failure to take the medication. There is evidence that poor compliance is a major problem, at least amongst patients attending hospital clinics, and it is probably more common in patients with psychological or other handicaps (Reynolds & Shorvon 1981).

Compliance can be improved by administering the drugs no more than twice daily, thus avoiding embarrassing or easily forgotten middle of the day doses; by avoiding complicated regimes of polypharmacy; by tablet counting; and by monitoring the blood level of the drug. Compliance is always important but no more so than in the early stages of treatment, when the pattern of what is to follow may be set, when the greatest potential for seizure control may exist, when the infrequency of seizures may lead to greatest complacency, and when patients are still having understandable difficulty in adjusting both to the diagnosis of epilepsy and the need for long-term treatment.

Not uncommonly in the past some patients have been started on treatment with a small dose of *two* drugs (e.g. phenobarbitone and phenytoin), either in the hope of obtaining synergism, or avoiding undesirable effects of bigger doses of either drug used singly. However, there is no evidence to support either belief and there is no justification for the practice as it already condemns the patient to polytherapy with all its problems (Reynolds & Shorvon 1981).

If seizures recur on the starting dose of the first drug, blood level monitoring will help to decide whether this is due to poor compliance (in which case the patient is encouraged to continue with the same dose more reliably) or whether the dose should be increased by small increments until seizures are controlled or the upper end of the optimum range for that drug (Table 23.1) has been achieved. As many as a further one third of patients may be controlled by this process. If seizures continue despite the constant achievement of high optimum blood levels of the starting drug this should be regarded as true failure of single drug therapy, which may occur in 15–20 per cent of adolescent or adult outpatients (Reynolds & Shorvon 1981). There is a further small group of up to 10 per cent of patients who, although they may occasionally achieve an optimum level, never adequately comply with treatment for a variety of personal and social reasons, and should not be regarded as failures of monotherapy. They are at particular risk of unnecessary polypharmacy. The percentage of patients with true failure of monotherapy, or apparent failure due to poor compliance, may prove to be slightly higher in selected groups of patients with brain damage and psychological handicaps of the type discussed in this book, but only further studies will clarify this.

In the event of true failure of single drug therapy two strategies are available. There is a case for trying the addition of a second drug, although the extent, if any, to which this may provide further protection is uncertain at the present time. The second drug should also be started in a small dose, following the same policy of small incremental increases, as dictated by clinical progress, into the optimum range for that drug, while maintaining the first drug in the optimum range. An alternative and possibly preferable strategy is substitution of another drug for the first drug. In this case the objective is to achieve an optimum level of the new drug as soon as possible and then slowly withdraw the first drug by small increments to minimise possible withdrawal effects.

There can be no doubt that either of the above two strategies in response to failure of the first drug will still leave some patients' seizures uncontrolled. There is no case, however, for adding a third or fourth drug. It should be accepted that some patients will continue to have seizures despite an optimum level of one or two drugs. The administration of further polytherapy should be avoided while attempts to improve seizure control by non-pharmacological methods should be continued (see below).

One exception to the strategy outlined above is the patient with more than one seizure type, e.g. grand mal and petit mal, each of which may require separate specific drugs, although it should also be noted that some of the drugs in Table 23.1 such as valproate and clonazepam do have a broad range of anti-epileptic activity.

CHRONIC EPILEPTIC PATIENTS WITH PSYCHOLOGICAL DISORDERS

There is no doubt that the combination of seizures and psychological disorders is most often to be found in chronic epileptic patients who have already been taking one or usually more drugs for several years. The reasons for the evolution of mental symptoms in these epileptic patients are many and complex as reviewed in several chapters in this book, and include anticonvulsant therapy itself as discussed in Chapter 19. There is also little doubt that the drug treatment of such patients presents much more formidable problems than those posed by the new, previously untreated, referrals discussed above. Indeed many of the pharmacological problems of the chronic patient arise because of the poor quality of their drug management in earlier years.

The typical anticonvulsant profile of the chronic patient with psychiatric disorder is that of polytherapy, usually anything from two to four or more drugs! The aim of future treatment should be to simplify and rationalise this polytherapy by cautious reduction to two or possibly one drug, each maintained in the optimum range under blood level guidance. However, this may be a very difficult and sometimes impossible task, which carries with it certain risks. On the other hand if the difficult withdrawal phase is successfully negotiated it may be of considerable benefit to the patient not only in terms of improved mental function and reduced toxicity, but also sometimes better seizure control. Shorvon & Reynolds (1979) were able to reduce polytherapy to monotherapy in 72 per cent of 40 chronic outpatients. A striking feature was the improvement in alertness, concentration, mood, behaviour and sociability in many, especially on withdrawal of barbiturates, and sometimes phenytoin therapy. More surprising was the significant improvement in seizure control in 55 per cent. Six patients actually became seizure free. However seizure control was worse in 17 per cent. Further, the attempt to reduce polytherapy failed in 28 per cent of the original 40 patients, either because of exacerbation of seizures during the withdrawal phase, or because of pressure on the authors (or failing them, other physicians) to do something in the face of continuing seizures, although there was no evidence that attacks were more frequent. Reduction in polytherapy was more difficult in patients with brain damage or other psychological handicaps, with more severe epilepsy, or on the most drugs. The Milano Collaborative Group (1977) also attempted to rationalise therapy in a particularly difficult institutionalised population, in whom they succeeded in reducing the mean number of anticonvulsant drugs from 2.5 to 2 while at the same time reducing the overall seizure frequency by 50 per cent, and improving alertness and psychomotor performance in many.

The major problem in rationalising chronic polytherapy is the risk of exacerbation of seizures or even occasionally precipitating status epilepticus during the withdrawal phase. This phenomenon amounts to more than simply the release of the underlying seizure tendency. Many patients are in any case already having frequent seizures. In all probability it represents a temporary decrease in seizure threshold as a result of drug withdrawal. This view is supported by the evidence that if the withdrawal phase is eventually negotiated seizure frequency may then actually improve on the pre-withdrawal rate in some patients. It is also well known that withdrawal from chronic barbiturate therapy in non-epileptic subjects may precipitate withdrawal seizures. The type of epileptic patients under consideration in this chapter are at particular risk of this withdrawal complication, especially if they are brain-damaged with severe epilepsy. However, it is also in the psychologically handicapped group in whom the rewards for improved mental health and seizure control can be most striking. This poses a dilemma as to how determined an effort should be made to rationalise therapy, and at what point should the attempt be abandoned if it seems not to be succeeding and the hazards appear to be outweighing any possible longer-term advantage? Such questions are not easily answered in general and the decision must be guided by all the individual circumstances.

How can the risks of withdrawal be minimised and the advantages maximised? Which drugs and at what rate should be withdrawn? Again these questions are not easily answered, partly for lack of sufficient study. Prudence suggests that drugs should be withdrawn one at a time and slowly, even if the whole process should take several months. However, I am not aware of any investigation to confirm the advantages of this cautious approach. There may sometimes be a case for admitting the patient, especially if the risks of exacerbation are thought to be high, or if one wishes to speed up the withdrawal process under careful supervision. As to which drugs to withdraw and which to continue, the choice will be very much influenced by the particular combination already being taken or tried in the past, as well as the suitability of the drugs for the type of epilepsy in question. Preference will usually be given to maintaining one or two of the drugs listed in Table 23.1 especially if they are easily monitored. However, if one of the older or less widely used drugs has suited a patient well for many years there may be no particular merit in switching him to a newer or more fashionable drug. The longer a patient has tolerated a drug the more difficult it may be to withdraw it. Drugs which are already being taken in inadequate dosage may perhaps be withdrawn first. Particular drug combinations such as two barbiturates or two benzodiazepines should be readily recognised as undesirable, justifying the withdrawal of one of them. Surprisingly, such irrational combinations are not uncommonly found, for example, but by no means exclusively, in mental hospital patients where little attention may have been paid to anticonvulsant therapy over the years. Preparations containing two or more drugs (e.g. combined capsules of phenobarbitone and phenytoin) may need to be split into two separate preparations in order to withdraw one of them or to facilitate the monitoring of each of them. Of all the drugs listed in Table 23.1 there are distinct advantages in maintaining carbamazepine as the drug of choice in patients with psychological problems, for the reasons already discussed (see also Chapter 19). I have observed striking improvement in mental function in some chronic patients with intellectual, personality or psychiatric problems when reduced to this drug alone (unpublished observations). The advantages of withdrawing barbiturate drugs and, to a lesser extent, phenytoin, will also be understood from their adverse effects on mental function (Chapter 19), although the withdrawal effects of barbiturates may be particularly troublesome. It should be emphasised that perhaps the most important gains come simply from reducing unnecessary polypharmacy with any drugs, especially if the polypharmacy is aggravating the epilepsy as well as mental function. On the other hand if reduction of therapy is followed by deterioration in seizure control this could have an injurious effect on the mental state. Herein lies the dilemma and the challenge of chronic anticonvulsant polytherapy. It emphasises again the need to *avoid* polytherapy if possible by more careful therapy at the onset, along the lines already discussed.

MONOTHERAPY OR POLYTHERAPY?

A central theme in the preceding discussion of the management of both new and chronic patients has been the emphasis on avoiding or reducing polytherapy while using one or at most two drugs per seizure type, if necessary to their optimum capacity with blood level guidance. The question of monotherapy or polytherapy for seizures has been reviewed by Reynolds & Shorvon (1981) but requires some amplification here.

Polytherapy seems to have been the traditional approach to treatment throughout the ages. Paradoxically it seems to have increased in this century with the advent of drugs of undoubted efficacy. Guelen et al (1975) showed in a survey of four European countries that the mean number of drugs per patient was 3.2 of which 84 per cent were anticonvulsants. There are many reasons for this polytherapy, including: the early age of onset of seizures; the natural tendency to add more and newer drugs in the face of continuing seizures, of which some types have a relatively poorer prognosis; the failure to recognise the limits of effective drug control, other than those imposed by toxicity; the poor quality of the evaluation and use of the drugs in recent decades; and the large numbers of drugs available, sometimes including two or three in a single preparation. More recently however it has become clearer that there are many undesirable consequences to unbridled polytherapy, such as subtle chronic toxic effects (including mental symptoms), drug interactions, failure to adequately evaluate new drugs, and possibly the most serious of all, aggravation of seizures in some patients. Further, despite the widespread practice of polytherapy, with all its problems, there is surprisingly little evidence to justify it. Since the availability of drug level monitoring, studies in new patients have shown there is considerable potential for monotherapy. In the 20 per cent or so of new patients who fail to respond to the optimum use of a single anticonvulsant drug, the value, if any, of a second drug remains uncertain at the present time, although it is clearly worth trying. It is highly questionable however whether more than two drugs should be given for any seizure type. In chronic patients there is considerable scope for reduction of polytherapy at least to two and sometimes to one drug. Although this may have many advantages for some patients both in terms of reduced toxicity, especially mental symptoms, and ultimately improved seizure control, it also carries the risk of deterioration in seizure control, mainly due to withdrawal effects, a phenomenon which has played a major role in perpetuating polytherapy. It is clearly more difficult to reduce polytherapy than to avoid it which is why I have emphasised more careful attention to pharmacological control of seizures from the beginning, which is also the time when the best control of seizures can be achieved.

There are advantages in this more simple and rational approach to drug therapy which extend beyond the pharmacological control of seizures. If seizures are treated in the most effective way with one or at the most two drugs with clearly defined limits, then more time and attention can be devoted to other important non-pharmacological aspects of management.

THERAPEUTIC OR OPTIMUM BLOOD DRUG LEVELS

Another major component of the approach to drug treatment discussed here is the use of blood drug levels. The reader has already been referred to reviews of our expanding knowledge of the clinical pharmacology of the drugs, but certain aspects of the use of drug level monitoring deserve more detailed discussion, as they are sometimes a source of misunderstanding.

We are fortunate that for several anticonvulsant drugs there is a good correlation between the blood and the brain level (which is presumably where the drug acts), and in turn with the antiepileptic efficacy and, to a lesser extent, some aspects of toxicity. However the widespread quotation or application of certain 'therapeutic' or optimum blood level ranges (as in Table 23.1) has sometimes given rise to the misconception that all patients should have their blood levels within these ranges for the desired antiepileptic effect. However it is clear that there is no such thing as a therapeutic range applicable to *all* epileptic patients, unless it be from just above zero to the top end of the ranges quoted. Epilepsy, like most disorders, is of variable severity. Less frequent seizures can certainly be controlled with low blood levels, below those quoted in Table 23.1, as may occur in up to one third of new referrals. The value of the ranges quoted, which are thought to encompass maximum or optimum antiepileptic capacity without intolerable toxicity, is that they are useful guidelines for the more severe epileptic patient. Of course there will still be some patients whose seizures are not controlled despite optimum levels of one or even two drugs, but at least the physician will know that each drug is being used to its maximum (optimum) effect and he can avoid polytherapy, while concentrating on non-pharmacological measures.

The most important aspect of the optimum range is perhaps its upper limit and there is certainly a need for more research into the careful delineation of this point for all the drugs discussed. The upper limit should not be applied too rigidly, as it may indeed vary between patients. Nor should it be regarded as the point at which toxic symptoms develop, because there is often some degree of overlap between optimum and toxic ranges, not only for acute toxicity but especially for chronic effects. Although above the upper limit there is an increasing prevalence of toxicity it may also be true there is little or no further antiepileptic action. Indeed, there is a suspicion that any further increase may be counter productive and in some patients lead to actual deterioration in seizure control. This concept also requires further research.

Finally I would emphasize that blood level monitoring is not a substitute for clinical judgement, but should be used as an aid to clinical management. The management of epilepsy is a complex, often multidisciplinary, affair which involves attention to many aspects of the patient including metabolic, neurological, psychological and social problems. At all stages it should be remembered that it is the patient that is being treated, not the blood level. Slavish adherence to blood level guidelines must not be allowed to replace careful attention to all aspects of treatment. Rather the judicious use of blood level monitoring should make it possible to pay more attention to the latter.

PSYCHIATRIC REASONS FOR REDUCING OR WITHDRAWING ANTICONVULSANT MEDICATION

The principles of pharmacological management discussed in the preceding sections have been orientated towards obtaining the maximum seizure control with the minimum of undesirable effects, especially of a mental kind. They are applicable to the great majority of epileptic patients with or without existing psychological handicaps. However there are some specific clinical situations in which adjustment of anticonvulsant medication will be dictated primarily by the objective of improving mental function or behaviour, while recognising that this may involve risk of exacerbation of seizures or even, rarely, with the deliberate intention of provoking one or more seizures.

Anticonvulsant intoxication
Acute intoxication with most of the drugs in Table 23.1 may present with mental symptoms ('encephalopathy', 'confusion', 'psychosis'), sometimes in the absence of other clinical signs, such as nystagmus or ataxia. It must of course be reversed by the appropriate reduction of the offending drug to a more suitable (optimum) blood level, even if there may be some risk of exacerbation of seizures (almost certainly a withdrawal phenomenon) in so doing.

Subacute encephalopathy
Less well recognised is the subacute deterioration in mental function ('subacute encephalopathy', 'dementia', 'pseudo-degenerative disorder') without more classical signs of toxicity, which is associated with phenytoin in particular, but probably also with barbiturates (Chapter 19). It also is reversible unless it has been allowed to continue unrecognised for too long. Although the blood drug level is usually high it may occasionally occur with more modest, even optimum, blood levels and it is probably advisable to withdraw the drug altogether and substitute carbamazepine.

Hyperkinetic syndrome
It is well known that this syndrome may be provoked in children by barbiturates, especially phenobarbitone (Ounsted 1955), but there has been remarkably little study of the problem. The offending drug should be withdrawn. Irritable, aggressive and disturbed behaviour in adults may also be an indication for withdrawal of barbiturate therapy and substitution of a more suitable drug, such as carbamazepine.

Schizophrenia-like psychoses
There is a subgroup of patients with usually short-lived episodes of psychosis, which seem to appear (alternate) at times of good control of seizures, sometimes,

but not always, associated with 'forced normalisation' of the EEG (see Chapter 19). In these patients the recurrence of seizures can be associated with a remarkable improvement in the mental state. It may therefore be justifiable in such patients to reduce or even withdraw therapy temporarily with the object of allowing the occurrence of one or more seizures. Some of the more chronic schizophrenia-like psychoses may also be associated with a tendency to reduced seizure frequency, but withdrawing or reducing anticonvulsant therapy has less predictable effects on the mental state. There may, however, be a case for substituting carbamazepine for barbiturate or hydantoin therapy, as indeed in other chronic psychiatric disorders associated with epilepsy, for the reasons already discussed (see also Chapter 19).

INTERACTION OF ANTICONVULSANT AND PSYCHOTROPIC DRUGS

The extensive literature on interactions between different anticonvulsants, and between anticonvulsant and non-anticonvulsant drugs is reviewed by Perucca (1981). A few interactions between anticonvulsant and psychotropic drugs have been reported, but for most of these the clinical significance is slight or uncertain. The influence of benzodiazepines on phenytoin has proved variable or contradictory, with reports of both elevation and depression of phenytoin blood levels. Both imipramine and chlorpromazine may depress serum phenytoin slightly due to inhibition of metabolism. Phenytoin, barbiturates and carbamazepine may also stimulate the metabolism of imipramine, desmethyl imipramine, nortryptyline or chlorpromazepine, but there is no clear evidence that the psychotropic effects of the latter drugs are significantly impaired. Potentially important are two case reports of lithium toxicity in the presence of phenytoin, despite therapeutic levels of the former (Spiers & Hirsch 1978, MacCallum 1980). The implication is that the clinical interpretation of lithium levels may be unreliable in the presence of phenytoin.

NON-PHARMACOLOGICAL APPROACHES TO MANAGEMENT

Drug treatment is only one of several important aspects of the management of seizures, the more so in patients with psychological disorders. It is not the purpose of this chapter to discuss these non-pharmacological approaches, many of which are covered in other chapters of this book. It is appropriate however to make brief reference to them so that the pharmacological measures discussed here may be seen in their proper perspective.

Precipitating factors

This subject is discussed by Fenwick in Chapter 22 with special emphasis on environmental and internal stimuli which may evoke seizures in otherwise predisposed individuals, including the conscious capacity of some patients to precipitate or inhibit their own seizures. Fenwick rightly emphasises the importance of such knowledge in treatment, whether by avoiding the provoking stimulus when possible, or by the development of behavioural or related techniques of inhibition.

Metabolic factors

It is assumed that patients will have been carefully investigated for treatable metabolic factors (Meldrum 1981) prior to the institution of treatment. Some have to be borne in mind during long-term management e.g. fluid retention or excessive fluid intake, hypoglycaemia, hypocalcaemia (sometimes drug-induced), menstrual irregularities and other hormonal disturbances. It is well known that such factors may precipitate or aggravate psychological symptoms, as well as seizures. Toxic factors such as alcohol, other drugs, or their withdrawal, should be considered during inexplicable exacerbations of epilepsy.

Regrettably however metabolic approaches to treatment play only a small role at present, mainly due to our ignorance of neurochemical mechanisms underlying seizure disorders. There is still a place, for example, for ACTH or steroid treatment, or ketogenic diet, in certain types of childhood epilepsy (O'Donoghue 1979). In view of the long-term nature of anticonvulsant treatment, with its inevitable accompaniment of chronic toxicity (Reynolds 1975), it is to be hoped in the future that metabolic treatment may have a more prominent place, as our understanding of neurotransmission and other possible neurochemical distur-bances grows. There has been recent interest, for example, in the manipulation of monoamine metabolism by the use of the relevant precursors, encouraged by the effect of 5-hydroxytryptophan on certain types of myoclonus (Chadwick et al 1978).

Neurosurgery

Temporal lobectomy has been shown to be of value in carefully selected patients with temporal lobe epilepsy of unilateral origin and resistant to medical treatment (Taylor & Falconer 1968, Falconer 1973; see Chapter 17). Most of these patients also have psychological handicaps. Indeed only 13.4 per cent were rated as psychiatrically normal pre-operatively in the series of Taylor & Falconer (1968). This figure rose to 32 per cent post-operatively. The psychological features which stand to benefit most from successful surgery are social adjustment and behaviour disorders, including aggression. Neurotic and psychotic features are much less commonly improved, and indeed some patients have developed psychoses for the first time post-operatively, as occurred in nine out of 74 patients reported by Jensen & Larsen (1979).

Psychosocial factors

It is appropriate to end this chapter by emphasising, as at the beginning, that I have been discussing the management of only one of the patient's problems, namely the seizures. The management of the associated psychological disorders is discussed in several other chapters in this book. However it should hardly need stressing that, even in the absence of overt psychological disorders, due attention to emotional, psychological and social factors is essential for the best control of seizures. This is even more true in the presence of such disorders, when the prognosis for seizure control is usually worse (Rodin 1968). Sympathetic handling of these problems often provides the best chance of optimum seizure control, which in turn is necessary for optimum emotional and psychological adjustment (see Chapter 5).

One reason for discussing the pharmacological control of seizures in such detail here is that too often in the past, as at present, too much attention has been paid to frequent and fruitless changes of anticonvulsant therapy, while the more time-consuming psychosocial problems of the patient are overlooked. The more simple and rational strategy for anticonvulsant use discussed here should make it possible to avoid unnecessary drug manipulation and accumulation, while releasing more time for consideration of the equally important psychosocial aspects of management.

References

Chadwick D, Trimble M, Jenner P, Driver M, Reynolds E H 1978 Manipulation of cerebral monoamines in the treatment of human epilepsy: a pilot study. Epilepsia 19:3–10

Coatsworth J J 1971 Studies on the clinical efficacy of marketed antiepileptic drugs. NINDS Monograph no 12, US Government Printing Office, Washington DC

Corbett J, Driver M, Reynolds E H 1981 Valproate encephalopathy. Communication to British Branch of the International League Against Epilepsy, April 1980 (in preparation)

Eadie M J, Tyrer J H 1980 Anticonvulsant therapy. Pharmacological basis and practice. Churchill Livingstone, Edinburgh

Falconer M A 1973 Reversibility by temporal lobe resection of the behavioural abnormalities of temporal lobe epilepsy. New Engl J Med 289:451–455

Gastaut H, Osuntokun B O 1976 Proposals on antiepileptic pharmacotherapy for use in developing countries. Epilepsia 17:355–360

Gowers W R 1881 Epilepsy and other chronic convulsive diseases. Churchill, London

Guelan P J M, Van der Kleijn E, Woudstra U 1975 Statistical analysis of pharmacokinetic parameters in epileptic patients chronically treated with antiepileptic drugs. In: Schneider H, Janz D, Gardner-Thorpe C, Meinardi H, Sherwin A L (eds) Clinical pharmacology of antiepileptic drugs. Springer-Verlag, Berlin, p 2–10

Jensen I, Larsen J K 1979 Mental aspects of temporal lobe epilepsy. J Neurol Neurosurg Psychiat 42:256–265

MacCallum W A G 1980 Interaction of lithium and phenytoin. Br med J 280:610–611

Meldrum B 1981 Pathology and pathophysiology. In: Laidlaw J, Richens A (eds) A textbook of epilepsy. Churchill Livingstone, Edinburgh

Milano collaborative group for studies on epilepsy 1977 Long-term monitoring in the difficult patient. Preliminary results of 16 months of observations — usefulness and limitations. In: Gardner-Thorpe C, Janz D, Meinardi H, Pippinger C E (eds) Antiepileptic drug monitoring. Pitman, Tunbridge Wells, p 197–213

O'Donohoe N V 1979 Epilepsies in childhood. Butterworths, London

Ounsted C 1955 The hyperkinetic syndrome in epileptic children. Lancet 2:303–311

Parnas J, Flachs H, Gram L 1979 Psychotropic effect of antiepileptic drugs. Acta neurol scand 80:329–343

Perucca E 1981 Drug interactions. In: Laidlaw J, Richens A (eds) A textbook of epilepsy. Churchill Livingstone, Edinburgh

Reynolds E H 1975 Chronic antiepileptic toxicity: a review. Epilepsia 16:319–352

Reynolds E H 1978 Drug treatment of epilepsy. Lancet 2:721–725

Reynolds E H 1980 Serum levels of anticonvulsant drugs: interpretation and clinical value. Pharmac Ther 8:217–235

Reynolds E H, Shorvon S D 1981 Monotherapy or polytherapy for epilepsy? Epilepsia 22:1–10

Richens A 1976 Drug treatment of epilepsy. Henry Kimpton Publishers, London

Rodin E A 1968 The prognosis of patients with epilepsy. Thomas, Springfield

Shorvon S D, Reynolds E H 1979 Reduction of polypharmacy for epilepsy. Br med J 2:1023–1025

Speirs J, Hirsch S R 1978 Severe lithium toxicity with 'normal' serum concentrations. Br med J 1:815–816

Taylor D C, Falconer M A 1968 Clinical , socioeconomic and psychological changes after temporal lobectomy for epilepsy. Br J Psychiat 114:1247–1261

Trimble M R, Reynolds E H 1976 Anticonvulsant drugs and mental symptoms. A review. Psychol Med 6:169–178

Woodbury D M, Penry J K, Schmidt R P (eds) 1972 Antiepileptic drugs. Raven Press, New York

Psychotropic drugs in the management of epilepsy

INTRODUCTION

While the mainstay of treatment in epilepsy tends to concentrate on anticonvulsant drugs, the psychiatric complications often require alternative prescriptions, and these include a wide variety of psychotropic drugs. At the outset, however, it should be again emphasised that prescriptions are only one aspect of the care and management of epileptic patients, and many problems, especially the presentation of minor forms of psychopathology, will clear up without the use of psychotropic drugs. The passage of time, and the institution of well-timed psychotherapeutic management, is important. Certain aspects of this have already been outlined by some other authors in this book, especially Chapters 5, 6 and 20. Psychosocial factors can never be underestimated, and must be taken into account when planning treatment for patients. It continually has to be emphasised that epileptic patients have a large number of difficulties to cope with, in addition to their seizures. The prejudice and stigma of epilepsy, plus the sudden unpredictable loss of consciousness which occurs, leads to gross restriction in life-style, and an inability of many people with epilepsy to fulfil their potential. With such a disorder, chronic and continuing, the full burden of the condition is often not recognised, but it comes to the surface at particular times of life when severe crises may result. Notable among these are the initiation of education, the starting of work, the falling in love, at getting married, on having children and at parental death. Such times as these in the life of an epileptic patient require specific support, often in excess of the regular supportive psychotherapy which should be offered to all patients with epilepsy who need it. While formal psychoanalysis is rarely recommended, it is suggested that at all times patients should have access to professional people who understand their difficulties, and who are willing to give them time in solving their problems.

The relationship of stress to seizures often needs clarification, and subtle changes in the patient's life-style that will diminish stress may also diminish seizures. It is important to recognise that psychiatric illness itself modifies epilepsy, such that a vicious circle is easily initiated. Increasing stress leads to increasing fits, which in turn lead to increasing stress. Breaking such a cycle can sometimes be an acute medical emergency in which immediate admission to hospital is required. Particularly difficult cases may benefit from admission to one of the specialised centres, as described in Chapter 25.

Anticonvulsant drugs in their own right can lead to psychopathology, and modification of a patient's anticonvulsant treatment may be helpful in dealing with the psychiatric difficulties. The impact of anticonvulsant drugs on the mental state has been discussed in Chapter 19. More detailed reviews are available which indicate that some drugs, such as phenytoin, are interlinked with cognitive deterioration in patients, and that several of the anticonvulsants, most notably phenytoin and phenobarbitone, lead to a variety of behaviour disturbances including aggression and hyperactivity in children, and depression and psychosis in adults (Stores 1975, Trimble & Reynolds 1976).

In addition it has been suggested that some anticonvulsant drugs actually possess psychotropic properties (see Trimble & Richens 1981). Although methodological difficulties, in particular measurement of behaviour itself, and the interplay between several factors including seizure frequency, all of which influence behaviour, have led to conflicting results in various studies, it is possible to come to some consensus of opinion from the available data. Some investigations, which may be said to be appropriately designed and attempt some objective method of quantification, have been carried out, mainly with sulthiame and carbamazepine. With sulthiame there are two studies which indicate that it reduces the incidence of disturbed behaviour in children, in particular aggressiveness, hyperactivity and destructiveness, although they were both carried out on subnormal patients (Moffat et al 1970, Al-Kaisi & McGuire 1974). Similar improvements were noted in both epileptic and non-epileptic children, suggesting that the drug's effect was not dependent on its having suppressed seizures. With regard to carbamazepine, there are a large number of anecdotes in the literature indicating that the drug has beneficial psychotropic effects. Dalby (1975) noted that 90 per cent of reports using the drug mention a psychotropic effect, and in 40 reports of over 2500 patients, improvement in seizures occurred in 60 per cent of cases and a beneficial psychotropic effect in 50 per cent. The psychotropic action was described as

'an increase in psychic tempo in patients with the so-called epileptic personality. The slowness, sluggishness and stickiness, the perseverations and the stereotypes, the apathy and lack of initiative of the patient with long-standing severe epilepsy, usually uncontrolled on large doses of phenobarbital, phenytoin and primidone, diminishes and a quickening of thought and action occurs. The affective changes, such as irritability, aggressive tendencies, impulsivity, dysphoric episodes, and states of depression and anxiety, are reduced or abolished, giving way to an elevation of mood. An improvement in intellectual capacities, in attention and concentration as well as perseverance has often been the impressionistic result of such improvements, leading to better adaptation at home, work, and school.'

In his own study he evaluated the effect on 93 patients with psychomotor epilepsy. Improvement of psychiatric symptoms was noted in 24 of 59 patients with psychiatric disturbances, and 11 of 18 with periodic depression had only occasional or brief episodes while on carbamazepine. Two of four patients with confusional paranoid episodes were 'normalised' psychiatrically, and in two cases of schizophreniform psychosis benefit was noted. A number of improvements occurred in spite of continued seizures.

These results are complemented by other studies of the effects of carbamazepine on the behaviour of epileptic and non-epileptic patients. Most, however, have been carried out on children with behaviour disorders, but the results suggest benefit in hyperactivity, impulsivity, aggression, and learning problems (see Trimble & Richens 1981). Of five controlled trials in patients with epilepsy, carbamazepine led to improvements in behaviour compared to phenytoin and phenobarbitone, although two studies of institutionalised epileptic patients failed to detect changes (Bird et al 1966, Pryse-Philips & Jeavons 1970). Recently Singh et al (1977), in a study of 20 patients with epilepsy and behaviour disorders, noted improvements in behaviour over three months following the initiation of carbamazepine to their treatment. Item analysis of the results revealed significant improvement, particularly for irritability, hostility, uncooperativeness and excitement. Trimble & Corbett (1979), using the Rutter rating scales to assess behaviour in disturbed children with epilepsy, noted significant negative correlations between the serum anticonvulsant levels of carbamazepine and conduct disturbance. This relationship to behaviour was significantly different from that of phenobarbitone, the latter drug being highly associated with conduct abnormalities.

In the light of these findings, it seems likely that some anticonvulsants are less likely to provoke or exacerbate psychopathology than others, and in treatment it is germane to consider that, in some patients with epilepsy and psychiatric disability, alteration of the anticonvulsant regime (in particular with the institution of drugs like carbamazepine) may lead to beneficial effects on behaviour and mood. Any changeover is most effectively carried out slowly, preferably by adding carbamazepine to the existing prescription and then withdrawing the alternative drugs. It is clear that such manoeuvres are preferable to adding psychotropic drugs to a patient's treatment, especially if the psychiatric disability is persistent and more severe than the problem of seizure frequency.

An alternative is to lower the number of different anticonvulsant drugs patients with psychiatric disability are receiving, preferably to monotherapy. There is now convincing evidence that this is followed by improvements in the mental state, not only with regard to mood but also with regard to cognitive abilities (Shorvon & Reynolds 1979, Trimble & Thompson 1980).

In many cases, however, the clinical situation is such that alteration of anticonvulsant therapy is not indicated, and psychotropic drugs may be needed in addition to the patient's existing treatment. A classification of those currently available is shown in Table 24.1.

While the most commonly used are probably the hypnotics and the minor tranquillisers, it is the major tranquillisers and the antidepressants that are of most concern in the management of epilepsy, in that the vast majority of both these groups lower the seizure threshold and are convulsant.

ANTIDEPRESSANTS

The antidepressants may be divided into two major categories, the monoamine oxidase inhibitors (MAOI), and the non-monoamine oxidase inhibitors. The latter drugs, which include the traditional tricyclic drugs, also include a number of new compounds which vary from the tricyclic structure. Some of these non-tricyclic non-MAOI drugs are shown in Table 24.2. Although the tricyclics are the most widely prescribed, in particular amitriptyline and imipramine, there are several claims that these newer antidepressants have less in the way of side effects

Table 24.1 A classification of psychotropic drugs

Antidepressants	1. MAOI	
	2. Non-MAOI	a. tricyclic
		b. non-tricyclic
Major tranquillisers		
Minor tranquillisers		
Hypnotics	a. barbiturate	
	b. other	
Anticonvulsants e.g. carbamazepine		
Psychostimulants e.g. amphetamine		
Lithium		

Table 24.2 Some non-tricyclic non-MAOI antidepressant drugs

1. L-tryptophan
2. Nomifensine
3. Mianserin
4. Iprindole
5. Viloxazine
6. Flupenthixol
7. Zimelidine
8. Trazodone

Rapid speed of onset 6	Decreased suicide risk 1, 2, 3, 6	Decreased cardiotoxicity 1, 2, 3, 8

than their predecessors, and therefore offer therapeutic advantages. Some of these are also indicated in Table 24.2. Drugs such as mianserin and nomifensine have little in the way of anticholinergic activity, and thus are less inclined to be cardiotoxic, particularly with overdose. Decreased suicide risk is noted for several of them, clearly an important indication in the management of depression, especially in epilepsy where an increased incidence rate for suicide has been shown to occur (see Chapter 7).

There is now a sizable body of data on the effects of these non-MAOI drugs on the seizure threshold. Shortly after the introduction of the tricyclic compounds there were clinical reports which indicated that convulsions occurred as a consequence of overdose, although this was soon followed by a series of reports of documented seizures which occurred following therapeutic doses (for full review see Trimble 1978). Betts et al (1968) reported on seven patients in whom amitriptyline precipitated epileptic fits at normal dosage. The seizures occurred within a few days of starting the drug, or changing to a higher dose, and several of their patients had received intramuscular preparations. Four showed some evidence of a low convulsive threshold prior to treatment. Dallos & Heathfield (1969) reported on nine patients who developed fits shortly after starting on a variety of tricyclic drugs. Four had either a family history or previous personal history of epilepsy, and five others had grounds for the suspicion of a lowered seizure threshold, which may have been an important factor in the precipitation of fits. The EEGs of six patients were normal, although in two, the findings suggested epilepsy.

Toone & Fenton (1977) compared 41 patients who had fits induced by psychotropic drugs with a controlled sample, noting biographical details which could be relevant to the aetiology of the fits. They were unable to confirm that a family history of epilepsy was of significance, but did note significantly more of the seizure patients were first born, had post-natal brain damage, and that the precipitation of seizures was associated with polytherapy and a change of the prescription with increasing drug dose.

Kiloh et al (1961) compared the effect of intravenous imipramine on the electroencephalogram of both epileptic and non-epileptic subjects. None of 24 non-epileptic patients had abnormalities provoked on the EEG, while 18 of 36 epileptic patients had activation of their EEGs to varying degrees, which was greater in those that showed electroencephalographic abnormalities prior to the injection. In this experiment, although no actual seizures were produced, the authors felt that imipramine was similar to bemegride as an EEG activating agent. Similar results have been obtained for amitriptyline (Davison 1965).

These results, and other studies (see Trimble 1978) show that tricyclic antidepressants lower the seizure threshold and can precipitate seizures clinically. While this is most likely to occur in patients with a lowered seizure threshold, this does not seem inevitably to be the case, and factors, such as polypharmacy and a sudden rapid change of dose with high dose regimes, seem also to be implicated.

With regard to the non-tricyclic non-MAOI antidepressants, less work has been carried out on the relationship of these to the seizure threshold. In an early clinical report, Burley (1977) reported that the incidence of seizures for a variety of antidepressants was 3.0 per cent for clomipramine, 0.7 per cent for imipramine, and 0.2 per cent for maprotiline. Crome & Newman (1977) assessed the incidence of convulsions following overdose with maprotiline and mianserin, and noted nine out of 41 cases with maprotiline, and none with the latter drug. Edwards (1979) commented on the number of clinical case reports of seizures that had been reported to the Committee on the Safety of Medicines following a number of different antidepressants. These data revealed that, with the exception of drugs that have a very small share of the market, the only non-MAOI antidepressants that had not at that time been associated with seizures were L-tryptophan and nomifensine.

This brief review of the clinical literature suggests that some of the non-tricyclic non-MAOI antidepressants have less of an effect on the seizure threshold than the traditional tricyclic drugs. Experimental evidence for this was reported by Trimble et al (1977). They gave clomipramine, imipramine, maprotiline and nomifensine intravenously to the photosensitive baboon, *Papio papio*, and noted any effect on the seizure threshold. In this animal model, following 10 mg/kg marked lowering of the seizure threshold was reported for the tricyclic drugs and maprotiline; however, following nomifensine no seizures were reported, and several of the animals actually had diminished myoclonic responsiveness during the first hour of the experiment when compared to saline results.

Thus most of the data have indicated that, with the exception of L-tryptophan and nomifensine, all of the non-tricyclic non-MAOI antidepressants appear to lower the seizure threshold and have a potential to produce convulsions. Nawishy et al (1980) used nomifensine clinically in epileptic patients to assess its safety. No change in the mean frequency of seizures in the month before, and in the month after administration of the drug was noted, and the compound did appear to be antidepressant in some patients. Pharmacokinetic interactions were assessed between nomifensine and phenytoin, and apart from a constant rise in phenytoin levels in the first week of treatment, which was greater in those with higher initial phenytoin levels, insidious development of anticonvulsant toxicity, as had been reported following some tricyclic drugs (Perucca & Richens 1977) did not occur. Their work raised the possibility, however, that patients taking anticonvulsant drugs may metabolise antidepressants more efficiently than others, with consequent lower serum antidepressant levels than might be anticipated. Similar metabolic problems have been reported with a variety of psychotropic drugs (Richens 1976), although specific interactions have not at the time of writing been worked out.

From the data available, therefore, it seems reasonable to suggest that, in patients with epilepsy, antidepressants should be chosen that are least likely to interfere with the seizure threshold, and the tricyclic drugs should preferably be avoided. At present only nomifensine and L-tryptophan have not been associated with seizures, and the antidepressant activity of L-tryptophan has not been clearly established (Cooper 1979). Whatever drug is chosen, patients should be started on low doses, which can be increased gradually to avoid sudden changes in serum levels. Following the institution of the antidepressant drugs, serum level monitoring should be carried out, especially if before therapy patients have levels near the upper limits of tolerance. Failure to achieve an antidepressant effect may well be due to low serum levels of the antidepressant, and dosage regimes may ultimately need to be higher than in non-epileptic patients. Clinical experience also suggests a further caution, namely that a rebound effect on the serum anticonvulsant levels may occur following the withdrawal of antidepressants in epileptic patients. Again, patients should be carefully assessed following such a change of prescription, and serum anticonvulsant levels monitored as necessary.

There is little data available on the MAOI antidepressants and epilepsy, although in therapeutic doses seizures are rarely reported as a side effect. Certainly, following overdoses they can provoke seizures, although which of the various compounds are most likely to do this is not known. Generally, they are not recommended for the management of primary depressive illness, but more for atypical depression including patients presenting with hypochondriasis, somatic anxiety, irritability, dysphoria and agoraphobia. A number of patients do not tolerate these compounds well, and because of the interaction with various food-stuffs and other medications, patient selection has to be carefully made. There is only one report of their use in patients with epilepsy, in which five patients with complex partial epilepsy were given both isocarboxazid and isocarboxazid plus L-tryptophan. These regimes were without effect on seizure frequency, only one patient showing a decrease of greater than 50 per cent. Serum carbamazepine levels were significantly lower than pre-trial values, in spite of no changes being made in the prescribing of the anticonvulsant drug (Chadwick et al 1978).

MAJOR TRANQUILLISERS

Major tranquillisers are distinguished from minor tranquillisers by their specific

Table 24.3   Major tranquillisers

Phenothiazines — side chain	a.	aliphatic (e.g. chlorpromazine)
	b.	piperadine (e.g. thioridazine)
	c.	piperazine (e.g. perphenazine)

Butyrophenones —e.g. haloperidol, pimozide

Thioxanthines

Others, e.g. Molindone: substituted benzamides

antipsychotic action. It is now virtually certain that this is related to their ability to block post-synaptic dopamine receptors, but as a consequence of this, the majority also provoke a number of side effects which include extrapyramidal disorders, and a lowering of the seizure threshold and thus seizures. Table 24.3 shows a classification of the major tranquillisers and some of their properties. The phenothiazines are the most commonly used, and dependent upon their side-chain, their properties slightly differ. The aliphatic compounds are less potent on a milligram for milligram basis than the others, and are therefore prescribed in higher doses. The butyrophenones, which include haloperidol and pimozide, are increasingly used in the management of psychotic disorders, tending to be less sedative than the phenothiazines, although extrapyramidal side effects are more common following their use. The thioxanthines are not widely used in this country, although flupenthixol is used as an intramuscular long-acting antipsychotic, and in small doses as an antidepressant. Substituted benzamides are attracting increasing attention as potentially useful antipsychotic drugs on account of their ability to preferentially block only certain dopamine receptors, and the possibility therefore that they will be associated with less side effects than some of the other major tranquillisers.

There are several studies which have assessed the effect of major tranquillisers on the seizure threshold. The effects of chlorpromazine on the electro-encephalogram are similar to those of the tricyclic antidepressants, and a number of authors have used it as an EEG activating agent in doses between 25 and 100 mg intravenously (Kiloh et al 1961). There is considerable evidence from animals, and other data, regarding the potential for these compounds to lower seizure threshold, with some suggestion that, as with the antidepressants, a spectrum of activity may be seen. Generally following administration there is a synchronising action with increased slow activity. The more sedative the compound the greater the EEG changes. Experiments with butyrophenones indicate that from the EEG point of view they produce similar patterns to the phenothiazines, including synchronisation and seizure activity. Studies in epileptic patients indicate that even small doses of chlorpromazine intravenously lead to a marked increase in paroxysmal dysrhythmic activity, with increased spikes on the EEG. As with the non-MAOI antidepressants, an increase in epileptic seizures following chlorpromazine has been related to the presence of low convulsive threshold in affected patients, and to the dosage of drug given.

Differences between drugs have been suggested by several authors (see Itil 1970). Of the phenothiazines, thioridazine, which produces EEG effects similar to chlorpromazine, results in less change of amplitude and synchronisation and there are only a few reports of increased epileptic activity following its administration. The incidence of seizures clinically reported is less than with chlorpromazine, and it has been used effectively in the management of behaviour disorders in epilepsy without an obvious increase in epileptic seizures occurring (Pauig et al 1961). Amongst the piperazine group, activation of epileptic seizures is less commonly seen with trifluperazine, perphenazine, and long-acting fluphenazines such as the decanoate preparation.

Haloperidol has also been reported to have little effect on seizure facilitation in human studies, inducing less paroxysmal dysrhythmic patterns than the phenothiazines. Meldrum et al (1975) compared the effect of haloperidol and pimozide on the epileptic threshold of the photosensitive baboon, *Papio papio*. Both drugs led to an increase in spike-wave and slow-wave activity, although less enhancement of myoclonic epileptic responses was seen following the pimozide. These reports suggest that generally the butyrophenones are less epileptogenic than the phenothiazines, with the possible exception of thioridazine, and that of the former, derivatives such as pimozide may be the least epileptogenic of all.

There are reports in the literature showing increases and decreases of both neuroleptic and anticonvulsant drug levels when these compounds are used together, suggesting that metabolic interactions are of importance, and emphasising that clinically, if these drugs are administered to patients with epilepsy, close attention should be paid to the possibility of anticonvulsant toxicity which may be induced. In the management of psychosis, the choice to use major tranquillisers will depend on the relationship of the psychiatric disease to both the timing of the ictus, and the seizure frequency. Thus, in peri-ictal psychotic disturbances the patient should be observed during the episode to make sure that he comes to no harm, but the use of psychotropic drugs is often not indicated. In these situations major tranquillisers may be contraindicated, because they may lead to further seizures which can aggravate the behaviour difficulty. If tranquillisation is required, a minor tranquilliser, such as a benzodiazepine, or chlormethiazole are probably more appropriate. During the interictal phase, the mental state may appear perfectly normal, and in these situations control of the epilepsy with judicious use of anticonvulsants to prevent further attacks is more important than long-term major tranquilliser therapy.

For the interictal psychoses, psychotropic drugs will be required in some instances. However, in those cases where there appears to be a reciprocal relationship between the onset of the psychosis and the seizure frequency, then gradual reduction of anticonvulsant drugs with the addition of psychotropic drugs may be undertaken. It is possible that in these situations the epileptogenic potential of the major tranquillisers is an important part of their therapeutic action. Drugs such as chlorpromazine and haloperidol are therefore not contraindicated, although clinically patients often respond to quite small doses, and large loading doses should be avoided.

OTHER PSYCHOTROPIC DRUGS

Drugs that fall into the category of minor tranquillisers often find use in the treatment of epilepsy and its problems, although not necessarily for their psychotropic properties. Barbiturates in particular have played a part in management, and more recently the benzodiazepines have found a place, particularly with clonazepam and clobazam. The value of intravenous diazepam in status epilepticus is well-known. In epileptic patients who are prone to anxiety neurosis, these drugs are cleary of value, and generally benzodiazepines are to be preferred to the barbiturates on account of producing less tolerance, and having less risk of suicide with overdose. On account of their muscle relaxant properties benzodiazepines are often found useful in patients who, because of tension states, present with non-epileptic seizures. For some reason not all benzodiazepines possess the same therapeutic potential in this regard; lorazepam seems to be preferred by a number of patients, and is often effective in relieving fits that have previously been difficult to control.

Amphetamine still has a place in the management of epilepsy, and probably possesses some anticonvulsant activity in its own right. Occasionally it is used to counteract the sedative effect of more traditional anticonvulsants, although with the wide range of drugs that are now available, in particular the introduction of newer less sedative drugs, such practice should be discouraged.

Lithium, which now is established for the prophylaxis of manic-depressive illness, and more recently has become used in the management of cyclical depressive illness even where bouts of mania do not occur, has not been studied in epilepsy, and little is known about its interaction with anticonvulsants. It does, however, produce seizures as a toxic side-effect, and in view of its potential to impair cognitive function, it is probably best avoided where possible. Manic-depressive psychoses in epilepsy, which are not uncommonly interlinked with electrophysical factors such as seizure frequency (Flor-Henry 1969), often require the same juggling act as do the other major psychoses with regard to obtaining a balance between the lowering of the seizure threshold with major tranquillisers, and raising of seizure threshold with anticonvulsants.

References

Al-Kaisi A M, McGuire R J 1974 The effect of sulthiame on disturbed behaviour in mentally subnormal patients. Br J Psychiat 124:45–49

Betts T, Kalra P, Cooper R, Jeavons P 1968 Epileptic fits as a probable side effect of amitriptyline. Lancet 1:390–392

Bird C A K, Griffin B P, Miklascewska J M, Galbraith A W 1966 Tegretol: a controlled trial of a new anticonvulsant. Br J Psychiat 112:737–742

Borenstein P et al 1970 Clinical and experimental electroencephalography. In: The neuroleptics. Mod Probl Pharmacopsychiat 5:109–125

Burley D M 1977 A brief note on the problem of epilepsy in antidepressant treatment. In: Jukes A (ed) Depression — the biochemical and physiological role of ludiomil. Ciba, Horsham, p 201–203

Chadwick D, Trimble M, Jenner P, Driver M V, Reynolds E H 1978 Manipulation of cerebral monoamines in the treatment of human epilepsy: a pilot study. Epilepsia 19:3–10

Cooper A J 1979 Tryptophan antidepressant 'physiological sedative': factor fancy? Psychopharmacology 61:77–102

Crome P, Newman B 1977 Poisoning with maprotiline and mianserin. Br med J 2:260

Dalby M A 1975 Behavioural effects of carbamazepine. In: Penry J K, Daly D D (eds) Advances in neurology II. Raven Press, New York, p 331–334

Dallos U, Heathfield K 1969 Iatrogenic epilepsy due to antidepressant drugs. Br med J 4:80–82

Davison K 1965 EEG activation after intravenous amitriptyline. Electroenceph Clin Neurophysiol 19:298–300

Edwards G 1979 Antidepressants and convulsions. Lancet 2:1368–1369

Flor-Henry P 1969 Psychosis and temporal lobe epilepsy. Epilepsia 10:363–395

Itil T M 1970 Convulsive and anticonvulsive properties of neuro-psychopharmaca. Mod Probl Pharmacopsychiat 4:270–300

Kiloh L, Davison K, Osselton J 1961 An EEG study of the analeptic effects of imipramine. Electroenceph Clin Neurophysiol 13:216–223

Moffatt W R, Siddiqui A R, Mackay D W 1970 The use of sulthiame with disturbed mentally subnormal patients. Br J Psychiat 117:673–678

Meldrum B, Anlezark G, Trimble M R 1975 Drugs modifying dopaminergic activity and behaviour, the EEG and epilepsy in *Papio papio*. European J Pharmacol 32:203–213

Nawishy S, Trimble M R, Richens A 1980 Antidepressants and epilepsy: the place of nomifensine. In: Nomifensine. R Soc Med Int Congress and Symposium Series no 25, Academic Press, London p 11–16

Pauig P M, Deluca M A, Osterheld R G 1961 Thioridazine hydrochloride in the treatment of behaviour disorders in epileptics. Am J Psychiat 117:832–833

Perucca E, Richens A 1977 Interaction between phenytoin and imipramine. Br J Clin Pharmacol 4:485

Pryse-Phillips W E M, Jeavons P M 1970 Effect of carbamazepine on the electroencephalographic and ward behaviour of patients with chronic epilepsy. Epilepsia 11:263–273

Richens A 1976 Clinical pharmacology and medical treatment. In: Laidlaw J, Richens A (eds) A textbook of epilepsy. Churchill Livingstone, London

Shorvon S D, Reynolds E H 1979 Reduction in polypharmacy for epilepsy. Br med J 2:1023–1025

Singh A M, Saxena B M, Germain M 1977 Anticonvulsant and psychotropic effects of carbamazepine in hospitalised epileptic patients: a long-term study. In: Penry J K (ed) Epilepsy: the eighth international symposium. Raven Press, New York, p 47–56

Stores G 1975 Behavioural effects of anti-epileptic drugs. Devel Med Child Neurol 17:647–658

Toone B K, Fenton G W 1977 Epileptic seizures induced by psychotropic drugs. Psychol Med 7:265–270

Trimble M R 1978 Non-MAOI antidepressants and epilepsy: a review. Epilepsia 19:241–250

Trimble M R, Anlezark G, Meldrum B 1977 Seizure activity in photosensitive baboons following antidepressant drugs and the role of serotoninergic mechanisms. Psychopharmacology 51:159–164

Trimble M R, Corbett J 1979 Anticonvulsant drugs and behaviour. Proceedings of the 11th International Epilepsy Symposium, Florence, Italy

Trimble M R, Reynolds E H 1976 Anticonvulsant drugs and mental symptoms: a review. Psychol Med 6:169–178

Trimble M R, Richens A 1981 Psychotropic effects of anticonvulsant drugs. In: Burrows G D, Werry J S (eds) Advances in human psychopharmacology, vol 2. Jai Press (in press)

Trimble M R, Thompson P, Huppert F 1980 Anticonvulsant drugs and cognitive abilities. In: Canger et al (eds) Advances in epileptology. Raven Press, New York, p 199–204

Special centres

PROLOGUE

This book is the centenary celebration of Sir William Gowers' classic work on epilepsy and other chronic convulsive disorders, and during the course of research for this chapter I found an anecdote relevant to the psychiatric aspects of the 'falling sickness', which have been covered extensively in previous chapters. It is well known that Gowers was a personal friend of that master of English literature, Rudyard Kipling. Dr Macdonald Critchley (1949) believed that Kipling consulted Gowers for medical advice when writing a short story entitled *Love o' Women* — a fictional description of tabes dorsalis — and also his poem *The post that fitted*. This tells the story of a young subaltern called Sleary, who loves a girl called Carrie but is too poor to marry her. When sent to the East, Sleary becomes engaged to Minnie Bofkin, whose father obtains for him a remunerative political job. To induce Minnie Bofkin to break the engagement, he simulates epileptic seizures, for which Pears' shaving stick provides the froth. Minnie returns the ring, and:

> 'Sleary bore the information with a chastened holy joy,
> Epileptic fits don't matter in political employ,
> Wired three short words to Carrie — took his ticket, packed his kit,
> Bade farewell to Minnie Bofkin in one last, long, lingering fit.
> Four weeks later, Carrie Sleary read — and laughed until she wept —
> Mrs Bofkin's warning letter on the 'wretched epilept'.
> Year by year, in pious patience, vengeful Mrs Bofkin sits
> Waiting for the Sleary babies to develop Sleary's fits.'

As Temkin (1971) points out, this contains nothing unknown to the imposters of old, but it is rather a nice description of some of the psychosocial problems of epilepsy.

INTRODUCTION

The Oxford English Dictionary carries at least ten definitions of the word 'special', including 'that which excels at something of common occurrence'. During the last decade, there has been much discussion concerning special centres for epilepsy in many countries of the world, particularly in Western Europe and the United States of America. In this chapter, I propose to discuss the wider implications of a special centre for epilepsy than the strictly limited definition of the so-called Reid Report published in 1969 (Department of Health and Social Security and Welsh Office) although the importance of that excellent Report in the future development of services for people with epilepsy cannot be overemphasised.

Historical background

Throughout the centuries, the 'falling sickness' has occupied a position of some importance, if the surviving medical writings are a reliable indication. Lennox (1960) has calculated that 2.6 per cent of all the Hippocratic writings are concerned with epilepsy, but Hippocrates was exceeded by Aretaeus with 3.4 per cent. This compared with the 1959 edition of Cecil's *Medicine*, which contained only 0.5 per cent about epilepsy. The major contribution by Hippocrates was to dissociate epilepsy from the concept of possession by evil spirits but, unfortunately, his hypothesis was largely ignored by the medical fraternity for some 2000 years. Because of the widespread ignorance and prejudice over the centuries, the person with epilepsy has had more than his fair share of adversity, and although much improved, this state of affairs still exists today.

Gradually, the kindlier elements of society provided places where people with epilepsy could escape from a hostile world intolerant of their condition. It seems that the earliest recorded expression of this was at the end of the 15th century when a 'hospice for epileptics' was established by monks at the Priory of Saint Valentine at Rufach, in Alsace. With the spread of Christianity over the previous millenium, people had come to expect help from saints and relics, and some saints lent their names to the disease and became its patrons (Temkin 1971). It is likely, at least initially, that fear of epilepsy as a contagious disease may have been a prominent consideration, as well as philanthropy. In 1773 the Bishop of Wurzburg established a home for people with epilepsy, and this survived for many years. By the 19th century, the practice of putting the insane in chains was discontinued, and because epileptics had often been confined with the insane, this was of benefit to them as well. In general, it was only from the time of Pinel (1745–1826), in France, and the Tukes, in England, that people with epilepsy confined to institutions became the object of systematic medical attention (Temkin 1971). In 1815, Esquirol made a strong plea for the establishment of special provisions for epileptics, but his motivation was suspect. He thought that the sight of an epileptic attack might be sufficient to make a healthy person epileptic, and be even more epileptogenic for the mentally deranged! About 1850 it became the practice in England to confine epileptic patients to separate wards in lunatic asylums, and when this segregation had become an established fact, the logical sequence was a demand for special institutions for people with epilepsy.

This demand began to be fulfilled from 1860, when the National Hospital for the Paralysed and Epileptic was opened in Queen Square, London. In Germany, in 1867, four people with epilepsy were taken into custodial care by a pastor in a farmhouse outside the town of Bielefeld. In 1872, Pastor Friedrich von Bodelschwingh took over what became the institution of Bethel, today, in some respects, one of the leading special centres for epilepsy in the world. This was followed, in 1882, by the colony at 'Meer en Bosch', in Heemstede, The Netherlands; and the Filadelfia Colony at Dianalund, in Denmark. In England, the first special institution for epileptics was established at Maghull, near Liverpool. This was followed by the Chalfont Colony for Epileptics in Buckinghamshire in 1894, due to the efforts of a lady called Miss Burden-Sanderson who had visited Bethel with a group of friends in 1891. When she returned to England an appeal was lauched so successfully that, within six months, the National Society for the Employment of Epileptics (later the National Society for Epileptics) was formed and a pilot scheme was started at Skippings Farm, Chalfont St Peter, and named the Chalfont Colony. The David Lewis Epileptic Colony, near Alderley Edge, Cheshire, was opened in September 1904 under the Trust Deed of Mr David Lewis, who founded a department store now widespread in the north of England. Altogether, some 17 homes or institutions for people with epilepsy developed in Great Britain between 1888 and 1933, with one in Scotland, the Colony for Epileptics, Bridge of Weir, founded in 1902 (Epilepsia 2nd Series 1:1937–1940).

Meanwhile, in the United States of America, similar developments were taking place initially at Gallipolis, Ohio, in 1891, followed, the next year, by a colony at Sonyea, New York State. Ultimately, 14 institutions were developed in various States which, by 1933, provided a bed capacity of 10 342. Today, only the New Castle State Hospital, in Indiana, survives.

I do not intend to mention all the colonies or centres that evolved in different parts of the world between the middle of the 19th and early 20th century. Basically, they developed to provide a haven of retreat from an increasingly industrialised and hostile world, and were originally intended to provide custodial care for many years, or for life. To this end, they were largely self-supporting communities and it is significant that many of the centres in Britain, Europe and the USA were deliberately established away from the urban areas of industry and employment. They performed a much-needed service that most of society had neglected, but by the middle of this century, a new role was necessary.

Present trends

In England, during the 1950s, two reports concerning people with epilepsy were published. The first (Ministry of Health 1953) concerned their special welfare needs. Amongst many recommendations, it was advised that separate accommodation should be provided in the epileptic colonies for (a) the 'low grade', (b) the 'difficult' and (c) those requiring short-term stabilisation. Of more importance was the subsequent report of the Cohen Committee (Ministry of Health 1956), which recommended that the epileptic colonies should be as much therapeutic as custodial, and that they should be concerned with the medical care and also with the rehabilitation of patients, ultimately returning them to a normal life in the community.

I am bound to say that very little action was taken over the more fundamental recommendations of these two reports, and it was not until the Reid Report (Department of Health and Social Security and Welsh Office 1969) that progress began to take place. The proposals have been well summarised by Reid himself

(Reid 1972). Of a total of 56 recommendations, 12 concerned the epileptic colonies and the proposed new concept of special centres, but the Report contains much wider implications and recommendations concerning the general management and care of people with epilepsy.

Meanwhile, progress was being made elsewhere, particularly in Europe and the USA. In France, a day hospital specifically for epileptic patients was established at Créteil, near Paris (Vidart 1966). In The Netherlands, in conjunction with the Instituut voor Epilepsiebestrijding, outpatient clinics and special centres for epilepsy had been established, not only at Heemstede, but in The Hague, Breda, Rotterdam, Heeze, Utrecht, Arnhem, Apeldoorn and Leeuwarden (Meinardi 1972). In Norway, a country which had never had epileptic colonies, a bill was passed in Parliament in 1970–1971, for the further development of the care of patients with epilepsy in that country, based on the developments in Britain (Henriksen 1972). Up to then there had been one National Hospital for Epileptics, the Statens Sykehus for Epileptikere, at Sandvika, which is associated with the department of neurology at Oslo University. In Denmark, the Filadelfia Colony remained functional at Dianalund, and the Danish Epilepsy Association founded a day centre for severely handicapped people with epilepsy in a suburb of Copenhagen (Lund & Randrup 1972).

In the United States of America the general trend had been to close the epileptic colonies and replace them with institutions and training schools for the mentally retarded, the concept being that epileptics with psychiatric illness should be admitted to psychiatric institutions, and those with severe brain damage and mental retardation should be placed in hospitals for the mentally subnormal. This arrangement did not appear to deal with people whose predominant problem was epilepsy. However, one colony remained; the Indiana Village for Epileptics was established in 1905, and was primarily intended for long-term custodial care. In 1955, the name of this institution was changed to New Castle State Hospital, and the emphasis was changed to intensive medical treatment, rehabilitation and return to the community. In addition, an outpatient service was provided for people with epilepsy. Later, The National Institute of Neurological and Communicative Disorders and Stroke (NINCDS) established five Comprehensive Epilepsy Programmes (CEP), or centres of excellence, with the function of providing a service of diagnosis, treatment and rehabilitation. They were also charged with developing an educational service for professional and lay groups, and sponsoring and co-ordinating clinical and social investigations concerned with epilepsy.

The next development in the USA occurred on July 29th 1975 when, under Public Law 94–63, The Commission for the Control of Epilepsy and its Consequences was established, under the executive direction of Dr Richard L. Masland of Columbia University, New York. The four-volume report was sent to the President at The White House on August 1st 1977 (US Department of Health, Education and Welfare 1978). The first volume is similar to, but considerably longer than, the Reid Report in England and Wales. Out of 418 recommendations, the Commission included nine on the development of a Comprehensive Epilepsy Service Network with the CEPs acting as supra-regional special centres. It was envisaged that this network would be fully established by 1982.

THE ESTABLISHMENT OF SPECIAL CENTRES
IN ENGLAND AND WALES

I have already referred to the Reid Report on which the present Special Centres in England are based (Department of Health and Social Security and Welsh Office 1969, Reid 1972). It was stressed that, with good co-ordination between family doctors and the hospital and local authority services, the vast majority of people with epilepsy could be given a high standard of care in the community, based on a multi-disciplinary approach, and including an extension of special epilepsy clinics. It was recommended that the latter should be at district general hospital level as well as in regional neurological and neurosurgical centres, and they should not be in isolation, but rather as parts of appropriate departments, such as neurology, psychiatry or paediatrics.

It was, nevertheless, recognised that however good these services turned out to be, there still remained a small but significant number of people with epilepsy who required even more specialised attention because of continued seizures, and also those who require medical supervision under ordinary living and working conditions. The concept of 'special centres' was introduced and it was recommended that they should comprise the following:

1. A hospital neurological and neurosurgical unit containing all the necessary facilities for diagnosis and treatment, which today would include CAT brain scan and serum anti-epileptic drug monitoring.

2. A residential unit to which *appropriate* people with epilepsy could be admitted for a period of care, after an established diagnosis and assessment has been made. I stress the word 'appropriate' because the danger was clearly seen that such residential components might become dumping grounds of convenience, in the same way that part of the epileptic colonies had been used during the first half of the 20th century.

The ideal concept is that special centres should be purpose-built, with residential and workshop components in close proximity to the neurological department, but it was realised that this would involve heavy capital expenditure. It was therefore suggested that the residential component might be situated in an existing epileptic colony, or psychiatric unit, provided that the need for assessment and rehabilitation could be separated from the long-term care function. It was also essential that full social work support and workshop facilities should be available. The Reid Report, on the basis of experience in The Netherlands, suggested that some five or six regional centres should be established in England and Wales. Since 1972, there have been two 'official' centres for adults. The special centre at Chalfont Colony was designated as the National Hospital—Chalfont Centre for Epilepsy, administered jointly by the two respective organisations and opened with a 45-bed unit. In the north of England, the Special Centre for Epilepsy at Bootham Park Hospital, York was designated. In fact, the latter was an ongoing development of the Neuropsychiatric Unit established in 1966 as a 20-bed unit in Bootham Park Psychiatric Hospital already staffed by a multi-disciplinary team (Parsonage 1974). I will refer to the special centre for children at the Park Hospital, Oxford, later. In addition, there is a 'special centre' at the David Lewis Centre for

Epilepsy, in association with the North West Regional Health Authority. These are currently under investigation by the Department of Health and Social Security.

It is frequently argued that people with epilepsy should not be segregated as this might reinforce the feeling of being special, and outcast, and might cause neurotic reaction. Like Meinardi (1972), it is my daily experience that this argument is not correct except in a very few cases and has, in any case, not been formally substantiated. I think the centres have a useful part to play in the management of a proportion of people with epilepsy, and that this will continue for a long time, but consider that they have not yet been used to their full potential.

THE PRESENT STATE OF SPECIAL CENTRES

Their role in the management of epilepsy

I would suggest that the following functions should be considered an integral part of a special centre for epilepsy, regardless of the country:

1. Comprehensive assessment of the patient is of paramount importance, including a detailed neurological, neurophysiological and psychiatric examination and assessment by a clinical psychologist. This is closely followed by a full social assessment, including educational, domestic and employment problems. Experienced social workers are mandatory in this respect. The majority of the work should, of course, have been carried out in the epilepsy clinic, but I agree strongly with Parsonage (1974, 1976), who has found that a significant proportion of patients admitted to the special centre have, in fact, turned out not to have epilepsy at all. This particularly applies to those patients with outpatient records weighing at least 1 kg and heavily marked with the words 'known epileptic'. This label requires highly critical consideration.

The advantages of the residential component of a special centre are several. Paramount of these is the fact that repeated and detailed observation of seizure patterns can be made by staff experienced in the finer nuances of seizures, supplemented, when necessary, by the more sophisticated techniques of intensive monitoring (Grant 1980, Penry & Porter 1977, Stores 1979). Such observation can be carried out in an environment much closer to normality than the sterility of a hospital ward and this, in itself, can help towards a more realistic appraisal of the epileptic state.

2. Control of seizures with the minimum of side effects is also fundamental, and admission to a residential special centre should be considered in all patients who have failed to respond to seemingly adequate treatment as outpatients. The uncertain relationship between the type of epilepsy and medication often demands lengthy trials of different drugs, especially in those slow to achieve steady-state blood levels. A higher rate of compliance with treatment can be obtained and serum drug level monitoring can, if necessary, be carried out much more frequently than in outpatients. It is common to find that patients are taking several drugs, many of which may be interacting with each other, and that reduction of medication is not only necessary, but beneficial (Parsonage 1974). Clearly, this can often be done on an outpatient basis, but by no means always,

particularly in those cases where there is doubt about correct administration of treatment.

3. Social adjustment. It cannot be denied that many people with epilepsy have considerable difficulty with social relationships, both within the family situation and also the community. Social rejection of epileptic patients appears to be widespread, even in so-called advanced societies (Bagley 1972), and this may be more marked than in the case of mental illness or ethnic minorities. Bagley suggests that this may be largely, or at least in part, responsible for the increased prevalence of behaviour disorders in the epileptic population. I believe there is a great deal of truth in this because, in the accepting environment of a special centre, some behavioural abnormalities disappear without the need for change in medication. Admission to the residential component of a special centre can often lead to considerable improvement in social adjustment in a relatively short time. Indeed, this also happens in the main epilepsy centres (updated colonies), provided that appropriate individual accommodation is provided and independence encouraged, in spite of the apparent paradox of segregation mentioned by Meinardi (1972).

4. Associated disorders are usually psychiatric. Depressive states usually respond well to treatment, but long-standing personality disorders may require a longer period of residential treatment than is appropriate in a special centre, and referral to a longer-term centre for epilepsy may be required.

5. Occupational training is essential. Many of the patients who are appropriate for treatment in a special centre have a history of problems with employment—sometimes simply because of seizure frequency, but often for multi-factorial reasons. The main need appears simply to get back into a daily working routine. The actual occupation is of less significance, but it must be seen as meaningful and constructive to the patient and, if possible, relevant to prospective employment in the community. There are advantages in an industrial workshop environment, either in the special centre itself or within reasonable reach by public transport. In the workshop, a more accurate assessment of seizure type and frequency is possible than in many other situations. In addition, the patient's abilities, attitude to work, time-keeping, flexibility, relations with 'management' and peer groups can be repeatedly assessed, and appropriate guidance given when necessary.

6. Rehabilitation must be the ultimate aim of all special centres, and can only be achieved if the foregoing factors are properly managed. It is clear that a multi-disciplinary approach is essential and regular case conferences between all personnel involved should be held on each patient. It is also important to ensure that those patients requiring longer-term treatment in a centre or hospital for epilepsy should be transferred as soon as possible, when it is certain that no further improvement can be achieved. This point was stressed in the Reid Report paragraph 112, and is one advantage of having the residential component of a special centre within the campus of a main centre for epilepsy.

During the patient's stay in the special centre, every effort should be made to eliminate dependence on 'the system', with minimum restrictions on social activities, consistent with medical needs. In fact, many of the patients admitted to a residential centre have been subjected to various forms of over-protection for many years, and find a relaxed, informal, non-hospitalised environment very beneficial. The minimum of 'nursing' techniques should be applied, and although there must be a structure of discipline, it should be unobtrusive.

Contact with the community, and especially family, must be maintained, and this can be most effectively supervised by experienced social workers, whether the patient is in the residential component or being treated as an outpatient. Good communication is vital — a facility notoriously denied to members of the medical profession. If the patient is in residence and already has employment, the employer should be contacted immediately and an outline of the therapeutic programme explained. Employment for some people with epilepsy is difficult enough as it is, without running the risk of losing it because of a treatment which is supposed to help! Liaison with a Disablement Resettlement Officer (DRO) particularly interested in epilepsy is important, but not always easy to achieve. The DRO must be involved early on in the assessment of those patients who have not been employed for some time, but who appear to have reasonable prospects, after treatment. Attendance at an Employment Rehabilitation Centre may be advisable before returning straight to open employment.

Finally, arrangements must be made for continued supervision for those patients discharged from the residential centre, and I think the ideal is for this to be done from the neurological or other outpatient component of the special centre — at least, for a period of time — to ensure that improvement is maintained. It is important that this should be done with the co-operation of the patient's family doctor who is, and should remain, the first line manager of the person with epilepsy.

7. Research programmes should be included whenever practical, particularly linked with the appropriate university department. The extent of such programmes will obviously depend on the resources, both financial and temporal, of the individual centres but, at the very least, could include short-term clinical trials of anti-epileptic drugs, both new and established. However, it is not only drug treatment that needs evaluation, because there is no doubt that some people with epilepsy are not only handicapped by the occurrence of seizures but by social problems, failure to work at adequate speed, neurotic behaviour, etc., and the environment of a special centre is suitable for the investigation of such factors.

8. Teaching is another function of a special centre so that greater appreciation of the problem of epilepsy at all levels of training can be achieved. Although primarily directed at the personnel of the special centre itself, it should include sessions for other groups such as visiting doctors, medical students, social workers, disablement resettlement officers, youth employment officers and, if possible, employers. Lastly, but by no means least, members of the patient's family can be included in some discussion groups to ease the transition of the patient back to the community.

9. Provision of longer-term accommodation. The Reid Report (Department of Health and Social Security and Welsh Office 1969) envisaged that the special centre should have facilities for those people with severe epilepsy, whose seizures cannot be adequately controlled, and who require longer-term accommodation purely on account of this, although the accommodation for this purpose should be in a separate part of the residential unit. Furthermore, if sited in one of the main

centres (colonies), the needs of the patients must be recognised as being different from the long stay resident who is there for other reasons, mainly custodial care. Dr and Mrs Laidlaw, formerly of Chalfont Centre for Epilepsy, Buckinghamshire, eloquently describe the need of those people with epilepsy who, *very nearly but not quite*, can manage on their own, who are employable but break down under external environmental stresses, and who, given just a little bit of support, can be most successful (Laidlaw & Richens 1976). The philosophy of today is that disabled people should be 'maintained in the community' but this assumes that the community is, firstly, willing and, secondly, able to carry out this function. Very often it is not, and the patient becomes 'contained' in the community with increasing isolation, frustration and no real opportunity for achievement, however limited. Thus, although apparently maintained in the community, one feels that this is more for the convenience of doctors and social workers, who can then pass on to the next problem. The Laidlaws suggest therapeutic communities for people with epilepsy, but correctly stress that the attitude within such a community must be radically different from that of the original colonies. I think it *is* practical to form a limited number of such units within the structure of a main centre for epilepsy, but it is not easy because of entrenched attitudes, mostly on the part of senior staff, from previous decades. At the present time, however, this might offer an alternative and better solution to the problem of some people with epilepsy than merely existing, unemployed and forgotten, in a so-called open community that neither cares not understands the problems peculiar to the condition.

At the David Lewis Centre we have started a project which approximates to the Laidlaws' concept, although there are still many deficiencies. One of the existing buildings in the main centre has been completely refurbished to modern standards, exceeding the quality of most university accommodation, including individual bedrooms with a high standard of furnishing. There is accommodation for 19 patients, two of whom share a large double room. This is a mixed sex house and is run on the principle of a minimum support group with only one full-time staff member supported by the senior social worker, and directly responsible to myself. There is no night staff and no real 'supervision' — only guidance. The patients who are admitted must agree in writing to take responsibility for themselves, collect, store and prepare their own food and be entirely responsible for their medication, which is obtainable on prescription from the nearby town's, and not from the centre's pharmacy. No member of the staff is allowed to enter the unit except by invitation, and this includes medical and nursing staff. Originally, it was anticipated that all patients would be discharged within 12–18 months but this criterion has now been relaxed, and it is possible that some patients will remain there for several years. An additional group of four patients have been accommodated in a three-bedroomed house, originally designed for one of the Centre medical staff. These patients are entirely responsible for themselves, with no staff intervention of any kind except on specific request, and even this is viewed with some reluctance.

Although most of these patients work in the Centre workshops or at other occupations, some are in normal employment in the local community. Although the latter is the ideal for all, it is likely to be limited in practice, because of the general unemployment problem and the geographical situation of the Centre in relation to public transport. Nevertheless, on the basis of only 12 months' experience, we are taking active steps to establish a second, probably slightly modified, unit in the immediate future. The principle is to remove the 'medical model' as far as possible, giving medical advice only on the specific request of the individual patient, although regular reviews of the epileptic state are carried out in the usual way in the clinic. In this way, we hope to provide small communities within a main centre for epilepsy, which will fill a need for those people who 'very nearly but not quite' can manage on their own to cope with the 'falling sickness'.

THE SPECIAL NEEDS OF CHILDREN

So far, I have made no particular reference to epilepsy in children, and it is not my purpose to enlarge on the epilepsies peculiar to, or predominantly seen in, childhood. The general indications for the establishment of special centres for children with epilepsy are broadly the same as for adults with an important difference — namely that they should be based on firm educational principles. Learning difficulties of one kind or another are common in epileptic children, and it is important that teachers are aware of these and able to deal with them. Some of the problems are related to the underlying cerebral damage that is responsible for epilepsy, and the effect of medication also has to be taken into account. Problems at school are not necessarily due to seizures and they can occur in children whose seizures are well controlled. For example, the attitude of the teacher can be important if the teacher does not understand epilepsy and believes that the child is slow or inattentive, or just plain lazy, or is simply frightened that the child may have a seizure in the classroom and disturb the routine. The reaction of peer group children can also provide considerable problems. Whitmore & Holdsworth (1971), in their investigation of children with epilepsy attending normal schools, found that 42 per cent of these children were described as 'markedly inattentive' with unsatisfactory educational progress. The various descriptions applied to these children included lethargic, absent-minded, sleepy, doped, lacking in concentration or otherwise unresponsive. Stores (1973) has emphasised the difficulty of the exact definition of 'inattentive' but agrees that the concept is of great clinical and educational importance in children with epilepsy (Chapter 4).

Faced with these and many other problems, it is hardly surprising that some children with epilepsy make sub-optimal progress at school. Few authorities would disagree with the general policy in the United Kingdom of educating all children, including those with disabilities of all kinds, in normal schools whenever possible. Nearly 40 years ago, the following statement was made in the British Parliament by Mr Chuter Ede, the Parliamentary Secretary for Education, during a debate on the Education Bill 1943, which subsequently became the Education Act 1944:

'May I say that I do not want to insert in the Bill any words which make it appear that the normal way to deal with a child who suffers from any of these disabilities is to be put into a special school where he will be segregated. Whilst we desire to see adequate provision of special schools, we also desire to see as many children as possible retained in the normal stream of school life.' (Hansard Vol. 398, Col. 703, 21 March 1944).

Forty years later, the continuing need for special and residential education for children with disabilities, including epilepsy, is recognised in the recent Warnock Report (Special Educational Needs 1978) and, of course, in the earlier Reid Report (Department of Health and Social Security and Welsh Office 1969).

In the United States of America, the Commission on the Control of Epilepsy and its Consequences (US Department of Health, Education and Welfare 1978) came to much the same conclusion, and laid strong emphasis on education in normal schools but, perhaps, went to the extreme in that no positive recommendation was made for the establishment of special schools or centres specifically for children with epilepsy. A survey of special education in Denmark (Jørgensen 1979) revealed that only 30 children with epilepsy, out of a total of 129 734 children receiving special education, were in special schools specifically for epilepsy, in spite of an earlier plea for special institutions for epileptic children (Lund 1972). In The Netherlands, there are no schools specifically designated for children with epilepsy as such, but children admitted to The Instituut voor Epilepsiebistrijding, in Heemstede, are educated during their period of investigation. Almost all these children have multiple handicaps. In 1972 Siegenthaler reported that 200 of a total of 1000 beds in the four centres for epilepsy in Switzerland were for children, and the concept appeared to be similar to that in the United Kingdom.

Present status of special centres for children in England and Wales

At the present time there is only one officially designated special centre for children with epilepsy, namely the Park Hospital, Oxford, to which children of all ages are referred with problems of diagnosis, seizure control and educational and behavioural difficulties. In addition, there are five residential schools which cater specifically for children with epilepsy.* Of these, two (David Lewis and Lingfield) come nearest to the concept of special centres, and it was envisaged by the Reid Report (Deparment of Health and Social Security and Welsh Office 1969) that, as the services for epilepsy developed, there would be an increasing need for short-term admissions for assessment and stabilisation of epilepsy. Subsequently, this was supported by the Warnock Report (Special Educational Needs 1978). Paragraph 8.14 of this Report reads as follows:

'We see a need for another kind of resource centre, also based in a special school, which would be developed in collaboration between local authorities and would specialise in relatively rare or particularly complex disabilities such as severe visual, hearing or physical disabilities, severe speech or language disorders, severe epilepsy and severe conduct disorders. Centres of this kind would provide facilities for specialist assessment, short- and long-term day and residential education and specialist advice and support to teachers and pupils in other schools as well as to other professionals. They would also be places where parents of children with the same type of disability could meet together.'

---

* Chilton House School, The Maghull Homes, Maghull, Lancashire
  David Lewis School, David Lewis Centre, Alderley Edge, Cheshire
  Lingfield Hospital School, Lingfield, Surrey
  Sedgwick House School, near Kendal, Cumbria
  St Elizabeth's School, Much Hadham, Hertfordshire

It was recognised that some special schools already carry out these functions, to which I would add the words '... at least in part'. With the present economic climate in Britain, I think it likely that special services for children with epilepsy will be concentrated in two or three of the existing residential schools. As I have already indicated, the basic principles for admission and management are the same as for adults, with the addition of a formal educational structure. These need not conflict with the wider need for special education of the child with epilepsy who has severe seizures requiring a combination of medical treatment, education and care beyond the combined resources of the family and day school, or when learning difficulties or other barriers to educational progress are so severe that the whole life of the child needs to be under continuous and consistent medical and educational control.

THE OUTCOME OF SPECIAL CENTRE TREATMENT

1. The long-term centres (colonies)

Throughout their history of about 100 years, the epileptic colonies satisfied a very real need which had not been adequately provided for since the origins of man. They served their residents and the community well. Some of them were well to the fore of medical treatment in their day, and provided opportunities for the study of epilepsy on a formal basis; for example, William Aldren Turner's classic book was based partly on work carried out at the Chalfont Colony, Buckinghamshire, England (Turner 1907). In spite of the fact that they were institutions, the attitudes within were often quite liberal and unrestrictive. In his annual report dated November 1911, Dr Alan McDougall, the first Director of the David Lewis Colony, Cheshire, England, wrote:

'It is seven years since this Colony began its work. Those years have taught us this: that unless misunderstood and improperly treated, the epileptic is a pleasant and very likeable person. The troublesome features that many of them show at the time of admission have arisen less from the disease than from the mishandling that the patient has received in the past from those most anxious to help him ... they must be allowed to run some risk; to protect them completely from risk would be to promote mental and physical degeneration and early decay.'

The majority of patients admitted to these colonies improved so long as they remained resident, but detailed analysis of the long-term outcome is impossible. I believe they did their job well until the wind of change began to affect the approach to epilepsy in the last two or three decades.

2. The modern special centres

There are considerable difficulties in the evaluation of the results of treatment in special centres in Europe and the USA — largely because insufficient time has elapsed since their inception, and little has been published in the medical literature. Review of Cumulated Index Medicus from 1973 through 1978 reveals a total of only 29 papers concerned with rehabilitation in epilepsy over the six-year period, and none of these concerned special centres. Parsonage (1974) has reported his experiences in an English Centre for Epilepsy shortly after its official designation as a National Special Centre for Epilepsy, although the survey covered the period 1966–1972 and concerned patients with a range of neuropsychiatric disabilities. During 1972 a total of 133 patients with epilepsy were seen at the Special Centre, 79 outpatients and 54 inpatients. Of the latter, 40 had psychiatric handicaps in addition to their epilepsy, including impaired intellect in 15 and personality disorders in 14. Seven patients had affective disorder and four psychosis. The average duration of treatment in the residential special centre was 2 months for males and 3 months for females. Two patients required 5 months' treatment and one nearly 7 months to stabilise the epilepsy.

The final outcome in Parsonage's series of 54 inpatients is interesting. 21 (38 per cent) returned to employment or resumed education at school or university and four were suitable for sheltered employment or residential training courses. Thus 25 (46 per cent) of the total had good prospects after discharge from the centre. On the other hand, 23 (42.5 per cent) were unemployable, usually because of impaired intellect or personality disorder. Only two of the total 54 patients failed because of uncontrolled epilepsy. In general, those who were employed before admission to the Special Centre were able to return to work but those previously unemployed remained so after discharge. This experience was confirmed in a later report by Parsonage (1976) and he also drew attention to the significant number of patients admitted to the Centre with a diagnosis of epilepsy who were subsequently shown not to be suffering from the condition. In 1975 this proportion was 24 per cent.

My own experience at the David Lewis Centre is similar. A total of 155 patients have been admitted to the small six-bed residential 'special centre' since 1973. The duration of stay has ranged from 1–46 weeks with a mean of 17.3 weeks. The higher average duration of treatment compared to Parsonage's series is partly accounted for by the fact that some patients admitted for assessment were then 'abandoned' by relatives and sponsoring authorities and the process of transferring them to alternative accommodation was lengthy. The staffing ratio is also lower than at the Special Centre in York. Of the 149 patients discharged, 70 (47 per cent) were placed either in open employment, sheltered workshops or residential training establishments. 37 patients (25 per cent) were considered totally unemployable, usually because of intellectual retardation, and 19 (13 per cent) were assessed as requiring longer-term residential treatment in the main centre. The remaining patients had very indefinite futures and I have not classified them. 11 patients who had been treated for up to 10 years (7.4 per cent) were found not to have epilepsy at all. No figures are available for long-term follow-up.

For the last four years the Department of Health has commissioned a team under the leadership of Professor E. Bennett of St George's Hospital Medical School, London, to investigate the services for people with epilepsy, in particular the long stay centres and special centres. At the time of writing the results are not available but should be published in 1981. Much of the investigation is concerned with facts and figures and whether the final results will justify the existence of special centres must be left for future judgement. My personal opinion is that whatever the figures say, there are, and probably will be for some time to come, a proportion of people with epilepsy who can *only* be adequately assessed in a special centre for epilepsy because of the need for a multi-disciplinary approach by professionals who are dedicated to the problem. This may be an old-fashioned concept but in few conditions in medicine is it more appropriate than in epilepsy. Many of the patients admitted to special centres have never been properly assessed by the ordinary medical services available. I believe the Special Centres for Epilepsy will be with us for quite a long time to come.

EPILOGUE

I have briefly drawn attention elsewhere to the long history of the treatment of epilepsy (Grant 1976). We have been amused by the efforts of our predecessors over four millennia and think we have most of the answers today. Yet we have still not explained why people have seizures when they do, and not when they don't, why some respond and some don't. That great epileptologist and humanist, William Gordon Lennox (1960), wrote 'Often, if all the factors are in the patient's favour, attacks may persist. On the other hand, if chances of relief seem against him, seizures may greatly diminish or even vanish. This unpredictability is a part of the interest in the puzzle of epilepsy'.

My good friend Dr Ernst Rodin, Director of the Epilepsy Centre of Michigan, commented on Lennox's words, as follows (Rodin 1968): 'With all the experience that Lennox had accumulated in a lifelong effort to understand the nature of epilepsy, the last sentences strike one as particularly sad. They had to be written because they correspond to the facts, but they are also testimony to our abysmal ignorance of the true nature of the disorder.'

Such is the fascination of the 'falling sickness'.

References

Bagley C 1972 Social prejudice and the adjustment of people with epilepsy. Epilepsia 13:33–45
Critchley M 1949 Sir William Gowers 1845–1915. William Heinemann, London, p 56
Department of Health and Social Security and Welsh Office 1969 People with epilepsy (Report of a joint sub-committee of the Standing Medical Advisory Committee on the health and welfare of handicapped persons). Her Majesty's Stationery Office, London
Grant R H E 1976 The management of epilepsy. Scottish Medical Journal 21:11–22
Grant R H E 1980 Intensive monitoring of patients with epilepsy. Irish Medical Journal Supplement 73:7–11
Henriksen G F 1972 The role of special centres in the care of epileptics in Norway. Epilepsia 13:199–204
Jørgensen I S 1979 Special education in Denmark. Det. Danske Selskab, Copenhagen
Laidlaw J, Richens A (eds) 1976 A textbook of epilepsy. Churchill Livingstone, Edinburgh
Lennox W G 1960 Epilepsy and related disorders. Little, Brown and Company, Boston
Lund M 1972 Epilepsy centres in Denmark. Epilepsia 13:219–220
Lund M, Randrup J 1972 A day-centre for severely handicapped people with epilepsy. Epilepsia 13:245–247
Meinardi H 1972 Special centres in The Netherlands. Epilepsia 13:191–197
Ministry of Health 1953 Welfare of handicapped persons. The special needs of epileptics and spastics. Circular 26/53, Her Majesty's Stationery Office, London
Ministry of Health 1956 Central Health Services Council. Report of the sub-committee on the medical care of epileptics. Her Majesty's Stationery Office, London
Parsonage M J 1974 Experience in an English centre for epilepsy. In: Harris P, Mawdsley C (eds) Epilepsy: proceedings of the Hans Berger centenary symposium. Churchill Livingstone, Edinburgh, p 286–291
Parsonage M J 1976 Experience in an English special centre for epilepsy, 1972–1975. 2nd South African international conference on epilepsy, Cape Town, 28–30 June 1976

Penry J K, Porter R J 1977 Intensive monitoring of patients with intractable seizures. In: Penry J K (ed) Epilepsy: the 8th international symposium. Raven Press, New York, p 95–101

Reid J J A 1972 The need for special centres for epilepsy in England and Wales. Epilepsia 13:211–217

Rodin E A 1968 Prognosis of patients with epilepsy. Charles C Thomas, Springfield, Illinois

Siegenthaler M 1972 The need for specialised centres for epileptics with 'scientific special education', (Heilpädagogik). Epilepsia 13:221–224

Special educational needs 1978 Report of the committee of enquiry into the education of handicapped children and young people. Her Majesty's Stationery Office, London

Stores G 1973 Studies of attention and seizure disorders. Developmental Medicine and Child Neurology 15:376–382

Stores G 1979 Ambulatory EEG monitoring in the diagnosis of attacks of uncertain origin. In: Stott F D, Raftery E B, Sleight P, Golding L (eds) ISAM 1979 Proceedings of the 3rd international symposium on ambulatory monitoring. Academic Press, London

Temkin O 1971 The falling sickness. A history of epilepsy from the Greeks to the beginnings of modern neurology, 2nd edn. The Johns Hopkins Press, Baltimore and London, p 255

Turner W A 1907 Epilepsy—a study of the idiopathic disease. Facsimile edn Raven Press, New York, 1973

US Department of Health, Education and Welfare 1978 The commission for the control of epilepsy and its consequences. Public Health Service, National Institutes of Health, Bethesda, Maryland. DHEW Publication no (NIH) 78-276

Vidart L 1966 Hôpital de jour pour épileptiques. Annales médico-psychologiques 124:343–367

Whitmore K, Holdsworth L 1971 Some observations from a study of children with epilepsy who were attending ordinary schools. Spastics Society Study Group on medical aspects of children with school difficulties, Durham

Multi-disciplinary aspects

INTRODUCTION

The concept of a multi-disciplinary team can hardly be regarded as a new one in its broadest sense. Indeed, the need for groups of people with differing trades or qualifications to work together to achieve a common aim must surely be as old as the history of mankind. Even the most primitive societies found it advantageous to devise a division of labour. More recently, as scientific methods have increasingly pervaded our lives, it has become imperative for individuals with diverse scientific backgrounds to work together in co-operation to achieve a common aim. Such a need becomes a matter of survival during wartime and it is probable that only under such circumstances is the greatest possible co-operation achievable. In peacetime the motives may be financial, enhancement of personal status, or even just the pleasure of the work itself, but in these circumstances co-operativeness may be tempered by competitiveness.

The idea of teams of workers operating together is long established in the practice of medicine both in hospital life and in family general practice. Medicine could scarcely be practised otherwise nowadays, but it only seems to be comparatively recently that the term multi-disciplinary team has come into vogue in relation to the management of epilepsy (De Boer & Donkers 1972, Henriksen 1972, Lund 1972, Meinardi 1972, Reid 1972, Siegenthaler 1972, Parsonage 1974, 1975).

In considering the functioning of a multi-disciplinary team in the care of patients with epilepsy (or with other conditions for that matter) it is perhaps helpful to remember that the word 'discipline' has two main meanings, one related to training and the other to the maintenance of orderly human behaviour. However, these meanings overlap and we are here concerned with the disciplines that are trainings in orderliness, obedience and self-control on the basis of a scientific education in medical and para-medical disciplines. Nevertheless, if the members of a multi-disciplinary team of this kind are to work effectively, they too should perhaps remember the need for orderliness, obedience and self-control.

THE NEED FOR A MULTI-DISCIPLINARY
TEAM (Table 26.1)

There is a sizable proportion of patients with chronic epilepsy whose treatment can only be regarded as either unsatisfactory or a failure. At worst this might apply to as many as 50 per cent of cases, depending on the excellence or otherwise of local epilepsy services, whatever their form. The essential aim of treatment is to enable such individuals to lead as near normal lives as possible; that is to say, they should be capable of earning their livings and of enjoying their leisure in a reasonably normal manner. This is, in fact, rehabilitation which does not necessarily mean the complete abolition of seizures, even if this were possible. Equally important is the avoidance of unacceptable adverse effects of treatment, whether they be medical or surgical. Potentially, these may be more disabling than the epilepsy itself and their maintenance at an acceptable level is essential for the patient irrespective of whether seizures occur or not.

The fact that there are patients with chronic epilepsy whose treatment has failed is due to many factors. For example, the epilepsy itself may be of a peculiarly intractable kind, as in the case of many instances of secondary generalised or bilateral temporal lobe epilepsies, or it may be because treatment has been inadequate. Quite often however failures are due to the fact that associated psychological disturbances have not been recognised or, if they have, to their unsuccessful treatment. Disorders of this kind can often be far more disabling than the epilepsy itself and may sometimes completely overshadow it.

Inadequacies related to drug therapy should be easily identifiable and correctable, given a sound working knowledge of the correct application of such treatment. Unfortunately, such expertise may be lacking and the result is poor control of seizures often associated with the effects of drug interaction. The failure to identify associated psychological disorders is more understandable since they can be so easily overlooked both in general practice and in hospital outpatient clinics; moreover, even if they are recognized, their treatment may be no easy matter, even in the hands of the most experienced clinicians.

Unfortunately the organisation of both general practitioners' surgeries and hospital clinics still seems to be unfavourable to the conduct of the kinds of interview that are necessary to elucidate the complex problems likely to be associated with chronic intractable epilepsy. Too little time is usually allowable, expertise may be insufficient and the epileptic patient is often unwilling or afraid to discuss the intimate details of his case when time is at a premium. Furthermore, his morale, often low in any case, is likely to fall progressively with his continuing

Table 26.1 The need for a multidisciplinary team (MDT) in the management of patients with chronic epilepsy

---

1. For those patients *whose seizures have not been controlled* via NHS general practitioner and hospital services

2. The *adequate assessment* of such patients in a comprehensive manner

3. The *identification and treatment of associated disorders and handicaps*

4. To *promote the training* and *enlarge the experience* of the members of the team

---

lack of progress and he may then cease attending his doctor's surgery or hospital clinic; or he may perhaps continue attending in the hope that some day things might improve. Only too often the scheduled appointments are made at too infrequent intervals to be effective and the result is a waste of time and resources.

Even if the services provided by general practitioners and hospitals could be more suitably organised in terms of more leisurely conducted interviews, etc., this would be unlikely to lead to satisfactory resolution of many of the problems posed by intractable cases of epilepsy. From my own experience it has become clear to me that they have little chance of being dealt with effectively unless they are submitted to the skills of a specialist multi-disciplinary team (MDT). This is because they have so many facets which cannot all be dealt with adequately by a single individual who would normally have neither the time nor the special training required. In short, I believe that the MDT offers the best means of both identifying the nature of the problems at issue and of solving them.

An important additional role of the MDT is to promote the training and enlarge the experience of its members and to initiate new methods of treatment and management. It can also play an important role in the training of new recruits who can learn much about its mode of operation by attending its meetings.

TYPES OF PATIENT NEEDING A MDT APPROACH

Patients whose treatment has failed for unknown reasons are the ones requiring an MDT approach (Table 26.2). This is particularly applicable to those with long-standing epilepsies and who have either never sought medical aid before or who have been attending general practitioner's surgeries or hospital outpatient clinics (or both) without apparently making any progress. Such patients are likely to have had long periods of unemployment and to be suffering from increasing social isolation.

In these circumstances it is imperative that a searching inquiry be made into the reasons for this state of affairs. I believe that this can only be done effectively through the agency of a MDT in view of the multiplicity and complexity of the

Table 26.2   Types of patient with chronic epilepsy requiring the services of the MDT

1. Those whose *medical treatment has been ineffective* for any reason—

e.g. poor compliance
     inadequate planning and administration
     unexplained poor response
     unmanageable drug toxicity

2. Those with *unusually difficult social problems*

3. Those with *associated disorders and handicaps*—

e.g. psychoneuroses
     personality disorders
     psychoses
     mental handicap
     physical handicap

4. Those with *combinations of 1, 2, and 3*

factors which have contributed to the failure of the patient's treatment. Most commonly these include inadequate drug therapy, poor compliance by the patient, an unusually poor response to or intolerance of drug therapy, chronic drug intoxication, intractable social problems and associated psychiatric disorders, or to combinations of two or more of these factors. Less often there may be associated physical handicaps but these are usually of relatively minor importance.

Quite often patients in these situations are reluctant to seek medical advice through feelings of hopelessness and rejection. Others who may have been under medical care for some time are apt to become disillusioned by their lack of progress and may then seek aid from such organisations as the British Epilepsy Association. The comparatively large number of calls for help which the latter receives every year is an indication of a need which is not being met by the facilities at present available in the National Health Service, a fact which appears to have been tacitly acknowledged by the Department of Health.

MEMBERSHIP OF THE MDT

Broadly speaking, the members of the MDT (Table 26.3) are those whose disciplines fall within the province of neuropsychiatry. These are neurophysicians, clinical neurophysiologists, psychiatrists, clinical psychologists and medical or psychiatric social workers. Apart from being experienced in their particular specialities they need to have special knowledge and interest in epilepsy and a willingness to undertake work in which they will encounter widespread prejudice against the patients with which they have to deal. Furthermore, the rewards of such work are intangible, effectiveness is not readily demonstrable or measurable, if at all, and success and failure will be encountered in varying degree in a field of endeavour to which few are attracted.

The role of the *neurophysician* can generally be regarded as primary in the sense that he begins the work of the team by investigating the epilepsy as such. He must search for causes that can be removed or modified and should be the initiator and controller of drug therapy, keeping a careful watch for adverse effects of all kinds. In many respects he is probably best equipped to be the leader of the team but this need not necessarily always be the case.

Table 26.3 Composition of the MDT in the management of patients with chronic epilepsy

All disciplines concerned with the *investigation and management of neuropsychiatric disorders* —
Neurophysicians
Neurophysiologists
Neuroradiologists
Psychiatrists
Clinical psychologists
Nursing staff
Social workers — medical and/or psychiatric
Physiotherapists
Occupational therapists
Technicians
Secretaries

The *clinical neurophysiologist* is primarily concerned with determining the type of epilepsy coupled with observations on the extent and distribution of seizure discharge. In particularly difficult cases he will undoubtedly need to use EEG telemetry and continuous monitoring (Stores 1980). In addition, depending on his training and inclinations, he may also wish to contribute to the clinical care of patients and in the development of new forms of treatment.

The *psychiatrist* with a special interest in epilepsy has acquired an increasingly important role in the work of a MDT. This is because of the high incidence of associated psychiatric disorders in patients, especially those referred to special centres, and he therefore often has an important part to play in day-to-day management. Indeed, it cannot be over-emphasised that the success or failure in the handling of associated psychiatric disorders is usually decisive in regard to success or failure in rehabilitation. To be effective the psychiatrist will need particular expertise in the combined use of psychotropic and anti-epileptic drugs in view of their potential interactions (Trimble 1980).

It is fortunate for patients with chronic epilepsy that *clinical psychologists* have taken increasing interest in their problems in recent years. A clinical psychological assessment of all such patients is essential in defining suspected or unsuspected areas of cerebral dysfunction, in determining levels of intellectual functioning, in assessing progress and in providing educational and vocational guidance. These examinations are often also helpful by way of important observations which can be made of patients' attitudes and personalities; furthermore, valuable supplementary information may accrue from the searching but sympathetic interview which a clinical psychological examination entails. Finally, the clinical psychologist has an important role to play in the development of new methods of seizure control other than by drug therapy (Wyler et al 1979).

The services of a *social worker*, whether medically or psychiatrically trained or both, are almost invariably required in all cases of chronic intractable epilepsy since associated social problems are to be expected in virtually every case. These range from the very mild, which can be easily disposed of, to the severe which can only be partially resolved, if at all. The social worker with the right kind of interest and training must make a thorough inquiry into the patient's socio-domestic situation, supplementing this with interviews with relatives, employers, teachers, etc., and with home visits. Liaison with all relevant social services is essential, particularly when after-care is being arranged.

Much of the success of a MDT depends upon the contributions made by specially trained *nursing staff*. In many ways their role is the most difficult of all since they are responsible for the daily care of patients who are often resentful and bitter about their lot. Truculence, aggressiveness, passivity, apathy, personal inadequacies and unco-operativeness are frequently the features of behaviour with which they have to cope; however, those who undertake such work should appreciate how vital are their contributions in terms of the daily observations they make on the general behaviour of their patients in addition to more specific direct observations on the nature, features and incidence of their attacks.

Occupational therapists are able to give invaluable assistance in the day-to-day management of medium or long stay inpatients. Occupational therapy is needed not merely as a diversion but as a means of developing overt or latent skills which can often do much to raise morale and build up self-confidence. At the same time patients' attitudes and handicaps related to visuo-spatial and motor skills can be assessed in a practical manner. Usually patients begin with simple handicrafts and thereafter progress in stages to work in an industrial therapy unit. Furthermore, it is helpful if the latter requires short-distance travel by public transport at regular hours in order to re-establish the habit of regular time-keeping lost during long periods of unemployment.

Although the *physiotherapist* has a relatively limited role to perform in view of the comparative rarity of associated physical handicaps, the latter must of course receive their due when present. There are however other more general ways in which the physiotherapist can help. For example, the organisation of ball games, swimming, etc., can do much to improve impaired motor co-ordination and provide pleasant recreation for patients needing a boost to their morale and self-esteem.

Technicians and *secretaries* are important contributors to the work of the MDT which would virtually be impossible without their assistance. Furthermore, their interest in the care of patients is to be encouraged as a valuable aid to the successful functioning of the team as a whole.

Although I have included neuroradiologists in the list of team members (see Table 26.3) their involvement has become progressively less in recent years for two main reasons. First, with increasing experience it has become clear that the management of chronic epilepsy is related more to the psychosocial than to its purely neurological aspects. The second reason is that the neuroradiological investigation of epilepsy has become simplified and at the same time greatly advanced by the introduction of computerised axial tomography. There is thus less need to involve busy neuroradiologists directly in the discussions of a MDT.

MODE OF OPERATION OF THE MDT

For a MDT to operate a successful inpatient or outpatient service there are a number of basic prerequisites (Table 26.4). Each member must adapt his discipline and apply his resources to the problems in hand. In the approach to a new case, the leader of the team would normally invite the appropriate individual members to undertake whatever investigation is necessary when the case is first presented for discussion. Thereafter it is essential that the MDT should hold regular conferences so that management can be co-ordinated and progress assessed.

The main role of the leader of the team is to integrate the information and advice submitted by the members of the team, to resolve all differences of opinion as far

Table 26.4 How should the MDT operate in the management of patients with chronic epilepsy?

1. By the *application and adaptation of the resources of each discipline* to whatever problems are presented

2. By *co-operation and regular consultation* between the representatives of the various disciplines

3. By *the application of an agreed plan* of treatment and management

as possible and to act as the final arbiter when reconciliation of views is not possible. For their part, individual members of the team should be prepared to make reasonable concessions whenever this is in the best interests of the patient. At all times the leader should exercise tact and understanding in the interests of a smoothly working team and ensure that every contributor has a fair hearing.

The meetings of the team are naturally held in the absence of patients since individual members will have direct contact with them in the course of confidential interviews and when giving treatment. It is however most important to ensure that the advice of the team is properly communicated to the patient by a chosen member who must also seek his approval and co-operation.

Practical experience in the work of a MDT in a special centre for epilepsy (Table 26.5)

As a result of experience working as a leader of a MDT over a number of years (Parsonage 1974) I have become convinced that it offers the best and probably the only means of grappling effectively with the problems posed by intractable cases of epilepsy. It is the collective skills and efforts of the members that are so invaluable in minimising bias and guarding against individual errors of judgement.

For example, it may transpire that treatment has failed because of previous inadequate history-taking, or because new factors having a decisive effect on the understanding or management of a case have come to light as a result of intensive inquiry. Thorough scrutiny of previous records, repeated interrogations of patients by different members of the team and discussions with general practitioners will often shed entirely new light on a case, sometimes to the extent of completely overturning a diagnosis of epilepsy. Case notes beginning with the term 'this known epileptic' are notoriously misleading and should prompt a thorough re-appraisal of the whole case.

It has been uncommon for failures to be attributable to inadequate neurological investigation, although there have been rare occasions when timely contrast radiography and computerised axial tomography have revealed suspected or unsuspected cerebral lesions. More often previous EEG surveys have been found to be very incomplete, this resulting either in errors in the typing of the epilepsy or inadequate assessments of the extent and distribution of seizure discharge. Telemetry and continuous EEG monitoring have already begun to play an important role in cases of special difficulty.

The value of clinical psychological examinations as virtually routine procedures has become very evident from several points of view. Thus, time spent in the detailed study of patients' mental functioning has frequently resulted in the

Table 26.5   How does the MDT work in practice?

Generally very effectively *if the basic rules of procedure are observed*

It results in the identification of those cases which are *treatable and those which are not*

Apparently intractable cases become manageable *if the main problems can be treated effectively*

The various members of the MDT *learn from one another* and regular conferences *promote interest and enthusiasm in case management*

---

correction of erroneous impressions of intellectual level, in uncovering unsuspected areas of cerebral dysfunction and in highlighting underdeveloped or latent abilities. Information derived from these examinations has often been helpful in vocational guidance and in the assessment of attitudes as well as being instrumental in the identification of associated psychiatric disorders. In addition, the finding of deteriorating mental functioning has often prompted a review of cases in the hope, not always realised, that effective intervention could be undertaken.

The social worker's role has become increasingly important in the management of the patient with chronic epilepsy. Women are particularly suited to perform this role by their ability to conduct sympathetic and tactful enquiries into the intimate details of people's lives, thereby uncovering hidden strife and conflict within families. It has been very striking how often in intractable cases siblings, parents and spouses have reacted adversely to a family member with epilepsy, with devastating results. For example, I may quote the case of a young housewife and mother, who was also an experienced schoolteacher, whose morale and self-esteem had been destroyed by her family's attitude of unacceptance, disapproval and rejection. Social workers have however done a great deal more than merely explore family problems; they have also been able to do much towards modifying unhealthy attitudes, as well as giving support to the lonely and miserable and good advice about daily living and work. Their help has also been important in the arranging of after-care and in acting as a liaison officer between patients, their family practitioners and local social services.

Occupational therapists have been very successful both in keeping patients happily occupied while observing their performance and behaviour in their departments. Their observations in this respect have often either shed new light, or corroborated the observations of other members of the team, and have thus contributed significantly to the organisation of either general or specific management. For example, apathy, poor application to tasks, truculence, aggressiveness, social isolation, have been very evident in the occupational therapy department and have been duly reported at meetings of the MDT.

Despite the uncommonness of associated physical disabilities, experience has shown that physiotherapists can make significant contributions to the work of the MDT. In addition to making skilled assessments of motor disabilities, they can usually improve function in this sphere. They have also successfully organised courses of relaxation therapy and recreational pursuits with very evident benefit to patients. Their reports on progress and patients' behaviour have also been helpful in making overall assessments.

Specially trained nursing staff, living and working with patients on a day-to-day basis, as they do, have soon become very skilled in describing and recognising the nature of attacks, as well as in assessing their frequency and the effects of drug therapy. In addition, their commentaries on the behaviour both of patients and of their relatives during visiting hours have been invaluable. In recognition of the fact that they have the responsibility of the day-to-day care of patients, their opinions have always been regularly sought as regards patients' conditions and they have often been able to help in deciding which types of case are suitable for admission.

In order to bring the best out of a MDT it has been clear that each member should feel that he or she is a valued member whose work and opinions are given their proper due. It has proved essential therefore for the leader to keep this constantly in mind and for him to prevent arguments and disagreements getting out of hand. When a cordial atmosphere of co-operation is maintained, the members of the team have found their meetings both enjoyable and educative. Indeed, much enthusiasm has been engendered in these circumstances and quite often the difficulties of management of intractable cases have been overcome surprisingly easily.

Many examples could be cited in support of the effectiveness of a MDT. Particularly striking is that of a young single woman, who had been receiving anti-epileptic treatment for a number of years, in which patient inquiry and careful observation coupled with a psychiatric approach to her case over a period of several months not only demolished an erroneous diagnosis but also led eventually to complete resolution of her symptoms. Similar results have doubtless often been recorded in other contexts, but the point I wish to make is that it was only after the combined skills of a MDT were brought into action that a proper evaluation of this case became possible.

Results obtained by a MDT working in a special centre for epilepsy

It is very difficult, if not impossible, to make an adequate and realistic assessment of the results of treatment of patients suffering from chronic, intractable epilepsies because it is just as much a matter of quality of results as of quantity (see Total care in severe epilepsy 1976).

Experience has repeatedly confirmed that these patients, with their frequently associated multiple handicaps, have histories of long-continued social maladjustment, long spells of unemployment, low morale and poor self-esteem. Furthermore, if the aggravating effects of unsuccessful treatment are taken into account, the cost in terms of resources and human misery must be very considerable (Summer 1974). It must surely be worthwhile therefore to provide the necessary means whereby at least some of these patients can be offered the kind of help they need.

It cannot of course be denied that there are still some epilepsies which defy treatment even by the best of modern methods. On the other hand a sizable proportion of cases are severely handicapped, even totally disabled, by other disabilities, such as a mental handicap, personality disorder, chronic untreatable psychoneurosis and especially combinations of these. Adequate assessment is one of the most important functions of a MDT in a Special Centre in order that those for whom little can be done, or who can only live under very sheltered circumstances, can be identified and that those who can be helped to lead a more or less independent existence be singled out for treatment. In this way effort and resources can be directed into channels in which they are most likely to be effective.

The future of those patients who can be successfully treated or substantially improved while under specialised care depends on the quality of their after-care and the environment to which they return. Much good work may be readily undone if the patients' subsequent treatment is not properly supervised and if the environment to which they return is unfavourable. In these circumstances relapse and deterioration are common.

The removal of the label of epilepsy when it has been wrongly applied is in itself another important function which a MDT is well equipped to undertake. This has sometimes proved to be a matter of considerable difficulty requiring prolonged, painstaking investigation. Unfortunately, even when this has been achieved, some patients have been found to be reluctant to accept the idea that their problem is not epilepsy because they and their families have long become so accustomed to living with such a label. Indeed, they have sometimes been unable to face problems of a more personal nature and have preferred to seek medical advice elsewhere in the hope, sometimes realised, that they can have their diagnosis of epilepsy restored.

Bell (1979) has made a detailed study of the social problems of 182 patients (mainly young adults) admitted to the Special Centre at York for assessment during the three-year period 1972–74. Ninety per cent of them had social problems and these were multiple in just over half. For example, no less than 72 per cent of those employable had work problems of some kind and just over half the patients had difficulty in accepting their epilepsy. Nearly one-third were assessed as being socially isolated, 46 per cent had family difficulties, 34 per cent reported practical difficulties at home, 29 per cent were in financial straits and 14 per cent had problems with accommodation.

Nearly 60 per cent of the patients studied by Bell had at least one associated psychiatric disability such as a psychoneurotic or personality disorder (34 per cent), mental subnormality (17 per cent) or a psychosis (2 per cent). At the time of discharge, half the patients were improved so far as their epilepsy was concerned, some 15 per cent had been found not to have epilepsy, and of those with psychiatric disorders 40 per cent were assessed as having improved. Over 75 per cent of those who were given social work help were considered to have responded in the sense that one or more of their problems had been solved or ameliorated at the time when they were discharged. Bell concluded from these findings that a skilled multi-disciplinary team is clearly needed to confront the problems of people with epilepsy, and was dismayed to find that only a small proportion of the patients studied were known to their local Social Services Department.

CONCLUSION

Practical experience has shown that a worthwhile proportion of patients suffering from seemingly intractable epilepsies can benefit from the help given by a skilled multi-disciplinary team. Indeed, the problems which they present are so complex and have so many facets that it seems hardly conceivable that they could be dealt with adequately in any other way (see People with epilepsy 1969).

It may again be emphasised that the previous treatment of all the patients referred to in this chapter had failed, despite varying periods of care by way of the ordinary NHS general practitioner and hospital services. Since there seems to be no sign of a fall in the numbers of such patients there would appear to be a continuing need for the provision of the services of specially trained multi-disciplinary teams. Ideally, these can function to their fullest effect in Special

Centres for Epilepsy, although there is no reason why they should not work effectively in suitably modified form both in hospital and in general practice.

References

Bell M 1979 Some social problems of adults with epilepsy, part I. In: Epilepsy 1979. Perspectives on epilepsy. Compiled by the British Epilepsy Association. Palantype Organisation Limited, London, p 93–98

De Boer H M, Donkers J G H 1972 A vocational therapist's view of an English, a Scottish and two Dutch centres for epilepsy. Epilepsia 13:239–243

Henniksen G F 1972 The role of special centres in the care of epileptics in Norway. Epilepsia 13:199–204

Lund M 1972 Epilepsy centres in Denmark. Epilepsia 13:219–220

Meinardi H 1972 Special centres in the Netherlands. Epilepsia 13:191–197

Parsonage M J 1974 Experiences in an English centre for epilepsy. In: Harris P, Mawdsley C (eds) Epilepsy. Proceedings of the Hans Berger centenary symposium. Churchill Livingstone, Edinburgh, p 286–291

Parsonage M J 1975 An English special centre for epilepsy. International Bureau for Epilepsy Newsletter no 39

People with epilepsy 1969 Report of a joint subcommittee of the standing medical advisory committee on the health and welfare of handicapped persons. Her Majesty's Stationery Office, London, p 19–20, 33–35

Reid J J A 1972 The need for special centres for epilepsy in England and Wales. Epilepsia 13:211–217

Siegenthaler H 1972 The need for specialised centres for epileptics with 'scientific special education' (Heilpädagogik). Epilepsia 13:221–224

Stores G 1980 Ambulatory EEG monitoring in the diagnosis of epilepsy. In: Parsonage M J (ed) Aspects of epilepsy. Research and Clinical Forums 2(2):141–147

Sumner D, Verna K B Ç, Peasland A 1974 The epileptic; his call on community resources. In: Harris P, Mawdsley C (eds) Epilepsy. Proceedings of the Hans Berger centenary symposium. Churchill Livingstone, Edinburgh, p 309–312

Total care in severe epilepsy. Presentations of multi-disciplinary teams. 1976 In: Parsonage M J (ed) Proceedings of the sixth international symposium on epilepsy. International Bureau for Epilepsy p 17–27

Trimble M R 1980 In: Parsonage M J (ed) Aspects of epilepsy. Research and Clinical Forums 2(2):114–120

Wyler A R, Robbins C A, Dodrill C B 1979 EEG operant conditioning for control of epilepsy. Epilepsia 20:279–286

Index